T0318534

Quality Assurance Management

Quality Assurance Management

A Comprehensive Overview of Real-World Applications for High Risk Specialties

Gayathri De Lanerolle

Digital Evidence Based Medicine Lab, London, United Kingdom

Evette Sebastien Roberts

Partnership of East London Co London, Ilford, United Kingdom

Athar Haroon

Barts Health NHS Trust, London, United Kingdom

Ashish Shetty

University College London Hospitals, University College London, London, United Kingdom

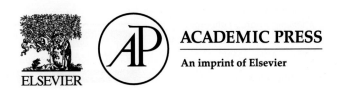

ELSEVIER

ACADEMIC PRESS

An imprint of Elsevier

ISBN: 978-0-12-822732-9

For information on all Academic Press publications visit our
website at https://www.elsevier.com/books-and-journals

Publisher: Stacy Masucci
Acquisitions Editor: Andre Wolff
Editorial Project Manager: Andrea Dulberger
Production Project Manager: Gomathi Sugumar
Cover Designer: Vicky Pearson Esser

Typeset by TNQ Technologies

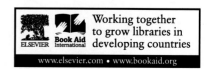

Contents

List of contributors

Author biographies

Gayathri Delanerolle is a Researcher. Her interests include women's health, aritificial intelligence and chronic conditions with a special focus on disease sequalae. She has experience in evidence synthesis, epidemiology and mixed-methods research. Gayathri's experience in quality assurance inspired her to develop the content for this book and co-author with others with a special focus on complex healthcare areas that is rapidly evolving.

Evette Sebastien Roberts is a practicing nurse and midwife in London, England. Evette has been pivotal in assisting healthcare organizations to better understand the principles of governance and quality assurance, leading them in achieving compliance during accreditation and audit programs. Her passion for risk management in healthcare has propelled her into seeking a number of roles, some of which include Risk Midwife, Clinical Governance Manager, and Regulatory and Compliance Lead. Having undertaken several inspections for the Care Quality Commission, Evette has knowledge and experience in what 'good' looks like and the factors which often impinge on the ability to match required standards. In addition to her clinical roles, Evette has embarked on a research journey, seeking to contribute new knowledge on the subject matter of midwives' experiences working with risk management frameworks. It is her enthusiasm for quality assurance which drives her appetite for research into this area which encompasses the patient safety agenda.

Dr. Athar Haroon is a Consultant Radionuclide Radiologist and has worked in an array of NHS organizations and academia, including United Lincolnshire Hospitals NHS Trust, the University of Leicester, the University Hospitals of Leicester NHS Trust, Nottingham University Hospitals NHS Trust, University College London Hospitals NHS Foundation Trust, and University College London, respectively. He has a special interest in hybrid imaging and utility of biomarkers for diagnosis, disease management, and treatment of a variety of clinical areas including neurology, oncology, endocrinology, and emergency Medicine. He has experience working with several biomarkers such as 18F FDG, 18F Choline, Ga 68 PSMA, Ga68 DOTATATE, and 18F Amyloid.

Dr. Ashish Shetty trained at Cambridge University Hospitals and underwent a clinical fellowship in pain management at Guy's & St Thomas Hospital in London. He is a Consultant in pain medicine at University College London Hospitals and Associate Professor at UCL. His private practice is located at Harley Street Clinic and London Bridge Hospital. His special interests relating to chronic pain include neuromodulation, spinal cord stimulators, sports medicine, pelvic pain, and CRPS.

Introduction

Abstract

Quality management is vital for clinical research and clinical practice. It is a costly aspect of clinical research and healthcare. The current interpretation of quality management is broad, where quality assurance and quality control methods vary based on a number of variables. Observing organizational functions to improve practices is paramount to ensuring the structure, process, and outcomes for patients are maintained at the highest quality, which leads to quality improvements.

Keywords: Data analytics; Data profiling; Electronic health records; Evidence-based medicine; Quality assurance; Quality management.

Key messages

- Quality assurance and quality control is integral to quality management
- Quality assurance management comprises a synergistic relationship between science, clinical, and administrative processes
- Compliance monitoring is important to ensure participant safety and study integrity
- Poor documentation and quality reporting of adverse events or documenting insufficient information to determine the efficacy of reporting a risk–benefit product
- Quality management includes multiple processes

1.1 Introduction

1.1.1 A brief history

Quality management is vital for clinical research and clinical practice. It is a costly aspect of clinical research and healthcare [1]. The current interpretation of quality management is broad, where quality assurance (QA) and quality control (QC) methods vary based on a number of variables [2]. Observing organizational functions to improve practices is paramount to ensuring the structure, process, and outcomes for patients are maintained at the highest quality, which leads to quality improvements (QI) [3,4].

Historically, healthcare quality goes back to the 19th century when the concept of evidence-based quality improvement was demonstrated in the 1850s when Florence

Nightingale showed basic sanitation and hygiene protocols could reduce mortality among wounded soldiers from the Crimean War [4,5]. In 1846, Hungarian Obstetrician, Dr. Ignaz Semmelweis also proposed handwashing to prevent the spread of disease and infections [6—8]. Abraham Flexner's 1910 report on medical education in the United States is one of the first quality reports that can be considered as an official document [9]. The emphasis of the report was on the significant role quality in healthcare plays directly and indirectly in medical education [10—12].

However, Dr. Ernest Amory Codman, a surgeon from Harvard Medical School and the Massachusetts General Hospital is credited with having founded outcomes studies where he kept track of his patients by way of an *"End Result Card"* system. These index cards included patient diagnosis, treatments, demographics, and outcomes that Dr. Codman believed to better understand treatment success. In 1913, Dr. Edward Martin, a renowned Gynecologist who cofounded the American College of Surgeons (ACS), and Dr. Codman formed the *"Committee for Hospital Standardisation"* [12,13]. Dr. Codman believes that each hospital has a duty of care to follow up with patients as much as possible to investigate every end result as much as possible by members of staff, trustees, the administration, or authorized personnel such as investigators or statisticians. In 1917, Dr. Codman's "End-Result-System" was adopted by hospitals based in the United States (US) that would provide the minimum standards required, including the following key features [14]:

- Medical staff organization
- Staff membership privileges were given to competent, educationally qualified, and licensed physicians and surgeons
- Establishing regular staff meetings and clinical reviews based on a set of regulations and framework
- Maintaining accurate medical records of all patients including their laboratory and physical examinations
- Establishing diagnostic and treatment facilities such as radiology departments and clinical laboratories with appropriate supervision

The American College of Physicians, American Hospital Association, American Medical Association, and Canadian Medical Association joined with the ACS in 1952 to form the Commission on Accreditation of Healthcare Organisations (JCAHO) [12,14,15]. The original Social Security Act established in 1935 by the Franklin D. Roosevelt presidency did not include medical benefits. This remained unaddressed till 1965, when amendments XIX and XVIII established Medicaid and Medicare, respectively, and led to healthcare in the United States falling within federal supervision. Within title XVIII, the US Congress established a set of rules called "Conditions of Participation," which mandated hospitals to have staff employed with appropriate credentials and 24-hour nursing services [16]. By the 1950s, medical audit models were used in hospitals. JCAHO furthered these standards by implementing a rigorous accreditation standard by the late 1980s that was based on the concepts demonstrated by Dr. Avedis Donabedian in his peer review publication titled Evaluating the Quality of Medical Care. Dr. Donabedian laid out three key components to evaluate and maintain care quality using structure, process, and outcomes. Each of these components was linked to measures that could assist with determining the quality standard of the care delivered and healthcare facilities linked to capacity, treatment processes, and healthcare outcomes. These were used when developing a framework for Medicare utilization and Quality Control Peer Review Organisation program that later transitioned to the Quality Improvement Organisation (QIO) program. By 1990, in the United States, a nonprofit organization called the National Committee for Quality Assurance (NCQA) was established by Margaret E. O'Kane to help advance quality care provided to patients. The mission of the NCQA was to provide accreditations and credentials to healthcare professionals and population health programs. Similar programs have been established globally.

In the United Kingdom (UK), post–World War II, the healthcare system experienced significant advancements, including the establishment of the National Health Service (NHS) in 1948. This marked a shift toward providing accessible and high-quality healthcare. The 1960s and 1970s saw the emergence of formal quality assurance programs in healthcare. These programs were influenced by the quality management principles developed in industries like manufacturing. The 1980s brought a growing emphasis on evidence-based medicine (EBM), where medical decisions were increasingly based on research evidence rather than solely on clinical intuition. This shift contributed to the foundation of quality assurance on scientific principles. Organizations started to implement quality control measures and develop guidelines for medical practices [17]. The concept of value-based healthcare gained prominence, focusing on delivering high-quality care at lower costs. This approach emphasizes outcomes that matter to patients while considering cost-effectiveness. Governments and healthcare accrediting bodies started implementing regulations and standards to ensure quality and patient safety. The Centers for Medicare and Medicaid Services (CMS) in the United States, for example, introduced value-based purchasing programs that tie reimbursement to quality metrics [17]. By the 1990s, the Care Quality Commission (CQC) was established with a view to operate independently to oversee all primary, secondary, and tertiary NHS. There are a variety of QA programs the NHS is subjected to, in particular for high-risk specialist areas such as maternity care, chronic conditions, radiology, and neuropsychiatry. The NHS newborn and infant physical examination (NIPE) screening program is one such example where QC steps have been processed to ensure safe and optimal screening pathways. Quality assurance and control procedures have advanced rapidly over the course of the last 5 years with the integration of technology into healthcare, such as electronic health records (EHRs) and data analytics, enabled more sophisticated monitoring of quality metrics, patient outcomes, and trends, allowing for data-driven quality improvement efforts [15–17].

Quality of healthcare is challenging to describe and measure, especially since this varies across all clinical areas; thus, the research conducted differs considerably.

A landmark quality management report published by the Institute of Medicine (IoM) referred to as *To err is human: building a safer health system* in 1999 influenced QA to become a mandatory component for healthcare systems globally. Within the United States, medical error is considered as one of the top 10 causes of mortality that continues to influence changes in legislation and safety protocols. Research continues to grow and proposes quality indicators and projects to develop a quality culture. The IoM released a second report, which emphasized the need to promote *change management* to improve six dimensions of healthcare: effectiveness, safety, efficiency, equity, accessibility and patient-centric approaches. These dimensions are mostly intertwined with quality that is driven by the use and completion of processes.

In the United Kingdom, the NHS comprises a centralized mainframe inclusive of standardized systems to ensure the quality of care delivered to all patients. The NHS has been under intense scrutiny for a number of years for a variety of reasons stemming from criticisms of its performance. The CQC is the independent authority in the United Kingdom that regularly inspects all NHS organizations and is held accountable for public inquiries in relation performance of the NHS organizations. The Francis Report in particular criticized a number of councils and committees, including the Department of Health for performance and governance issues pertaining to the NHS. Since the reporting of failures, a number of white papers by independent organizations have been published, calling for the need for better regulations, evolving approaches to managing the system and operational principles that should be built on the premise of QA. This approach could action intended effective for frontline and management staff.

There are a variety of facets that need to be linked to optimal healthcare quality efforts and are vital to meet sustainable value-based quality systems. These work on the premise of hierarchical quality management concepts that lead to the development of *Quality-Pyramids* (Fig. 1.1).

It is vital to combine QA assessments across physician leadership, infrastructure, and clinical approaches. Performance measures and indicators, as well as assessing these appropriately as part of a cyclical approach, are important. Historically, changing healthcare demands and resources has meant a paucity of resources have been available to gather insightful data to understand strengths and weaknesses in healthcare systems. However, such data are more commonly available over the last 2 decades, and the validity of clinical, administrative, and patient-reported outcomes has allowed better assessment of the care provided. Throughout its history, quality assurance in healthcare has evolved from a focus on individual clinical practices to a broader emphasis on patient safety, evidence-based practices, and overall healthcare system improvement. It is an ongoing journey driven by the collective effort of healthcare professionals, policymakers, researchers, and patients to ensure that healthcare services are safe, effective, patient-centered, timely, efficient, and equitable. To continue with these approaches, reliable evidence and analytical methods remain important.

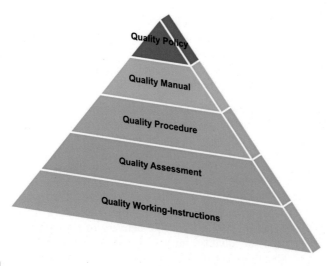

FIGURE 1.1

Hierarchy of quality management as part of the five-stage process. Basic quality concepts are engrained within this pyramid including quality attributes and metrics across the quality assurance plans.

1.2 **Quality assurance**

The definition of QA is broad and focuses on a standard setting with the specific aim of achieving compliance against set criteria. However, within healthcare, a universally accepted definition of quality is absent. Within the context of the NHS, a single broad definition of quality was developed where the focus remains on the provision of effective and safe care that allows patients to have a positive experience by way of being responsive, caring, and person-centered. As part of this definition, it is expected that care offered should fall within the remit of equitable, sustainable, and well-led hence these are measured during the course of any inspection or audit cycle. Healthcare organizations in the United Kingdom also look at the environmental impact services rendered can provide to ensure the efforts rendered to improve the quality of care provided alongside the experience.

The term *External Quality Assurance (EQA)* is another facet of QA with a variety of definitions. However, the most common definition is that of Donabedian, which outlines the implications of the cyclical nature of quality from a quality improvement perspective, as they affect patient care and outcomes including accountability. This is particularly vital for laboratory practices where the benefits of producing high-quality outputs have a direct impact on the clinical decision-making process. An interesting viewpoint was provided by Sandle et al. [17,18];

> *Management can have measurable effects on performance—an aspect that is usually only appreciated when things go wrong*
>
> **L.N. Sandle.**

The long-term integrated approach the NHS uses in the United Kingdom aims to ensure sustained improvements. The audit is central to the quality assurance agenda, as it aims to measure current practice, comparing it with set standards, identifying the gaps, and developing workable, measurable, and sensible action plans to close the gaps and enable sustainable improvement [4,5].

> *The aim is to allow quality improvement to take place where it will be most helpful and will improve outcomes for patients. Clinical audits can look at care nationwide (national clinical audits) and local clinical audits can also be performed locally in trusts, hospitals or GP practices anywhere healthcare is provided*
>
> **(NHS England, Ref. 9).**

The increasing focus on quality assurance in the healthcare industry seemed to have placed a shift from its vague and intangible nature to a more meaningful construct, relative to actual patients and the delivery of care [1]. The appeal has driven the movement of quality initiatives, which has remained consistent throughout the healthcare spectrum, which includes care delivered in all key healthcare settings. Essentially, at the core of this movement is the ultimate objective of patient safety, which goes hand in hand with quality as a deliverable.

The National Institute for Health and Care Excellence (NICE) has compromised a set of 200 QA standards and indicators that can be used to define and measure quality across the healthcare sector [14]. A QA indicator is a measurable element of performance that can be used to assess the quality of a certain service or process within a healthcare setting [12]. The NICE Indicators Menu outlines all outcomes that measure and reflect quality of care, exploring evidence that can be used to improve outcomes [15].

QA in healthcare covers a number of key categories linked to all aspects of clinical practice, laboratories, and electronic healthcare data. These categories can be subdivided based on clinical specialties and healthcare practices based on staffing groups. Medical doctors for example are assessed for their competency and continuous development requirements on a yearly basis although the specifics can differ across global healthcare systems. In the United Kingdom, revalidation appraisal is carried out for all doctors licensed to practice within the NHS. Responsible officers conduct the annual organizational audit (AOA) on behalf of designated organizations. All 862 designated bodies confirmed a 100% response rate affirming a level of assurance about the appraisal process supporting the revalidation to continue to provide clinical care to patients. Throughout this process, some of the differences noted were based on the requirement of the clinical area and the complexities surrounding its practice.

Data are fundamental to effective, evidence-based decision-making; however, data are of unknown or questionable quality [19,20]. Poor or unknown quality data weaken evidence, undermines trust, and ultimately leads to poor outcomes. Within database services, QA relates to the process of determining and screening anomalies by means of data profiling, removing obsolete information, and data cleaning [20]. Data are at risk of being distorted by individuals and external factors throughout its lifecycle. It is therefore vital to have robust QA strategies in place to protect the quality and value of the data. By ensuring there is data quality oversight within the managerial teams, organizations can track and monitor data management to ensure quality and compliance are maintained [21].

The UK Government Data Quality Framework focuses on assessing and improving the quality of data [19]. The framework asks organizations to develop a "culture" of data quality, by treating issues at source, and committing to ongoing monitoring and reporting. The National Data Strategy notes that by improving data quality ensured better insights and outcomes [19,22]. The Office for Statistics Regulation also provides a standard for QA of data [23]. This Standard recognizes the vital role of data and official statistics and hence provides guidance on procedures and practices that could be implemented to assure data quality [23].

QA in the global healthcare sense is another important facet to explore the systematic process of ensuring that healthcare services and interventions provided to patients around the world meet established standards of safety, effectiveness, and patient-centered care. It encompasses a set of activities, strategies, and practices aimed at continuously monitoring, evaluating, and improving healthcare services to deliver the best possible outcomes for patients and populations. Key components of quality assurance in global healthcare include a variety of standards and guidelines that define and adhere to internationally recognized best practices for healthcare delivery. These standards can cover a wide range of areas, including clinical practice, patient safety, infection control, data management, and more. Performance monitoring is another aspect that is vital to regularly measure and assess healthcare performance indicators to identify areas of improvement and track progress. This involves analyzing data related to clinical outcomes, patient satisfaction, adverse events, and other relevant metrics. Feedback and reporting develops mechanisms for patients, healthcare workers, and other stakeholders to provide feedback on their experiences with healthcare services. This feedback can help identify issues and drive improvements. To this effect, complex areas such as radiology, pain medicine, psychiatry, and maternity care were at the forefront due to a number of reasons including the diagnostic and treatment procedures used, risks pertaining to patients, qualifications, and training requirements. Radiology for example is well known as a high-risk clinical specialty due to the use of ionizing radiation and extensive use of medical equipment.

1.3 Behavioral quality assurance

Behavior-based quality assurance refers to an approach within quality assurance that focuses on assessing and improving the behaviors, actions, and interactions of healthcare professionals and staff. In healthcare, behaviors can significantly impact patient safety, outcomes, and the overall quality of care. Ensuring that healthcare providers adhere to proper protocols, follow guidelines, communicate effectively, and demonstrate patient-centered behavior could be a part of behavior-based quality assurance. Institutional productivity and sustainable performance by way of fostering a positive and blame-free culture is vital, especially within healthcare. Psychology plays an important role in workforce performance. In particular, organizational culture plays an important role, particularly in patient-centered QA. In this context, the term might imply an emphasis on the behaviors of healthcare providers that directly impact patient satisfaction and experience. Ensuring that healthcare professionals exhibit empathy, active listening, effective communication, and respect toward patients would be crucial for maintaining a patient-centered approach to care delivery.

Behavioral psychology, also known as behaviorism, has a significant impact on quality assurance in healthcare by influencing how healthcare professionals, patients, and organizations behave, interact, and make decisions. Understanding behavioral psychology principles can help design and implement effective quality assurance strategies that improve patient care, safety, and overall quality. For example, adherence to protocols or guidelines is linked to behavioral psychology, which emphasizes the importance of reinforcement and consequences in shaping behavior. Quality assurance efforts can use this principle to encourage healthcare professionals to consistently adhere to established protocols and guidelines. Positive reinforcement, such as recognition or rewards, can motivate healthcare workers to follow best practices, leading to better patient outcomes. Behavioral interventions are another facet to enhance QA that could provide insights into how behavior change occurs. Behavioral interventions to promote quality assurance in clinical practice involve strategies and approaches aimed at improving the behaviors and actions of healthcare professionals to ensure the delivery of high-quality care. Quality assurance in clinical practice refers to the systematic efforts to monitor, assess, and improve the quality of healthcare services provided to patients. In addition, it refers to developing and implementing clinical pathways and protocols that outline standardized procedures for specific medical conditions or procedures. This helps ensure consistency in care delivery, reduces variations, and promotes adherence to evidence-based practices. Establishing a peer review processes where healthcare professionals review each other's clinical practices. This can be done through case discussions, chart audits, and collaborative problem-solving. Peer review encourages accountability and knowledge sharing among colleagues and provides opportunities for everyone involved to share their views in a transparent manner. Recognition and incentivization can also be another strategic approach to reward healthcare professionals who consistently demonstrate high-quality care and adherence to best practices. Incentives can motivate professionals to maintain and enhance their quality of care. Behavioral psychology emphasizes ethical behavior and professionalism. Quality assurance initiatives can reinforce these principles by setting standards for ethical conduct, ensuring patient privacy, and promoting respectful interactions between healthcare providers and patients. Behavioral psychology highlights the importance of emotional and psychological well-being. Quality assurance strategies can address healthcare professionals' well-being to prevent burnout and promote a positive work environment, ultimately benefiting patient care. In addition, these approaches could also recognize that creating a safe environment encourages individuals to report errors without fear of punishment. Quality assurance initiatives can foster a culture of safety by promoting open communication about errors and near-misses. By addressing errors constructively, healthcare organizations can prevent recurrence and improve patient safety.

The Bologna Declaration of 1999 focused on quality assurance systems within European universities that showed the importance of engagement between students, academics, and administrative staff. This resulted in many organizations establishing quality assurance units that show different forms of measuring quality. Most organizations circulate annual surveys to assess a number of activities in addition to student or staff satisfaction. Loukkola and colleagues (2010) reported a high level of academic engagement with 90.5% completing the survey [24].

1.4 Quality control

QC in healthcare refers to the systematic processes, practices, and measures put in place to monitor, assess, and regulate the quality of healthcare services and products. The goal of quality control is to ensure that healthcare is delivered consistently, safely, and effectively, meeting established standards and guidelines. There are a few key definitions and concepts related to quality control in healthcare. Quality control in clinical care involves a systematic approach to monitoring, evaluating, and ensuring the delivery of safe, effective, and consistent healthcare services. Here are the steps and methods involved in quality-controlling clinical care. It is vital to establish a clear set of standards and guidelines that can be defined as evidence-based standards, guidelines, and best practices for clinical care. These should be based on the latest medical research and industry recommendations. As part of this developing effective clinical protocols is important especially for common medical procedures and treatments. These protocols outline step-by-step processes that healthcare providers should follow to ensure consistency and adherence to established standards. Missed steps within a protocol can often reduce the quality and integrity of clinical care offered. However, it does allow a root-cause analysis to be performed relatively quickly to identify the reasons for the missed steps and any additional steps required to ensure these errors are not repeated. This provides an opportunity for ongoing training and education to healthcare staff to ensure they are well versed in the latest clinical guidelines and protocols. The use of clinical protocols, training programs, standards, and guidelines assists with maintaining accurate and comprehensive patient records, including medical history, treatment plans, and progress notes. Clear documentation helps ensure continuity of care and allows for retrospective analysis. This could assist with implementing a peer review process where experienced clinicians evaluate and provide feedback on the clinical care provided by their colleagues. This promotes accountability and knowledge sharing. When adverse events occur, it is important to identify the underlying factors that led to the issue enabling corrective actions and compare clinical outcomes and, processes with established benchmarks and best-in-class institutions to identify gaps and opportunities for improvement. This is also vital for technology integration where EHRs and other health information technologies are used to track patient data, streamline communication among healthcare providers, and facilitate data-driven decision-making. This collective information allows continuous reviews to take place that aid with updating clinical guidelines and best practices based on the latest research and advancements in medical knowledge.

A definitive outcome of effective QC procedures is the management of risk. Risk is defined as ISO31000 as the impact of uncertainty on objectives that could result in patient harm or death [25]. Risk management is a systematic approach to management procedures and practices linked to specific tasks such as evaluations and analysis. Clinical tests such as those conducted in pathology laboratories and radiological investigations are procedures that require risk management. Verifying the performance of the mechanical tools used and the personnel operating these is vital to ensuring the responses provided are aligned with the clinical responses required for physicians to make informed decisions (Fig. 1.2). Quality control plans for clinical investigations can often be supported by working instructions, process maps, and standard operating procedures. Designing and developing these documents could also allow staff to consider weak steps during the preanalytical, analytical, and postanalytical phases that can primitively reduce the potential errors [26].

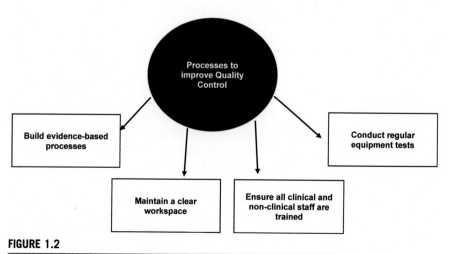

FIGURE 1.2

Four common quality control processes to ensure clinical practices are maintained at optimal levels.

1.5 **Quality management**

Quality management is a comprehensive approach to ensure that an organization consistently meets or exceeds the expectations of its customers, stakeholders, and regulatory bodies. It involves a set of principles, methodologies, processes, and practices aimed at achieving and maintaining high levels of quality in products, services, and processes. Quality management is applicable to various industries, including manufacturing, services, and healthcare [27,28]. Quality management frameworks such as ISO 9001 (for general quality management), ISO 13485 (for medical devices), and Joint Commission accreditation (for healthcare) provide structured guidelines for implementing quality management principles. Organizations adopt these frameworks and tailor them to their specific needs and industries.

Within clinical practice, all efforts aim to ensure the highest quality of care for each patient, without losing societal aspects such as cost control, and accessibility of care, out of sight [16]. Within clinical research, QA teams are responsible for providing oversight of the whole research process involving patient safety, data quality, and research integrity [17]. One core element of QA in clinical research is adhering to the Good Clinical Practice (GCP) guidelines, defined as [17]:

> *a set of internationally recognised ethical and scientific quality requirements which must be observed for designing, conducting, recording and reporting clinical trails that involve the participation of human subjects.*
>
> **EU Directive 2001/20/EC, Article 1, Clause 2.**

There are 13 Principles of the GCP guidelines which ensure [17]:

1. All research is carried out in accordance with the Declaration of Helsinki and ethical guidelines; conducted in compliance with protocol as reviewed by the institutional ethics board.
2. Risk–benefit ratio is appropriately assessed.
3. Rights, safety, and well-being of participants prevail over all other interests; informed consent.
4. All available information should be provided; scientifically sound, and in a clear protocol; all study information should be recorded and stored accurately.
5. Medical care and decisions made on behalf of the participant should be the responsibility of a qualified medic.
6. Each staff member should be adequately qualified and experienced.
7. Confidentiality and privacy should be maintained.
8. Investigational products should be manufactured and handled in accordance with Good Manufacturing Practice.
9. QA systems and procedures should be in place and implemented throughout the course of the study.

QA involves many different disciplines and should include procedures that can be conducted readily, should be able to identify and quantify variations in relevant parameters, should be able to detect and correct significant variations, and should be able to demonstrate an effect on the outcome of the trial [18,24]. The importance of properly established and managed quality control and quality assurance systems with their integral well-written SOPs and other quality documents cannot be ignored [18,24,25].

Quality improvement in clinical practice is important and underpinned by evidence-based practices driven by healthcare research. Hippocrates, the *"Father of Medicine"* was the first to diagnose and treat disease using systematic approaches which has led to the culture of evidence-based medicine. These efforts lead to reaching a common goal in an efficient and effective way, which allows sustainable development. Thus, successful QI ensures quality is engrained within healthcare systems, which would reduce the risk for patients and support the evolution of clinical practice. QI-based research is often conducted using qualitative methods. While it is important to utilize empirical studies to demonstrate causal relationships that can be generalized across clinical specialties and differing settings, populations, and outcome measures, it is important to develop pragmatic improved research that is applicable to the real world.

1.5.1 Quality management of clinical care

Managing quality in the context of clinical practice comprises using systems in place within the context of policies and frameworks. Systems used in clinical care are not restricted to electronic or paper-based records of patients but also any investigations conducted as part of a patient's care pathway. This means a holistic overview of details from conducting a particular test to the interpretation of the report and/or any recommendations to clinicians is recorded. In the United Kingdom, all healthcare professionals who immediately care for a patient are able to access the tests and their results (Fig. 1.3). As part of managing quality, quality management systems (QMS) are deployed across organizations and are a common tool used to organize, standardize, track, and improve activities related to clinical service. These can be accessed by any regulatory or governing organization as part of a clinical audit or inspection to ensure best practices have been used as part of the care delivery process.

For example, an NHS hospital that offers trauma services requires several optimal layers of safeguards to assess, stabilize, and treat a patient following a traumatic injury. Often, trauma-associated injuries are time critical and may require advanced trauma life support (ATLS) to address the life-threatening issues [27,28]. In this scenario, the quality management model (QMM) and approach can be highly specific due to the clinical requirements of the patient. Maritz and colleagues showed that there are approximately 64 different QMMs with 17 in clinical practice at present, which includes total quality management (TQM) systems [28]. TQMs comprise integrated processes involving all the systems and employees involved in the treatment pathway to continuously include information that allows effective care of the patient. TQMs can also provide information for any future regulatory or independent authorities to conduct an audit on how the clinical team

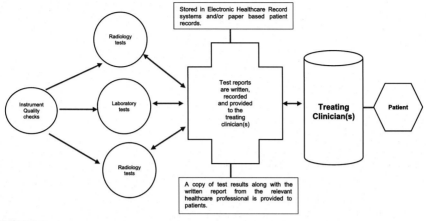

Independent oversight by regulatory and non-profit organisation such as the Care Quality Commission (CQC), Medicines and Healthcare Products Regulatory Agency (MHRA), European Medicines Agency and U.S. Food and Drug Administration (FDA)

Radiology tests

Stored in Electronic Healthcare Record systems and/or paper based patient records.

Instrument Quality checks

Laboratory tests

Test reports are written, recorded and provided to the treating clinician(s)

Treating Clinician(s)

Patient

Radiology tests

A copy of test results along with the written report from the relevant healthcare professional is provided to patients.

FIGURE 1.3

Chain of processes that develop a quality management system that clinicians can rely on as they make clinical decisions.

performed their role and verify their training and any other administrative records [29]. In addition to this, a key requirement is leadership at all levels to ensure the purpose and objectives of using a TQM are understood, such as the Trauma surgeon ensuring the ATLS protocol is followed and all interventional procedures used remain fit for purpose. The surgeon's role in this context in addition to perhaps performing the procedure is to ensure the team is encouraged and all tasks required are transparently communicated to all parties involved.

1.5.2 Quality in research using investigational medicinal products

Quality management in the context of research is often more complex in comparison to clinical practice, especially if it involves an investigational medicinal product (IMP) that is yet to be fully tested for its efficacy, safety profile, and effectiveness. First human clinical trials in particular are high risk and often require multiple layers of QC and QA steps to be embedded to ensure patient safety can be maintained.

In addition, it is vital to ensure that the drugs used within the clinical trial itself are able to maintain their quality and integrity throughout the clinical trial. While all IMPs are manufactured to the Good Manufacturer Practice (GMP) standard, this does not always guarantee high-quality drugs. Indindili and colleagues conducted a double-blind, randomized, 2-arm trial that compared the efficacy and safety of low-dose versus high-dose vitamin A supplements in Tanzanian infants [19]. The drugs were produced by companies in Italy and Canada. It was reported that all samples were regularly checked during the trial to ensure the capsules contained vitamin A. However, within 13 months of trial initiation, the 50,000 IU capsules degraded to 32% of the originally stipulated amount of vitamin A, despite following the storage recommendations. This was reported as a major confounder during the data analysis and the authors emphasized the need for QA and QC checks of IMPs during clinical trials and routine care. In another drug trial in 2011 consisting of antimalarial drug sulfadoxin pyrimethamine, pregnant women in six countries were meant to use four locally available brands. These brands were tested at the US Centers for Disease Control and Prevention where one of the brands showed sulfadoxine content at less than 90% of the manufacturer's recorded amount. However, the trial proceeded following the procuring of a good quality brand [20]. It is increasingly evident substandard formulations in medicinal products are a public health issue that impacts the developing world more commonly [21,22]. Clinical trial guidelines from the World Health Organisation and the International Conference on Harmonisation of Technical Requirements for registration of pharmaceuticals for human use (ICH) need compliance with GMP for all IMPs and any subsequent comparators [23,30]. However, these require urgent updating as the previous standards were deployed in the 1990s and additional considerations to the current drug market challenges including manufacturing, drug quality, and variability between similar formulations have not been considered [31,32].

Global clinical trials conducted in developing countries in particular have limited regulatory oversight and capacity for bioequivalence and pharmacovigilance procedures [33]. As a result, drugs with the same active pharmaceutical ingredients may differ in different batches. For example, clinical trials using different batches or brands of Digoxin and Mefloquine may provide different results that could be challenging to interpret results and lead to biases in any subsequent systematic reviews and meta-analyses that may be used for policy recommendations [34]. In 2007, a Clopidogrel batch labeled as Plavix with an estimated value of £1m ($1.5m) that was scheduled to be a comparator in a clinical trial in the United States was found to be counterfeited. Following initial tests, abnormal formulations were detected and contained only 50%−80% of Clopidogrel. The people responsible for this issue were linked to fraud and the further importation of two million doses of falsified olanzapine, bicalutamide, and clopidogrel in the United Kingdom [35].

In addition, globalization, the complexity of diseases and population demands, and outsourcing further purport quality challenges. To overcome these challenges, consignment verification checks can be a useful quality management approach to ensure authentic and high-quality drugs are used in research and thereafter. Ad hoc batch testing in particular can prevent patient harm and also erroneous results linked to clinical trials. Additionally, the MHRA published a set of guidelines in 2022 that showed risk-based clinical trial designs inclusive of risk assessments can address these challenges.

1.5.3 **Quality in research using medical devices**

Medical device clinical trials are more complex to design and conduct given the differences in device categories. Regulatory bodies globally have categorized medical devices in a variety of ways although the parity between the definitions is slowly closing the gap. This gap can introduce quality management challenges that could negatively impact clinical trial conduct.

Advancement of technologies has meant artificial intelligence (AI) techniques and data science methods are being used to develop digital technologies that either function to support patients with their clinical conditions and/or act as clinician-decision aids.

Regulating medical devices in the United Kingdom involves a comprehensive framework to ensure that these products are safe and effective for population use. The regulation of medical devices in the United Kingdom has undergone significant changes and updates following Brexit. Considering the last update in September 2021, the literature can provide an overview of how medical devices were regulated in the United Kingdom at that time [35].

1. **Regulatory Authorities**: In the United Kingdom, medical devices were regulated by the Medicines and Healthcare products Regulatory Agency (MHRA) before and after Brexit. The MHRA is responsible for ensuring the safety and quality of medical devices placed on the UK market.

2. **CE Marking**: Before Brexit, medical devices in the United Kingdom were regulated in alignment with the European Union (EU)'s regulations. The CE marking was used to indicate that a product complied with EU directives and could be legally placed on the market in the European Union and the United Kingdom.

3. **UKCA Marking**: Following Brexit, the United Kingdom introduced its own conformity assessment mark called UKCA (UK Conformity Assessed). Medical devices intended for the UK market should bear the UKCA mark. However, the CE marking was still accepted for a limited time, provided certain conditions were met.

4. **Regulatory Categories**: Medical devices are categorized into different classes based on their risk level, with Class I being the lowest risk and Class III being the highest. The classification determines the level of scrutiny and assessment required.

5. **Conformity Assessment**: Manufacturers are required to undergo a conformity assessment process for their medical devices. The level of assessment depends on the device's class. This process involves demonstrating that the device meets essential safety and performance requirements.

6. **Post-Market Surveillance**: Manufacturers and authorized representatives are obligated to monitor the performance of their medical devices once they are on the market and report any adverse events or safety concerns to the regulatory authority.

7. **Unique Device Identification (UDI)**: The United Kingdom has introduced a UDI system to improve the traceability of medical devices. Manufacturers must assign a unique identifier to each device to facilitate product recalls and monitoring.

8. **Clinical Investigations**: Clinical investigations may be required for certain medical devices to demonstrate their safety and efficacy. These studies must adhere to ethical and regulatory standards.

9. **Registration and Listing**: Manufacturers and authorized representatives must register with the MHRA and provide information about their devices. This information is used for regulatory oversight.

10. **Recalls and Safety Alerts**: If safety concerns arise, manufacturers and authorities can initiate recalls or issue safety alerts to protect patients and users.

1.5.4 Quality management using software

Corrective And Preventative Actions (CAPA) are the improvements and changes made to organizational processes to mitigate any nonconformities often related to quality assurance [36]. Corrective action explores the root cause for various issues and works to eliminate these to ensure similar issues do not arise again [36]. Preventive action involves identifying and removing possible sources of nonconformities before incidents or issues occur [36]. Organizations that offer CAPA Software include Intelex, MasterControl, and Ideagen [37,38].

Q-Pulse is a document management software developed by Ideagen Company Ltd and used in some organizations for managing policies and procedures [32]. For any QMS to succeed, it is fundamental to design and deliver an effective and extensive training program according to the appropriate level of staff. Even though the research of the study seems consistent with the case study findings, the lack of independent and nonbiased support raises the question of the efficiency and validity of Q-pulse as a quality improvement system.

Although it has been widely used in multiple trusts, research to prove its efficacy and efficiency has been scarce. Individual cases of different Trusts have been presented by Ideagen, outlining the benefits of using Q-pulse in different contexts and services [33]. Those benefits included automatization and increasing efficiency in document control and review in research at Southampton University Hospital, which generated significant extra time and resource cost reduction. Meaningful data collection and reporting of incidents in Clatterbridge Cancer Centre NHS Foundation Trust, as well as a reduction in report times, which is better for patient safety and staff time. Sharing of best practices between departments and usage of correct papers and procedures, standardization of processes in NHS Grampian, Royal Wolverhampton NHS Trust showed a significant reduction in time validating the system was facilitated by Q-pulse, huge savings in time, and associated staffing costs. Those case studies have also shown the initiatives of Ideagen to design and promote initiatives to address the requirements and needs of different trusts [33]. Finally, an independent study was conducted in KEMRI-Welcome Trust Research Laboratory to enhance effectiveness and efficiency by reducing the bureaucracy that comes with paper-based QMS implementation. Q-Pulse also achieved an increased involvement of staff participating in the QMS activities, which had a significant effect on operational efficiency.

The Production Part Approval Process (PPAP) outlines the process to ensure design and product specifications and objectives are met [34]. PPAP principles help reduce delays and nonconformances during part approval by providing a consistent approval process [34]. PPAP software supports the ability to make informed decisions at the right time by enabling the use of Design Failure Mode Effect Analyses (DFMEA) and Process Failure Mode Effect Analyses (PFMEA). These run crucial risk assessments into the possible failures surrounding both the design of the product and the overall manufacturing process [35]. Other elements of PPAP include Safety and Regulatory Issues, Process Flow Diagram, and Control Plans. The PPAP process is a detailed and lengthy process [24]. The PPAP package includes documentation of various multiple cross-functional tools and documents the ability to meet all requirements. PPAP software applications are offered by various companies, including Ideagen, PPAP Manager, and EHS Insights.

1.6 System thinking

System thinking is defined mostly as the assessment of system errors which would be inclusive of human errors and recognition of limitations. Limitations could be addressed in different ways [37–39]. For example, human limitations such as laps in concentration, prolonged attention, and multitasking could increase system errors. This was acknowledged by Florence Nightingale in her attempts to standardize nursing practices in 1854, which has been reiterated across a number of quality management reports and training programs [37–41]. The system thinking approach recognizes rather than individual blame, a system error approach is used [42,43]. This does not prevent an individual from being held accountable but simultaneously emphasizes the entire system to rethink the failures in an active manner to adopt better practices [42,44–46]. To achieve this, investigating the systems regularly to better evaluate the active failures could help prevent errors from occurring in the future. Latent conditions in a system are characteristic of the *know-how* of employees that help develop suitable organizational policies which should cover considerations toward understaffing, work pressure, multiple software systems, unreliable checklists, and procedures to raise concerns [47–50]. The system approaches could also demonstrate the lack of processes and/or issues with existing processes that influence a clinical and/or management outcome that impacts the system as well as patients [51–54]. The collective assessment of system thinking could prevent fatal events. A program approach to system thinking would be to conduct a suitable audit program to emphasize a learning culture and promote better clinical practices [55–60]. This could also influence the quality research landscape.

1.7 Conclusion

Quality of clinical trials is a moving target, as such to maintain integrity and protect patients, active surveillance of QA and QC steps should be followed. Similar approaches could be beneficial in research and clinical practices.

References

[1] De Jonge V, Nicolaas JS, van Leerdam ME, Kuipers EJ. Overview of the quality assurance movement in health care. Best Pract Res Clin Gastroenterol June 1, 2011;25(3): 337−47. https://doi.org/10.1016/j.bpg.2011.05.001.

[2] Kohn LT, Corrigan J, Donaldson MS. To err is human: building a safer health system, xxi. Washington, D.C.: National Academy Press; 2000. p. 287.

[3] Berwick DM. A user's manual for the IOM's "Quality Chasm" report. Health Aff (Millwood) 2002;21:80−90.

[4] Kudzma EC. Florence Nightingale and healthcare reform. Nurs Sci Q 2006;19(1):61−4.

[5] System control centres NHS England. Available from: www.england.nhs.uk/wp-content/uploads/2022/10/BW2084-system-control-centres-october-22.pdf. [Accessed 21 August 2023].

[6] Our purpose and role - Care Quality Commission. Available from: https://www.cqc.org.uk/about-us/our-purpose-role/who-we-are. [Accessed 21 August 2023].

[7] About the francis inquiry (health.org.uk). Available from: https://www.health.org.uk/about-the-francis-inquiry. [Accessed 21 August 2023].

[8] Manghani K. Quality assurance: importance of systems and standard operating procedures. Perspec Clin Res January 2011;2(1):34.

[9] Clinical Audit. NHS England. https://www.england.nhs.uk/clinaudit/. [Accessed 27 May 2024].

[10] Busari JO. Comparative analysis of quality assurance in health care delivery and higher medical education. Adv Med Educ Pract December 3, 2012:121−7.

[11] Goldstone J. The role of quality assurance versus continuous quality improvement. J Vasc Surg August 1, 1998;28(2):378−80.

[12] Mallon B, Philadelphia PA, Saunders WB. Ernest amory codman: the end result of a life in medicine. 1999.

[13] Donabedian A. The end results of health care: Ernest Codman's contribution to quality assessment and beyond. Milbank Q 1989;672:233−56. discussion 257−267.

[14] Roberts JS, Coale JG, Redman RR. A history of the Joint commission on accreditation of hospitals. JAMA 1987;258(7):936−94.

[15] Neuhauser D. Ernest Amory Codman, M.D., and end results of medical care. Int J Technol Assess Health Care 1990;6(2):307−25.

[16] Institute of Medicine. Medicare: a Strategy for quality assurance, vols. I and II. Washington, DC: National Academy Press; 1990.

[17] Donabedian A. Evaluating the quality of medical care. Milbank Q 2005;83(4): 691−729.

[18] Sandle LN. The management of external quality assurance. J Clin Pathol 2005;58: 141−4.

[19] Idindili B, Masanja H, Urassa H, et al. Randomized controlled safety and efficacy trial of 2 vitamin A supplementation schedules in Tanzanian infants. Am J Clin Nutr 2007;85: 1312−9. https://www.researchgate.net/publication/6340875_Randomized_controlled_ safety_and_efficacy_trial_of_2_vitamin_A_supplementation_schedules_in_Tanzania_ infants#fullTextFileContent. [Accessed 23 February 2024].

[20] Newton PN, Schellenberg D, Ashley EA, Ravinetto R, Green MD, ter Kuile FO, et al. Quality assurance of drugs used in clinical trials: proposal for adapting guidelines. BMJ February 25, 2015;350:h602. https://doi.org/10.1136/bmj.h602.

[21] Mori M, Ravinetto R, Jacobs J. Quality of medical devices and in vitro diagnostics in resource-limited settings. Trop Med Int Health 2011;16:1439−49.

[22] Newton PN, Green MD, Fernández FM, Day NP, White NJ. Counterfeit anti-infective medicines. Lancet Infect Dis 2006;6:602−13.

[23] World Health Organization. Guidelines for good clinical practice (GCP) for trials on pharmaceutical products. WHO technical report series No. 850. 1995. Annex 3, http://apps.who.int/medicinedocs/pdf/whozip13e/whozip13e.pdf.

[24] Loukkola T, Zhang T. Examining quality culture: Part 1-Quality assurance processes in higher education institutions. Brussels: European University Association; 2010.

[25] International Organization for Standardization. ISO31000: risk management − principles and guidelines. Geneva, Switzerland: ISO; 2009. p. 24.

[26] Hubbard D. The failure of risk management: why it's broken and how to fix it. Indianapolis, IN: John Wiley & Sons; 2009. p. 46.

[27] Galvagno SM, Nahmias JT, Young DA. Advanced trauma life Support® update 2019: management and applications for adults and special populations. Anesthesiol Clin March 2019;37(1):13−32.

[28] Maritz R, Scheel-Sailer A, Schmitt K, Prodinger B. Overview of quality management models for inpatient healthcare settings. A scoping review. Int J Qual Health Care July 01, 2019;31(6):404−10.

[29] Mosadeghrad AM. Essentials of total quality management: a meta-analysis. Int J Health Care Qual Assur 2014;27(6):544−58.

[30] International conference on harmonisation of technical requirements for registration of pharmaceuticals for human use. ICH harmonized tripartite guideline. Guideline for good clinical practice E6(R1); 1996. http://www.ich.org/fileadmin/Public_Web_Site/ ICH_Products/Guidelines/Efficacy/E6/E6_R1_Guideline.pdf.

[31] Lang T, Cheah PY, White NJ. Clinical research: time for sensible global guidelines. Lancet 2011;377:1553−5.

[32] Caudron JM, Ford N, Henkens M, Macé C, Kiddle-Monroe R, Pinel J. Substandard medicines in resource-poor settings: a problem that can no longer be ignored. Trop Med Int Health 2008;13:1062−72.

[33] World Health Organization. Assessment of medicines regulatory systems in sub-Saharan African countries. An overview of findings from 26 assessment reports. 2010. http://apps.who.int/medicinedocs/en/d/Js17577en/.

[34] Gutman J, Green MD, Durand S, Rojas OV, Ganguly B, Quezada WM, et al. Mefloquine pharmacokinetics and mefloquine-artesunate effectiveness in Peruvian patients with uncomplicated plasmodium falciparum malaria. Malar J 2009;8:58.

[35] Medicines and Healthcare Products Regulatory Agency. Press release: four month trial concludes of Operation Singapore—the most serious known breach of counterfeit medicine in the regulated supply chain. April 2011. http://www.mhra.gov.uk/NewsCentre/ Pressreleases/CON114481.

[36] What is CAPA and why is it important? Available from: https://blog.falcony.io/en/what-is-capa. [Accessed 2 August 2023].

[37] CAPA Management Software. Available from: https://www.intelex.com/products/applications/capa-software-corrective-and-preventive-action. [Accessed 2 August 2023].

[38] CAPA Management Software. Available from: https://www.ideagen.com/solutions/quality/quality-management/capa-management. [Accessed 2 August 2023].

[39] Trends 2010: a decade of change in European higher education Europe University Association. 2010 [Accessed 2 August 2023], https://eua.eu/resources/publications/312:trends-2010-a-decade-of-change-in-european-higher-education.html.

[40] Continuous Quality Improvement (CQI) combines scientific methodologies with the management philosophy of continuously improving processes and services.

[41] Berwick DM, Godfrey AB, Roessner J. Curing health care: new strategies for quality improvement. San Francisco, CA: Jossey-Bass; 1990.

[42] de Jonge V, Nicolaas JS, van Leerdam ME, Kuipers EJ. Overview of the quality assurance movement in health care. Best Pract Res Clin Gastroenterol 2011;25(Issue 3):337–47.

[43] Lawrence M, Olesen F. Indicators of quality in health care. Eur J Gen Pract 1997;3(3):103–8. https://doi.org/10.3109/13814789709160336.

[44] Our indicators measure outcomes that reflect quality of care. They also look at processes that are linked by evidence to improved outcomes. Available from: https://www.nice.org.uk/standards-and-indicators/indicators. [Accessed 2 August 2023].

[45] Quality assurance in clinical trials — an introduction to GCP. Available from: https://www.quanticate.com/blog/bid/49734/quality-assurance-in-clinical-trials-an-introduction-to-gcp. [Accessed 2 August].

[46] Ibbott GS, Haworth A, Followill DS. Quality assurance for clinical trials. Front Oncol December 19, 2013;3:311. https://doi.org/10.3389/fonc.2013.00311.

[47] Van Tienhoven G, Mijnheer BJ, Bartelink H, Gonzalez DG. Quality assurance of the EORTC Trial 22881/10882: boost versus no boost in breast conserving therapy. An overview. Strahlenther Onkol 1997;173(4):201–7. https://doi.org/10.1007/BF03039289.

[48] Manghani K. Quality assurance: importance of systems and standard operating procedures. Perspect Clin Res January 2011;2(1):34–7. https://doi.org/10.4103/2229-3485.76288.

[49] Burnett D. Understanding accreditation in laboratory medicine. London: ACB Venture Publications; 1996.

[50] Pacey AA. Quality assurance and quality control in the laboratory andrology. Asian J Androl January 2010;12(1):21–5. https://doi.org/10.1038/aja.2009.16.

[51] Taverniers I, De Loose M, Van Bockstaele E. Trends in quality in the analytical laboratory. II. Analytical method validation and quality assurance. TrAC, Trends Anal Chem 2004;23(8):535–52. https://doi.org/10.1016/j.trac.2004.04.001.

[52] Guidance the government data quality framework. Available from: https://www.gov.uk/government/publications/the-government-data-quality-framework/the-government-data-quality-framework. [Accessed 2 August].

[53] A review of data quality assessment methods for public health information systems.

[54] Data quality assurance: importance and best practices in 2023. Available from: aimultiple.com. [Accessed 2 August].

[55] Available from: https://best-practice-and-impact.github.io/qa-of-code-guidance/data. html. [Accessed 2 August].

[56] Available from: https://osr.statisticsauthority.gov.uk/guidance/administrative-data-and-official-statistics/. [Accessed 2 August].

[57] Bashan A, Kordova S. Challenges in regulating the local and global needs of quality management systems. Int J Qual Reliab Manag August 18, 2021;39(8):1996−2019.

[58] Gumba H, Lowe B, Mosobo M, Njuguna S, Musyoki J. Implementation of an electronic quality management system using Q-pulse: the KEMRI-wellcome trust research laboratories experience. Annals of Clinical and Laboratory Research; 2019.

[59] Ideagen quality management - modular SaaS QMS solution. Ideagen.

[60] Case Studies | Resources. Ideagen. Available from: https://www.ideagen.com/resources/casestudies. [Accessed 2 August].

Further reading

[1] (PPAP) Production part approval process. Available from: https://www.aiag.org/quality/automotive-core-tools/ppap. [Accessed 2 August].

[2] Papp Software. Available from: https://www.ideagen.com/solutions/quality/quality-control/ppap-software. [Accessed 2 August].

[3] Introduction to production part approval process (PPAP). Available from: https://www.quality-one.com/ppap/. [Accessed 2 August].

Building a quality management system

2

Abstract

Quality management system (QMS) is defined as a formal system that includes documents procedures, processes, and responsibilities to ensure aims and objectives are met. A QMS can be designed for multiple levels: organizational, departmental, and specialty. The field of medicine in particular is a *learned profession* that rapidly changes its' approach to diagnosing, treating, and managing the clinical care offered to service users/patients. Organizations driven by clinical research and/or practice have knowledge management embedded within their core operational models. These models are a rich source of explicit and tacit knowledge, which is often fluid in healthcare and academic settings. The distinction between the two is fundamental to knowledge management and therefore any QMS developed and utilized. Tacit knowledge in particular comprises experiences endeavored by the workforce where the *"know-how"* and *"learning"* are embedded among routine practices. These practices evolve with wisdom and context-specific experiences including insights and intuitions felt by staff. This aspect of any role is crucial to document, in order to capture optimal versus suboptimal practices that could transform future practices. On the other hand, explicit knowledge is codified and documented within a variety of materials such as books, memoranda, reports, and other forms of publications to facilitate a process or a practice. The identified and articulated structured knowledge-base can be shared and reproduced in a variety of settings, to enhance decision-making and reduce duplication of efforts. For these reasons, the structure of the QMS needs to be adaptable and accommodative of both types of knowledge and driven by the need to *change* with features covering principles of reliability, responsiveness, and assurance aligned to healthcare outcomes such as recovery, survival, and restoration of function to prevent knowledge loss. Effective standard operating procedures, working instructions, and other guidelines could assist with developing a robust procedure and process led QMS, which would encompass seven pillars of quality.

Keywords: Assurance; Maternity; Quality management system; Radiology; Responsiveness.

Key messages

- Quality management systems (QMSs) are important to ensure the quality of a service or product, especially at the developmental stages.
- Lean healthcare is a subset of *Lean management ideologies* that are useful to minimize waste. Building these approaches into a QMS can improve operational efficiency.

Quality Assurance Management. https://doi.org/10.1016/B978-0-12-822732-9.00009-6

- QMSs are defined as systems comprising documents, procedures, processes, and responsibilities to ensure aims, objectives, and policies are adhered.
- A QMS can direct a team or organization to maintain compliance and fulfill regulatory requirements.
- QMSs can improve continuous efficacy and effectiveness in a team or the evaluation process of a product.
- A QMS can be developed to a variety of standards, for example, ISO 9001:2015, ISO 13485, ISO 14000 series, ISO 19011, or ISO 9000 series.

2.1 Introduction

Quality management system (QMS) is defined as a formal system that includes documents procedures, processes, and responsibilities to ensure aims and objectives are met. A QMS can be designed for multiple levels: organizational, departmental, and specialty. The field of medicine in particular is a *learned profession* that rapidly changes its' approach to diagnosing, treating, and managing the clinical care offered. Organizations driven by clinical research and/or practice have knowledge management embedded within their core operational models. These models are a rich source of explicit and tacit knowledge, which is often fluid in healthcare and academic settings. The distinction between the two is fundamental to knowledge management and therefore any QMS developed and utilized. Tacit knowledge in particular comprises experiences endeavored by the workforce where the *"know-how"* and *"learning"* are embedded among routine practices. These practices evolve with wisdom and context-specific experiences including insights and intuitions felt by staff. This aspect of any role is crucial to document to capture optimal versus suboptimal practices that could transform future practices. On the other hand, explicit knowledge is codified and documented within a variety of materials such as books, memos, reports, and other forms of publications to facilitate a process or a practice. The identified and articulated structured knowledge base can be shared and reproduced in a variety of settings to enhance decision making and reduce duplication of efforts. For these reasons, the structure of the QMS needs to be adaptable and accommodative of both types of knowledge and driven by the need to *change* with features covering principles of reliability, responsiveness, and assurance aligned to healthcare outcomes such as recovery, survival, and restoration of function to prevent knowledge loss. Effective standard operating procedures, working instructions, and other guidelines could assist with developing a robust procedure and process led QMS, which would encompass seven pillars of quality (Fig. 2.1).

The formalized system can also be adapted in many ways to provide flexibility if a healthcare or academic institution requires the processes to demonstrate the multifaceted nature of their routine work. Healthcare organizations in particular are complex given the intangible outcomes linked to a variety of services and professional groups. Fundamental to the processes is the relationship between a QMS and a

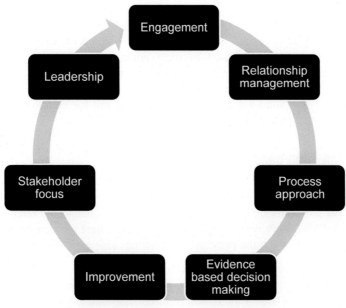

FIGURE 2.1

Indicates the seven principles of a quality management system.

healthcare organization which is a complex relationship with a variety of standard operating procedures, guidelines, and work instructions implicitly linking the routine functions. Hence, any QMS developed and implemented will need to demonstrate direct applicability to the rendered services, affordable, effective, efficient, and user related. A similar premise applies to clinical trial units (CTUs) that are hosted by academic or healthcare organizations. For CTUs, however, the need for processes and procedures related to delivering clinical research may require additional components as the QMS will need to reflect optimal risk management as clinical trials are testing either experimental treatments or repurposing treatments for diseases by way of off-label use.

Before developing a QMS, it is vital that an organization or an area of the organization that intends to use it identify the scope and purpose of the system to ensure the multifunction processes required can be managed. The QMS design should be able to influence the objectives, needs, services, and products used by way of quality processes. There are four main types of quality process-based standards used in healthcare, industry, and academia: ISO9001, AS9100, Six Sigma, and CMMI. However, ISO 9001:2015 is the most recognized and common QMS standard used globally. The flexibility this standard allows is an attractive feature for organizations, as internal programs can be developed within the constraints of this framework. In addition, ISO 9000 series also includes ISO 9000 and ISO 9004, which are used by healthcare organizations, while ISO 13485 is the standard QMS developed for developing, testing, and deploying medical devices. ISO 19011 is commonly used for regulatory purposes, in particular for conducting audits.

The most common format is based on *a plan—do—check—act (PDSA)* cycle, allowing continuous improvement to incur among all stakeholders within the QMS and the services rendered. The PDSA cycle is a useful method to use to ensure continuous improvements can be made at regular intervals, and the process can be documented at each time point. This audit trail is of use for monitoring tasks and improvements that can be completed.

2.1.1 Plan—do—check—act cycle

The origins of PDSA cycles are linked to industry and Edward Deming and Walter Shewhart, who discussed iterative processes that can be employed to improve methods and procedures. The terminology and the interchangeable references to a variety of methods were developed by Deming's [1]. There are many variations to the PDSA cycle although the principles remain the same as the following points:

- Plan: identify a problem and plan a change
- Do: Explore and assess the change by reviewing existing evidence
- Check: Evaluate and test the results from the evidence gathered.
- Act: Take a step to learn the problem and

A PDSA model specifically to assess and quality check improvements could be developed.

In the absence of a framework, four key principles can can be used to develop a suitable evidence-based scientific method that can be evaluated at multiple stages (Fig. 2.2).

This approach is not commonly used within healthcare but has been used in clinical trials. There are many commonalities between areas that conduct clinical trials and healthcare services. The same concept could also be used to develop a system to report quality assurance management. Similarly, simultaneous cycles can be used to assess changes in complex areas, especially within a single division that includes several departments or multiple teams. It is vital the PDSA cycles are representative of each of those departments or teams, and common features to showcase any potential interactions are also shown to indicate the evidence needed to measure the desired outcomes and continuous improvements. In such instances, it is imperative to coordinate the cycles and their outcomes (Fig. 2.3). These can be represented in a report or a digital dashboard that could be displayed in real time within the said department. Transparency of the findings could influence change management.

The evidence within the scientific literature and improvement programs is used to improve quality assurance management in smaller areas. The cancer services collaborative in the National Health Services (NHS) United Kingdom (UK) is a good example of using 28 change principles grouped within four areas to successfully improve services [2]. The four categories included mapping the process of a patient's journey, developing a team centered around the journey, centralizing

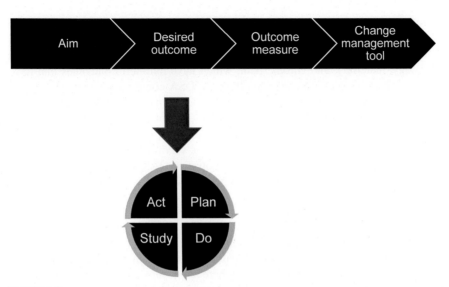

FIGURE 2.2

Key principles that need to be considered to develop a framework to develop a PDSA.

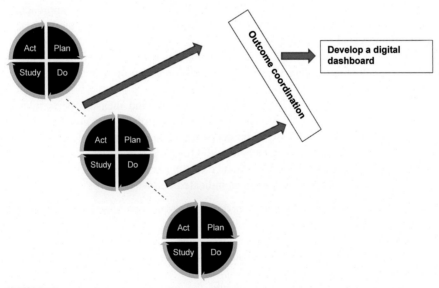

FIGURE 2.3

Combination of multiple PDSA cycles and the coordination of the desired outcomes to display over a digital dashboard.

patient and care experience, and the capacity to meet the needs of the patient at every stage. The use of multiple PDSA cycles was a benefical approach in this instance [3]. This approach can be translated to complex clinical specialties, in particular, such as radiology, maternity, and chronic pain, which have long-term outcomes that have several influences on the manner in which a PDSA could be adopted. This QAM approach can also be managed using project management principles that can then be displayed for leadership teams to review as part of their regular operation and strategic discussions. This level of oversight aids improvement and better design of QMSs, as well as transformation plans for services and the development of new quality indicators. This could further optimize QAM by way of developing a workforce that is more accepting of change.

2.1.2 Quality improvement

Quality improvement (QI) is a vital component in the management of QAM and in delivering safety and quality within healthcare. Although the most common QI method is considered to be PDSA cycles, there are novel adjunct methods that could aid with an overarching evaluation of a service rendered within a healthcare organization. Quality improvement in clinical practice is important and underpinned by evidence-based practices driven by healthcare research. Hippocrates, the *"Father of Medicine"* was the first to diagnose and treat disease using systematic approaches, which has led to the culture of evidence-based medicine. These efforts lead to reaching a common goal in an efficient and effective way that allows sustainable development. Thus, successful QI ensures quality is engrained within healthcare systems, which would reduce the risk for patients and support the evolution of clinical practice.

QA indicators are utensils developed to monitor and measure performance. These are often referred to as key performance indicators (KPIs) commonly used as part of management processes. The decision-making process could use KPIs as an indispensable benchmark that can aid with QI. QI is an important facet of healthcare management and the benefits influence continuous clinical practice.

There are five common indicators as indicated below:

- Efficiency or performance indicators demonstrate the operational throughput and output within an organization
- Impact indicators that demonstrate fidelity and patient satisfaction
- Effectiveness indicators to demonstrate service or product value that can influence patient-reported outcomes
- Patient-reported indicators demonstrate the increase or reduction in patient complaints
- Quality or safety indicators, which demonstrate the integrity of the service provided by the organization

There are a number of theoretical frameworks published although there is a paucity of testing, validation, and long-term QI outcomes of these in a variety of settings and organizations. Also, there are secondary challenges such as evaluating the validity of QI interventions and their alignment to any theoretical frameworks. Specificity to a setting may not be cost-effective although this may be the appropriate step to undertake. For example, clinical specialties within healthcare have specific requirements, and the processes followed will differ depending on the care offered to patients. In comparison, academic institutions may be significantly different as the organization may have ongoing teaching and research activities. This is further perplexing, if the academic organization functions alongside a teaching hospital where some staff have job-share roles. This is a common feature among teaching hospitals and large academic centers in the United Kingdom, where even the most basic processes differ vastly; therefore, any QMS will need to be broad, with specific PDSAs or localized components of the QMS. Any subsequent quality policies used will need to cover the broad QMS with localized policies as well. These alternations could influence complex social systems. The gathering of this data through either surveys or even qualitative interviews is useful to successfully implement QA and QC processes as part of a QI program. This can be an evidence-based approach to improve healthcare practice by way of complex multifaceted step-wise interventions in particular [4]. These can be iterative to adapt to the local context and gather unintended effects [5].

The paucity of research to enhance iterative methods to assess interventions is a significant limitation in complex clinical areas which are also considered as high-risk services offered to patients. Add to this burden are the financial constraints within these areas as often, the interventions used within complex areas are expensive to manage [6]. PDSA cycles can provide an iterative method to develop change as part of using a QI approach such as the Total Quality Management (TQM), Model for Improvement (MFI), Lean, Six Sigma, or Quality Improvement Collaborative (QIC). However, the theories and evidence base to analyze effectiveness are underreported, and formal evaluation of the objectives and outcomes remains underreported. Some PDSA approaches also report clinical and patient-reported outcomes, as shown by Pronovost et al. where a cohort study was conducted to test an evidence-based intervention to minimize the incidence of catheter-related blood infections [7]. Multilevel Poisson regression modeling was the statistical method of choice that was used to compare infection rates pre- and postimplementation of the intervention over a 18-month period. The study concluded by demonstrating a significant reduction in infection rates of up to 66% in catheter-related blood infections, which were sustained over 18 months with outcome measurements at 3-month intervals indicating the National Nosocomial Infections Surveillance System [7]. However, there were similar interventions that showed no improvement as shown by Landon et al. in their EQHIV study [8]. The EQHIV study (Effects of a quality improvement collaborative on the outcome of care of patients with HIV infection) assessed the effectiveness of a QI collaborative to improve the care provided to HIV-infected patients using a controlled pre- and postinterventional evaluation with 9986 patients. The difference in the change in quality was not statistically significant; therefore, the improvement program was unsuccessful. Another example of a failure of a QI program failure is a study that attempted to reduce in-hospital length by redesigning 18 project teams using a case study approach by Vos et al. [9]. The study team attempted to gather data using qualitative methods by way of question-naires, semistructured interviews, and observations documented during collaborative meetings. The QI method used for process redesign proved challenging as the members of the first team did not use the change management processes that were proposed and the customized solutions proposed by the researchers did not fit the context-specific issues linked to possible delays and waiting times. The second team had capacity issues around testing the idea within short time frames due to the complexities within the demand while their team did not receive a peer stimulus due to the lack of alignment between the project's proposed process and the actual tasks they did. The project teams also reported that there was a lack of external and internal support available [9]. These failures indicate it is vital to have staff engagement when QI programs are developed and, to understand the requirements of a department before any quality control and assurance measures are put in place when designing processes. Process mapping requires a real-time understanding of the activities conducted within a team and its alignment with any quality management procedures already in place. It is vital to fully understand the design process before any program is developed, in order to achieve any meaningful change.

2.1.3 Interpretation of outcomes from a PDSA cycle

Interpretation of outcomes from a PDSA cycle requires a true understanding of the processes, outcome measures, and quality control steps used within this system. Surface level results sometimes may not resonate with those of the actual service, for example, a pain management service's performance can be evaluated using multiple quality indicators. Interpreting the outcomes and measures linked to these indicators can be more complex as reporting and management of pain is challenging due to the high heterogeneity observed within the disease cohort. In addition, reporting pain is highly personal to a patient, and therefore the management of this is equally challenging. Although at the surface level, pain intensity is often considered an outcome measure, from the perspective of a quality indicator, this can be ambiguous. Yet, pain intensity is a valuable indicator within the context of patient-reported outcomes. The inclusion of this to a QMS as a quality indicator can be an important measure to determine the frequency of patient follow-up requirements and the overall quality of life of the said patient due to the care offered. The successful deployment of a PDSA cycle therefore needs adaptability and analyses of the data gathered in the wider context as opposed to the common thought that PDSA methods are a "black box" approach of QI. Complex interventions used to promote QI and QAM require the completion of specific QC and QA processes that are aligned to the key principles that inform the success or unsuccess of the application alongside a summarized explanation for failures detected [10,11]. Interpreting the outcomes also requires specific methodologies and SQUIRE guidelines. SQUIRE guidelines demonstrate a framework to report new knowledge about quality improvements within healthcare by way of safety, value for money, and quality of the methods used to assess the outcomes of any interventions. The guidelines also discuss an array of approaches authors should consider when explaining and elaborating on any improvements being reported within a scientifically appropriate method that can be based upon a theoretical framework. Comprehensive PDSA applications can be described and reported using SQUIRE guidelines.

More traditional healthcare methods such as randomized clinical trials (RCT) or evidence-based-medicine (EBM) methods have not been used to evaluate most complex interventions or assess QI applications. Moen and colleagues report that PDSA cycles are better as it is a pragmatic scientific method for assessing change in complex systems [12]. However, there is evidence to indicate that PDSA cycles are not always suitable for reporting quality improvement as it does not fully capture important granular details about the clinical and scientific aspects linked to procedures carried out in a department or organization. It is often perceived that PDSA provides more pragmatic methods to test complex systems than clinical trials although this would largely depend on the scope, purpose, and risks associated with stakeholders. For example, complex interventions developed for improving and quality assuring chronic noncancer pain management would benefit from a clinical trial due to the high heterogeneity of the patient population, long-term access to healthcare services, and healthcare cost implications. Using a pragmatic clinical trial with long-term follow-up could easily assess this form of complex intervention with a qualitative and quantitative synthesis of the findings. Iterative approaches used in this context could also demonstrate acceptability by healthcare professionals and patients alike, allowing better adaptability at the point of implementation if the intervention is demonstrated to be effective and purposeful. A feasibility clinical study is another option for assessing complex interventions, which could provide the opportunity to build evidence on the efficacy, acceptability, and engagement of all stakeholders to influence sustainable change. A PDSA approach could equally be embedded into either of these approaches to assess natural variation in a system, awareness, and overall impact of the intervention. Learning through robust scientific experimental methods is important to promote evidence-based healthcare approaches, which would be considered as an optimal quality assurance method to deliver safe clinical care, in particular, by independent authorities including regulators.

2.2 Quality improvement methodologies

There are many QI methodologies although their specificity and adaptability to healthcare, industry, and academia vary. For complex clinical specialties such as radiology or obstetrics, safety, effectiveness, and experience of care are paramount to service users and those who are delivering the care. This is further perplexed when applied to healthcare or academic environments that deliver research care, which is riddled with a variety of complexities ranging from risks pertaining to the intervention and/or the study population to managing human factors and the systematic approaches required to gather safety data at specific time intervals. The benefit of designing bespoke QI is primarily for patients, clinicians, and healthcare providers. However, this can be complicated due to challenges such as increasing costs and sustainability within an evolving workforce. Hence, designing, experimenting, and implementing real-time changes require flexible QI methodologies that may use both qualitative and quantitative measures.

The understanding of systems and practices is vital to designing QI methodologies suitable to answer a particular clinical question and measurement of the improvement model. Initiating a clinical audit with a SMART framework (specific, measurable, achievable, realistic, and timely) may be an effective starting point. The use of quantitative methods to report QI is not commonly used. However, it is an important and responsible method to report findings. There are similarities between QI methodologies, clinical audits, and empirical research especially based on common variables such as safety, frequency, efficiency, effectiveness, stakeholder outcomes, and equity.

2.2.1 Bibliometric statistical methodology

Bibliometric statistics are defined by the use of bibliometric indicators to map the frequency by which terms or words are used in publication databases. This was considered an imperfect tool although a variety of optimal applications and simple tools have been developed over the last decade. Simple methods such as the use of mesh terms and continuous development of a framework of mesh terms have optimized refinement and search algorithms used in many search engines such as PubMed. Bibliometric statistics are commonly used in research management to evaluate structured processes driven by peer review. This is similar to conducting a systematic review with or without a meta-analysis or network meta-analysis, which uses predefined variables to construct data tables for a suitable analysis. Bibliometric indicators can also be predefined variables or exposures that can be used as consistent measures to explore and disseminate *Lean thinking* or *Lean production* that can reflect societal shift to public sector or institutional accountability and managerialism. Langfeldt et al. stipulated [13]:

> Mechanisms for constituting research quality notions that were once reserved for highly professionalised knowledge communities have extended to encompass notions generated within policy and funding domains

Quality is still debated in the context of clinical and research practice often despite some concepts being mutually inclusive. Mutually inclusive probability would imply the following where

P is probability
and
Event X and Y

$$P\ (X \text{ or } Y) = P(X) + P(Y) - P\ (X \text{ and } Y)$$

Or

$$P\ (X \text{ or } Y) > 0$$

2.2.2 Six Sigma methodology

The Six Sigma is an improvement methodology developed in the 1980s by engineers at Motorola to improve the manufacturing process. It is defined as a method to reduce variability and waste in a system based on defining, measuring, analyzing, improving, and controlling by leveraging data to remove defects and improve overall quality and efficiency. Both quantitative and qualitative measurements can be gathered to conduct a statistical analysis, as demonstrated in Table 2.1.

A key challenge using Six Sigma is that human interactions are limited as the focus remains to be fact driven. In some instances, allowing a team or a unit to manage the problem is more effective than a complete operational overhaul. In addition, historically, this methodology used a one-size-fits-all approach, which may not be suitable for organizations that drive innovation. University hospitals or academic environments that thrive in conducting research, for example, may not benefit from using the standard Six Sigma methodology.

However, adapting the Six Sigma methodology to a particular organization or an area of an organization may be beneficial. For example, the use of a waterfall method where multiple sequential tasks are completed in a particular order can benefit a team developing and delivering research projects. Similarly, an agile method where the use of a scrum with an incremental approach to allow deliverables to be tracked and delivered with adjustments may be useful for those delivering clinical trials, in particular, in emergency medicine or communicable diseases. The agile and waterfall methods demonstrated their strength during the emergency licensing of COVID-19 vaccines. Kanban or dashboards could further assist with tracking the logistical aspects of the delivery of a product or its effectiveness by way of gathering safety information over a period of time that could further allow adjustments to be made to the product or the scrum in real time, in some instances. This can be a useful approach for artificial intelligence (AI) tool testing, in particular where there is either diagnostic accuracy or prediction of disease severity.

Statistical improvements within organizational processes can be an advantage to understanding functionality and management techniques required to optimize workflows and leadership strategies required for an organization. Six Sigma projects can demonstrate root-cause issues that can then be understood by way of their effect on the processes, which can be addressed by way of statistical processes controls and capability calculations that can act as quality control steps.

Table 2.1 Processes at each stage of a modified approach to the Six Sigma process.

Principle	Purpose	Process	Method
Define	Describe the issues and design a mandate to address the issues	Identify characteristics of the issue	Develop a charter and/or framework
		Develop a charter with a clear scope and purpose	Develop a milestone map with a trajectory dashboard
		Recognize improvement opportunities	Develop a project plan
		Discuss these in detail with stakeholders	Discussions with all stakeholders
		Process map end-to-end	Design process maps
		Consider quality control steps	Develop affinity diagrams and a tracker
Measure	Describe performance	Identify performance measures	Detailed map of the processes
		Develop definitions for operational terminologies	A measurement plan using a performance dashboard with existing and new data that is updated at a regular frequency
		Develop and implement a continuous measurement plan	
		Develop any further performance indicators	
		Develop outcome measures, where appropriate	
Analyze	Assess the effects of the processes used associated with the root causes	To identify and understand root causes	Quality control processes using statistical methods
		To validate root causes and any identifiable variation	Evaluate process capability
		Quality control of processes and capabilities	Evaluate gaps per million calculations
		Evaluate process maps to identify quality improvement indicators	Develop fishbone diagrams

Table 2.1 Processes at each stage of a modified approach to the Six Sigma process.—*cont'd*

Principle	Purpose	Process	Method
Improve	Develop, identify, and implement evidence-based solutions	Using analytics plot and analyze the data	Develop cause and effect matrices
		Evaluate any process variation to find the Sigma score	Use Pareto or any other suitable statistical analysis
		Design and develop solutions to the problems identified	Brainstorm and process map the ideas
		Assess and select the most appropriate evidence-based solutions	Use visual aids to demonstrate the identified problems and solutions
		Develop process maps and statistical inferences to report identified measurables	Conduct statistical analysis and solution screening
		Discuss the findings with stakeholders and obtain feedback	Conduct a pilot or feasibility study to test the solutions identified including any PDSA cycle
Control	Evaluate solutions, quality controls, and a suitable framework	Conduct a pre- and post-implementation to recalculate the Sigma score to report any possible variation	Use a performance and quality indicator-based dashboard
		Develop standard operating procedures	Check and monitor deviations from quality control processes
		Develop any evidence-based guidelines	Check and monitor deviations from the standards
		Develop working instructions	Check and monitor deviations from statistical process control
		Continuously monitor the performance and integrate findings with a lesson-learned approach	Check and monitor uptake from training and education
		Develop a recommendation plan with milestones and a monitoring plan	

Pragmatic composites of Six Sigma methodologies can be useful for healthcare and academic organizations. As this is a flexible methodology, it can be useful in clinical trial management. Regardless of the intervention, a clinical trial is testing, Six Sigma methods could improve quality assurance in the conduct of key tasks such as data collection and analysis. These can be built into an electronic data collection (EDC) system although some teams continue to use paper-based data collection forms in some parts of the world. Data-driven decision making in Six Sigma can uncover the root cause of a problem to apply Lean principles to resolve them and consequently improve operational performance and productivity. Conventionally, Lean and Six Sigma principles have been used as part of manufacturing and solidifies the good manufacturing practice (GMP) standard that regulators require. There is an established group that uses Lean Six Sigma at the independent review board level; Copernicus group, which was established in 1996. The Copernicus group's primary responsibility, like with any ethics committee, was to ensure the welfare and rights of human participants taking part in research studies remain protected. The group meets the standards for industry certification and became one of the first institutions to be accredited by the Association for the Accreditation of Human Research Protection Programs Inc. in 2007 and 2011. The program improvement has focused largely to commit to quality management, and in May 2010, they received ISO 9001; 2008 certification. The goal became to minimize nonvalue processes and reduce variations where possible to reduce costs and waste. This was achieved by way of employee team-based approaches and the development of a steering committee. Interestingly, clinical trial steering or management committees have been a long-standing practice when conducting clinical trials in academia and the NHS in the United Kingdom. Cross-functionality of Six Sigma methodologies especially in process development is a useful value-stream map for optimal workflow in relation to the following:

- Reducing time taken to review and approve amendments
- Improving delivery times for documentation, samples, and interventions
- Reducing errors when writing documents and data

This also emphasizes the need for a cultural shift toward consistent collaboration and continuous process improvements. Daily accountability and transparency would be provided as part of this approach using three steps:

- The use of an operational dashboard that allows all team members to visualize objectives, ongoing activities, and outcomes. This approach allows staff to understand the strengths and weaknesses of the processes they are completing making it easier for management and leadership teams to discuss improvements.
- The use of a correction database that can increase efficiency and reduce redundancies in data captured for analysis. This would be a quality control step to prevent internal and external errors as part of the data-capturing process that could demonstrate trends in errors and where training can be utilized.
- The use of matrices to demonstrate data accuracy and reduce the overall clinical trial life cycle.

In the United Kingdom, a centralized national process coordinated by the Health Research Authority aims to provide some of these attributes to reduce the time taken to secure a variety of approvals. However, the time taken for initial approvals and any subsequent amendment approvals vary due to a number of reasons including availability of resources, understanding of risk, and mitigation of risk. In addition, research associated with vulnerable populations takes longer to secure approvals. Although the UK approval process has been criticized, it still provides valuable oversight and comparatively better quality assurance than many other parts of the world. Culture shift also requires a greater and ongoing understanding of the novel intervention development landscape across all diseases to ensure the Six Sigma method application also evolves.

2.2.3 **Lean methodology**

Lean theory focuses on a number of principles that remove waste such as prolonged waiting times or overproduction. It is a typical process involving teams across an organization, and many healthcare systems have been using the Lean thinking principles since the early 2000s. Lean concepts have been successfully used in industry, particularly in manufacturing and engineering. There are three key features associated with Lean thinking of identifying value and developing workflow and systems that lead to efficiency and effectiveness [14]. The building blocks of using Lean methods within management highlight empowering and respecting the team to encourage a *blame-free* culture that focuses on problem-solving and continuous improvement. This aspect is referred to as the *Lead improvement* method that can provide structural approaches to improve the purposes, processes, and workforce.

Lean management approaches would therefore encourage responsible and shared leadership [15]. Achieving this in healthcare would require careful consideration to ensure relevant expertize, experience, and service requirements are taken into consideration. Initiating this change would require the implementation of *lean* ideologies to facilitate efficient healthcare practices to reduce waste at a process and procedures level, by way of using a continuous improvement system. This Lean thinking approach was first developed at Toyota in the 1950s to improve the Toyota Production System. This strategic approach improved workflow to improve the value stream and removed waste, hence leading to the development of a model.

This was further developed into the *Lean Thinking Model (LTM)* and implemented by the Virginia Mason Medical Centre in Washington, which showed quality improvement and reduced repeating works. The Virginia Mason approach was then piloted within five NHS Trusts in England that showed improvements. The *LTM* (Fig. 2.4) in essence requires a behavioral change that would require a rapport across the operational and strategic teams. Often, the most effective teams will have representatives from these teams within the senior management and leadership structures. Sustainability of these changes to continuously improve requires commitment from operational and strategic teams in organizations that can be challenging if there are changes within the workforce. For example, the COVID-19 pandemic changed the

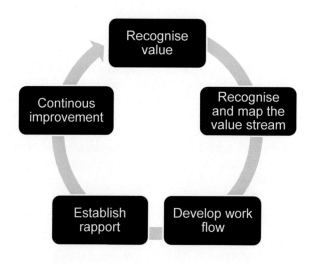

FIGURE 2.4

Diagrammatic representation of the Lean thinking model that can facilitate Lean ideologies in the practitioner domain.

way patients were cared for. The diversion of the majority of the resources toward emergency service requirements meant that challenges linked to managing the symptoms had a negative impact on the workforce that led to a higher level of occupational burnout. During this period, some healthcare systems demonstrated ongoing resourcing challenges including a high turnover, such as the NHS in the United Kingdom. In such a situation, an LTM may not be as optimal and efficacious as originally predicted and additional adaptable steps may need to be completed.

2.2.4 Lean Six Sigma methodology

Six Sigma and Lean are often used in tandem within healthcare improvement programs despite the different approaches. Lean focuses primarily on removing waste, whereas Six Sigma reduces variation by decreasing defects using quantifiable statistical measures with a metrics system. Over the last decade, the two systems have been combined to develop the hybrid *Lean Six Sigma* methodology.

Lean Six Sigma offers greater flexibility in comparison to Six Sigma in particular to reduce waste. There are eight types of waste according to Lean Six Sigma referred to as DOWNTIME. The acronym represents the following;

- Defects: defined as a defective product that does not meet the required quality standard
- Overproduction: defined by excessive production of a product that is beyond the scope of demand
- Waiting: defined by any unplanned breaks in a process or barriers to completing a particular process

- Nonutilized talent; defined by the lack or underuse of skills, expertize, and experience of the workforce.
- Transportation: defined by suboptimal transportation method used for the distribution or implementation of a product or method
- Inventory; defined by an excess of supply in comparison to the available demands.
- Motion; defined by excessive fluctuations of products or people.
- Extra processing: defined by the conduct of excessive tasks not necessarily required to complete a task or procedure.

2.2.5 Failure mode and effects analysis

Failure mode and effects analysis (FMEA) is a common methodology used to assess the risk of failure by way of quantifiable variables. The statistical weights of these variables are adjusted to ensure their suitability for real-world applications. As such, this approach can be considered an effective QC step that could aid quality audits at regular intervals. Therefore, FMEA is a quality assurance management tool that can analyze the failure of a profess or a product. This approach can also be then used as a learning objective to better design products and processes in the future. FMEAs use ordinal scale variables such as occurrence (A), Severity (B), and Detection (C). The definition of these variables differs. The risk priority number (RPN) used to characterize FMEA is as follows;

$$RPN = Y_o \times Y_B \times Y_c$$

where

- Y_o is defined as the probability of incurred defects
- Y_B is defined as the defect detection probability as part of the quality assurance process
- Y_c is defined as the severity of the defects

The scale of the assessment can vary from a level of low to high significance. The statistical significance and sensitivity of the findings can be useful to understand further adjustments that could be made to the FMEA. A clinical category-specific framework with key features can also be developed to ensure the RPN is completely aligned to a clinical area.

For example;

A clinical radiology category comprises multiple departments of molecular imaging, medical physics, radiology, and nuclear medicine. Each of these departments has a multitude of healthcare professionals who work concurrently to provide diagnostic and treatment support. Therefore, the RPN within this category will need to consider a large number of processes based procedures delivered as part of the diagnostic and/or treatments offered for a particular disease. Clinical radiology remains the brain child of diagnosis and monitor ongoing treatment effects among cancer patients. In this instance, patients may require molecular imaging techniques such as

Positron Emission Tomography Computed Tomography (PET CT) and nonradiation imaging methods such as Magnetic Resonance Imaging (MRI), which will require the involvement of radiographers, radiologists, radiology nurses, imaging technicians, and medical physicists.

$$\text{RPN in PET/CT} = Y_o \times Y_B \times Y_c$$

$$\text{RPN in MRI} = Y_o \times Y_B \times Y_c$$

Depending on the ranking of the RPN quality assurance management recommendations can be provided. The specificity of the quality improvements required can be determined based on the RPN scores and the process or procedure this was derived from. An inevitable occurrence, a low probability of detection, and a possible high statistical significance of the cause of the defects can be reported from an end-user and/or service-user and/or any other stakeholders' perspective. The higher the RPN score the need for optimization is greater. The equation and calculations can be adapted based on the needs and aims.

The urgency of improvement measures varies across clinical areas although the priorities often gravitate toward complex specialties such as pain medicine, radiology, uclear medicine, and obstetrics. Any issues around processes and products have financial, psychosocial, and ecological implications that could be addressed through modifications. FMEA could develop the required modifications although these have not been demonstrated as effectively as possible. A literature review by Wu and colleagues showed that FMEA's may not explicitly address modifications [16]. This may be due to the lack of testing the method in a real-world environment as opposed to the common academic approaches that have been used by a variety of researchers. Ahsen and colleagues showed a systematic review that indicated FMEA has been used in the automotive industry and the fragmented approaches used to report the FMEA [17].

2.2.6 Leadership for quality

Leadership is a key ingredient that enables and drives quality assurance by way of continuously improving quality management systems. Senior leadership and management teams should work in integrated formats to improve quality as part of operational and strategic planning processes at all levels of an organization. This is particularly important for promoting quality values and the practical input of introducing quality indicator techniques.

The most optimal forms would gather appropriate evidence and drive forward-thinking changes at the governance levels to ensure both healthcare staff and non-healthcare staff have a thorough understanding of activities that have been successful and unsuccessful. The generally accepted approach for quality history has been a *bottom-up* approach; while this may have advantages given the considerable practical experience that may be embedded into changes, influencing all levels of management and leadership may be cumbersome. As such, a more linear and collective approach could have a better impact on change that is sustainable as hospital management often requires flexibility due to the different clinical areas it houses.

The use of hybrid knowledge-based systems (KBS) is another approach that could aid the decision-making process. These approaches can be either artificial intelligence (AI)-based tools that can provide insightful information using real-world healthcare data or computer software-based analytical tools coupled with expert knowledge as an interphase to engineer pragmatic solutions to complex problems. The KBS approach in general is considered as an AI approach to drive performance that is patient focused. These AI tools have built-in parameters involving different scenarios and assumptions to provide varying outcomes that can act as a model for decision makers to discuss. A similar system has been proposed across a variety of healthcare systems, such as those in Oman. The KBS engine proposed by Khamisi et al. showed that the primary processing component of their KBS can show conclusions based on available knowledge. This included a KBS scheduler indicating the process that derived the proposed solution, which is a useful feature to ensure transparency when using qualitative and quantitative data. Benchmarking the KPIs and ensuring the Gauge absence perquisites are completed are useful processes that were completed by Khamisi et al. This could have been further advanced with a frequentist approach set aligned to the parameters of the KBS, which would allow the model to learn in real time. The use of *Super Decision Software* (SDS) is another optimal dimension completed to show pair-wise comparisons in the matrix when results are produced. This validated KBS appears to be effective in the context of the organizations in Oman and is a useful tool to be tested in other healthcare systems and settings. The rules and methodology can be adapted to suit the needs of clinical specialties as well and therefore has the potential to remain as a cost-effective quality improvement method that is suited to the clinical and clinical research workforce.

In addition, a KBS approach is useful for ongoing conversations and potentially improving the system itself by way of introducing new parameters or additional data. These types of systems appear to use the principles and some aspects of probabilistic learning that could be highly beneficial for disease prevention programs in healthcare organizations as preparedness can optimize the operational and clinical infrastructure and, patient experience. The *lived-learning* approaches can also avoid the use of a *black box* that can often raise ethical and governance implications in a variety of healthcare settings. Thus, the use of a KBS in conjunction with management and leadership teams can improve the development of future systems where *human-centered learning* becomes the foundation of its' functionality.

2.2.7 Quality improvement and assurance training programs

Training programs developed alongside stakeholders and available evidence could achieve improvements in clinical outcomes. The premise of quality improvement programs often relies on delivering assured or accredited training programs to the required workforce. Yet, only a fraction of the training programs meet the specific criteria that a specific group or clinical area may require. Therefore, the use of bespoke training programs that are quality assured and aligned to the needs of the improvement areas may be a better application to use. Specific and tailored training is vitally important especially for clinical satff who are new to the idea of QI. Specifically, in maternity care, QI is a fairly new concept and this will require time and resources to grapple with its concepts.

To develop bespoke training programs, it is vital to understand the knowledge and practice gaps. Mapping these gaps to the identified quality improvement targets would aid both the trainer and trainees maximize the opportunity to learn linear methods to improve practice. However, the use of evidence synthesis by way of systematic reviews and meta-analyses is not often discussed or used within the context of QI training programs. The use of research as a quality notion is important as professionalized knowledge is an important facet of training the workforce to think about ongoing changes needed to deliver optimal care. For example, the use of an evidence synthesis approach can be useful as a *living* approach that updates the systematically gathered evidence at specific time intervals and can be beneficial for updating local practice with prescribing pain medications. This approach allows clinicians and patients to have flexibility with titrating doses at safe and acceptable levels that are more catered to the clinical need. Some clinical guidelines may take longer to amend which could impact the patient's quality of life in negative manner. One such instance is pain management in endometriosis patients where chronic pelvic pain is a key feature yet it is challenging for patients and clinicians to manage long term. Although some patients report a reduction in pain following surgical intervention, others feel there has been either an exacerbation or no change in pain. As such, pain management may not always be aligned with the stage of endometriosis or the surgical treatment offered. Therefore the clinical guidelines themselves are challenging to develop and then to change as the ongoing evidence landscape is rapidly advancing. For such instance, quality improvement programs could address the complications around these issues and allow better adaptations to good practice in shorter timescales.

2.3 Developing a quality management system

Developing a QMS requires a clear understanding of the requirements for a given department or organization alongside of quality control (QC) and quality assurance (QA) steps aligned to the aims and expected outcomes in the form of quality assurance management. The use of QI methods is another facet of designing and developing a comprehensive QMS.

The starting point of developing a QMS should be using an evidence synthesis to understand the practice and other gaps within the department or organization. Such an approach would enable the development of a clear quality policy with a relevant scope and purpose. A high-quality evidence synthesis can be conducted by way of a systematic review or a SWOT (strengths, weaknesses, opportunities, and threats) analysis. SWOT is more commonly used as the framework evaluates internal and external factors, and it is more aligned to business and can be a useful tool to develop strategic and operational planning. Facilitating a SWOT analysis is more powerful in the presence of qualitative and quantitative data as it could assist with assessing current and future potential of services within an institution.

For example:

1. The components of the SWOT analysis would provide key outputs enabling an organization to understand its needs and thereby optimize existing processes where possible, and implement new ones
   - Strengths; this describes the areas that are managed well and meet the required key performance indicators within an organization. For example, if emergency services departments are managing their bed capacity aligned to their service user requirements, the processes in place may be working well. This will require limited immediate input but rather strategic points to continuously improve.
   - Weakness; this describes the areas of the organization that are suboptimal or performing poorly. These could negatively impact the business processes of the organization or department. For example, a high turnover of the workforce can be considered as a weakness and is also an indicator of management and/or leadership issues that require to be addressed.
   - Opportunities; this describes any favorable external factors that could provide an advantage to the organization. For example, the use of national statistics data for mortality to draw comparisons within an organization to reduce these within particular clinical areas such as maternity care. These insights could influence the conduct of quality improvement projects to improve patient care and the quality of care offered to reduce the mortality rates as well as overall outcomes for mother and child.
   - Threats: this describes factors that can cause harm to organizations. For example, minimal staffing levels could be unsafe for patients. These have significant implications for patients, the general public, and the organization in delivering safe and trustworthy care. Identifying these threats, and putting in place risk mitigation plans well in advance can be useful and trigger prevention programs where the healthcare workforce could learn to operate in a more optimal manner.

The SWOT analysis can be visualized with a segmentation table with four quadrants indicating each element. The visual arrangements can be a powerful tool and show the importance of presenting opportunities to address internal and external factors as well as priority areas organizations need to focus.

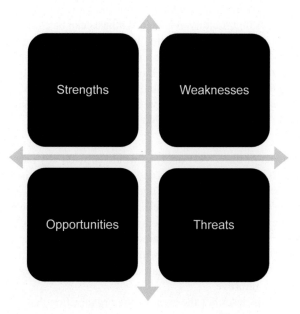

To achieve this, the SWOT analysis can be completed using the following steps;

Step 1:

Identify and characterize the primary and secondary objectives that need exploring. A common objective of a SWOT analysis can be to determine risk factors leading to bed capacity issues in busy emergency departments.

Step 2:

The analysis would vary depending on the dataset gathered for this excercise. However, information that is available for analysis should indicate the strengths and limitations of the data gathered, quality of the data, and best practices to improve this, if required at the end of the SWOT analysis.

Step 3:

This step focuses on compiling ideas using the four quadrants, incorporating the relevant key performance indicators and other details of the analysis to enable a team to develop a catalogue of the findings and any shortfalls. For example:

- Internal factors can serve as an important source of information to indicate strengths and weakness, especially for human resources where tangible and intangible components can provide an insightful outcome to highlight operational efficiencies and inefficiencies. Common queries included within the internal factors section could be:
  - What are we doing well?
  - What are we not doing well?
  - Who are our lowest-performing teams?

- Who are our strongest performing teams?
- Which area of the organization has the highest turnover?
- External factors are those that an organization may use to compare and contrast their performance, as well as optimize influencing capabilities and development of effective policies to create an environment that could thrive even in challenging circumstances. Potential questions that can be listed within the external factors section are as follows:
  - What policies are currently effective?
  - What are the efficiency trends linked to high performing organizations?
  - What are the key demographics that need to be targeted?
  - Are there any new regulations that will impact current processes in place?

Step 4:

Refine the findings gathered using the categories to demonstrate a clear focus and risks linked to the objective. This step requires extensive analysis and summarizing to ensure the priorities can be ranked based on evidence, and the raw data has been accurately interpreted.

Step 5:

This step focuses on developing the strategy based on the identified evidence and converting the SWOT outcomes into a strategic plan. This is a crucial step for management and leadership teams to ensure the plan can be synthesized in a realistic manner to complete the necessary objective.

The outcomes from the SWOT analysis could also be used to improve any existing QMS at an organization and/or department level. The use of quantitative risk assessments comprising numerical values that correspond to individual and general risk and their ranking can be another useful facet of a SWOT analysis. This could have a degree of influence to show the occurrence of risk events, and their consequences that would aid in reverse engineering any relevant steps. This approach can be a useful exercise to develop new processes, procedures, and policies and/or improve existing material. Collectively, during this process, guidelines or working instructions could improve the occurrence of a risk event or prevent it thereby positively impacting the organization. These improvements can then be used as an indicator to assess the efficiency and effectiveness of a QMS.

Similarly, qualitative risk assessments could assist with identifying intra- and/or inter-dependencies that could show valuable links between causation and risk factors that could cripple operational management outputs. This could help organizations better identify risks and their mitigation that can positively influence decision making. The subjectivity of qualitative assessment can be further mitigated when combined with the outcomes of quantitative assessments where the validity of the findings can be optimal. This approach can also reduce any potential biases thereby improving the overall reliability of the resulting approaches. The structuring of the quality management system can be furthered by way of tabulating the risk events with an appropriate scale that describes the probability of their occurrence (Table 2.2).

Table 2.2 Recommendations based on assessing risk probability and its association with quality.

Assessment of risk probability		Interpretation	Recommendation
Point	Quality		
1	Very low	Unlikely risk to appear although the probability of the event may be 1 in 4 years	A risk mitigation plan should be in place with clear key performance indicators and a milestone map to evaluate the assessments
2	Low	There is a possibility that this risk may or may not incur with a probability of 1 in 3 years	A risk mitigation plan should be in place with relevant key performance indicators with a milestone map and a review plan, including a frequency cycle
3	Average	This is a likely risk that may appear often	A risk mitigation plan should be in place with relevant key performance indicators with a milestone map and a regular review plan
4	High	There is a high probability that this risk may be incurred routinely	A risk mitigation plan should be in place with relevant key performance indicators with a milestone map and a regular review plan
5	Very high	This is a definite risk that will incur	A risk mitigation plan should be in place with relevant key performance indicators with a milestone map and a regular review plan

Actions to manage and identify the risks and opportunities should be discussed within the management and leadership teams. These aid with developing in-roads and process maps that could help design improvement programs. These aid with developing and finalizing a suitable QMS using a structured approach that encompasses prevention and mitigation as part of the operational approach.

References

[1] Imai M. Kaizen: the key to Japan's competitive success. New York: McGraw-Hill Education; 1986.

[2] This report details the work of the NHS Cancer Programme in the first six months of 2021 (covering Quarter 4, 20/21: Jan-Mar 21, and Quarter 1 21/22: Apr-Jun 21). It is part of an ongoing series of reports published by the NHS Cancer Programme.

[3] Langley K, Nolan K, Nolan T, et al. The improvement guide: a practical approach to enhancing organisational performance. San Francisco: Jossey-Bass; 1996.

[4] Damschroder LJ, Aron DC, Keith RE, et al. Fostering implementation of health services research findings into practice: a consolidated framework for advancing implementation science. Implem Sci 2009;4:50.

[5] Powell AE, Rushmer RK, Davies HTO. A systematic narrative review of quality improvement models in health care: NHS Quality Improvement Scotland. 2009. Report No. 1844045242.

[6] Boaden R, Harvey J, Moxham C, et al. Quality improvement: theory and practice in healthcare. NHS Institute for Innovation and Improvement; 2008.

[7] Pronovost P, Needham D, Berenholtz S, et al. An intervention to decrease catheter-related bloodstream infections in the ICU. N Engl J Med 2006;355:2725−32.

[8] Landon BE, Wilson IB, McInnes K, et al. Effects of a quality improvement collaborative on the outcome of care of patients with HIV infection: the EQHIV study. Ann Intern Med 2004;140:887−9.

[9] Vos L, Duckers ML, Wagner C, et al. Applying the quality improvement collaborative method to process redesign: a multiple case study. Implement Sci 2010;5:19.

[10] Walshe K. Pseudoinnovation: the development and spread of healthcare quality improvement methodologies. Int J Qual Health Care 2009;21:153−9.

[11] Deming WE. Out of the crisis. Cambridge, MA: Massachusetts Institute of Technology Center for Advanced Engineering Study; 1986. p. 507. xiii, 1991.

[12] Moen R, Norman C. The history of the PDCA cycle. In: Proceedings of the 7th ANQ congress, Tokyo. 2009; September 17, 2009.

[13] Langfeldt L, Nedeva M, Sörlin S, Thomas DA. Co-existing notions of research quality: a framework to study context-specific understandings of good research. Minerva 2020; 58:115−37. https://doi.org/10.1007/s11024-019-09385-2.

[14] Khalil SF, Mohktar MS, Ibrahim F. The theory and fundamentals of bioimpedance analysis in clinical status monitoring and diagnosis of diseases. Sensors June 19, 2014; 14(6):10895−928. https://doi.org/10.3390/s140610895.

[15] Ahmed S, Abd Manaf NH, Islam R. Measuring Lean Six Sigma and quality performance for healthcare organizations. Int J Qual Ser Sci 2018;10(3):267−78.

[16] Wu Z, Liu W, Nie W. Literature review and prospect of the development and application of FMEA in manufacturing industry. Int J Adv Des Manuf Technol 2021:1−28.

[17] Woodnutt S. Is Lean sustainable in today's NHS hospitals? A systematic literature review using the meta-narrative and integrative methods. Int J Qual Health Care October 1, 2018;30(8):578−86. https://doi.org/10.1093/intqhc/mzy070.

Audits and monitoring

3

Abstract

Auditing and monitoring are two related, but distinct processes often used in various contexts, including business, finance, healthcare, and information technology. Both processes are used to assess and evaluate activities, performance, or compliance with established standards or guidelines. In the context of clinical and research practices, auditing and monitoring can share a sequential relationship with dependencies specific to a particular context. For example, monitoring a clinical trial can be dependent on a number of factors such as risks, complexity of the disease participants may have, and potential adverse events linked to the therapeutic intervention, which can then be reflected in the type and frequency of monitoring completed throughout the study period. On the contrary, during clinical practice, the same population of patients may have a different schedule of clinical appointments to adhere to during their treatment phase. Monitoring is an ongoing process of observing and overseeing activities, processes, or systems to track their performance, progress, or compliance in real time or at regular intervals. Monitoring is proactive and helps identify any issues early on, allowing timely corrective action. Monitoring can be carried out by managers, supervisors, or dedicated monitoring teams within an organization. Real-time observations, performance tracking, and feedback loops are common monitoring methods that can be used in the context of research. Real-time monitoring provides continuous or regular updates on the subject being observed. Performance tracking: Monitoring tracks progress and performance against established targets or benchmarks. Therefore, this method is more action oriented where the issues or deviations are identified, and any triggers can prompt corrective action to be put in place almost immediately. Feedback loops are another useful monitoring method to feed information back into the decision-making process to improve performance and achieve goals.

Keywords: Auditing; Compliance; Enforcement; Molecular imaging; techniques; Performance tracking; Radiology.

Key messages

- Auditing is a systematic examination conducted periodically or at specific intervals to assess compliance and accuracy, while monitoring involves ongoing observation to track performance and identify issues in real time
- Crucial roles in ensuring accountability, efficiency, and compliance in various sectors

Quality Assurance Management. https://doi.org/10.1016/B978-0-12-822732-9.00003-5

• Monitoring can promote corrective action to be put in place relatively quickly and can be a positive step to prevent any potential escalations

3.1 Introduction

Auditing and monitoring are two related, but distinct processes often used in various contexts, including business, finance, healthcare, and information technology. Both processes are used to assess and evaluate activities, performance, or compliance with established standards or guidelines. In the context of clinical and research practices, auditing and monitoring can share a sequential relationship with dependencies specific to a particular context. For example, monitoring a clinical trial can be dependent on a number of factors such as risks, complexity of the disease participants may have, and potential adverse events linked to the therapeutic intervention, which can then be reflected in the type and frequency of monitoring completed throughout the study period. On the contrary, during clinical practice, the same population of patients may have a different schedule of clinical appointments to adhere to during their treatment phase. Monitoring is an ongoing process of observing and overseeing activities, processes, or systems to track their performance, progress, or compliance in real time or at regular intervals. Monitoring is proactive and helps identify any issues early on, allowing timely corrective action. Monitoring can be carried out by managers, supervisors, or dedicated monitoring teams within an organization. Real-time observations, performance tracking, and feedback loops are common monitoring methods that can be used in the context of research. Real-time monitoring provides continuous or regular updates on the subject being observed. Performance tracking: Monitoring tracks progress and performance against established targets or benchmarks. Therefore, this method is more action oriented where the issues or deviations are identified, and any triggers can prompt corrective action to be put in place almost immediately. Feedback loops are another useful monitoring method to feed information back into the decision-making process to improve performance and achieve goals.

On the other hand, auditing is a systematic and independent examination of records, processes, or activities to determine the accuracy, completeness, reliability, and adherence to predefined standards or regulations. The primary objective of an audit is to provide an objective assessment of the subject matter and to identify any discrepancies, errors, or noncompliance issues. Auditing can be conducted by internal auditors within an organization or by external auditors who are independent of the entity being audited. There are a few key features when conducting audits, such as:

• **Independence**: Auditors should be impartial and free from any conflicts of interest to maintain objectivity
• **Systematic approaches**: Auditing follows a well-defined and structured process to ensure comprehensive coverage and consistency

- **Documentation**: Audit findings, observations, and recommendations are documented in a formal report
- **Scope**: The audit's scope defines what is being examined and the timeframe covered
- **Verification**: Auditors collect evidence to verify the accuracy and compliance of the subject matter

There are many different types of audits that can be conducted, especially within the context of research. The most common type of audits includes study specific, which is based on the operational delivery, compliance, and information system specific. Operational audits focus on the efficiency and effectiveness of an organization's operations and processes, as well as the delivery of the said study protocol. Compliance audits focus on specific regulations and guidelines, such as Good Clinical Practice (GCP), Good Laboratory Practice (GCLP), and Good Manufacturer Practice (GMP). This form of audit ensures that an organization complies with relevant laws, regulations, and internal policies. Information system-based audits are common to explore the recording of data and management of data in line with the said protocol. As part of these audits, it is common to evaluate an organization's information technology systems, data security systems, and information handling processes.

3.2 How to prevent failures with audits/monitoring visits?

Audits within the clinical and non-clinical settings have the potential for huge benefits and can be used as an invaluable tool to improve the quality of care for patients [1]. In essence, conducting audits in a meaningful way provides accurate results, providing that the benchmarking process is robust. This gives staff the opportunity to review current practice in light of required standards and should induce a drive toward quality improvement for the benefit of patients. The importance of a good working knowledge of the standards relevant to the specific health setting cannot be understated, and emphasis must be placed on achieving the right equilibrium. During the past 2 decades, the health service has been extremely focused on what many see as a "tick-box exercise" when referring to success in audits and monitoring visits. Concerns grew around whether the emphasis was rather lopsided in that; the actual delivery of patient care through the provision of the right resources was outweighed by the need to complete checklists in readiness for audits and or inspections. The regular program of visits to healthcare settings was aimed at achieving a particular accreditation level or rating to secure a financial discount on the organization's healthcare insurance policy. Hospitals in particular were repeatedly preparing for those all-important and scary visits led by the National Health Litigation Authority (NHSLA), now known as National Health Service Resolution (NHSR) [2].

Healthcare standards are usually set with one specific goal in mind; largely to achieve maximum patient safety, by providing the highest standards of care. These objectives have been particularly evident in the content of the specific standards set out for different specialisms. For example, NHSR issued standards under the Clinical Negligence Scheme for Trusts (CNST), which were targeted for only maternity services. Conversely, for general medicine, a different set of deliverables, equally applicable to mental health, ambulance services, and other acute areas, were formulated.

Following the disbandment of the Health Care Commission and replacement with the Care Quality Commission is to some extent a replacement of one independent watchdog with another [3]. The idea of star ratings for health organizations continues, albeit in a different format and aimed at giving the public reassurance about the delivery of safe and effective care. Over the years, several inquiries have been the catalysts for the introduction of national drivers; mounting pressure on health organizations to achieve the requisite standards, which makes a bold public statement about the safety of their services. Having seen the dissolution of *Quangos* such as the Commission for Healthcare Audit and Inspection (CHAI), the Commission for Healthcare Improvement, and others in the early 2000s, health organizations continue to work with cloned versions to achieve similar outcomes. To some extent, this form of quality assurance in most recent years is supported under the underpinning principles of good governance, which less than a decade ago has found statutory footing [4]. This legal requirement requires auditing systems to be in place in conjunction with appropriate risk assessments, to ensure improvement in the quality of care, which must be on a continuum. It is interesting to note that the implications of such regulation extend beyond just a pass or fail at a healthcare standards' inspection, but enforcement can result in the form of prosecution for breach(es).

Barriers to successful audits and monitoring visits cannot be ignored, nor must little attention be placed on them in any healthcare organization, which genuinely has patients' safety at the core of its business. Although certain factors may raise challenges for organizations, audits must be seen as central to their operational framework as a conduit for the improvement of quality care to patients and users of healthcare services. Undoubtedly, any form of benchmarking against standards, whether in the form of conducting an incident investigation, complaint of mere review of documentation in healthcare records or local audits would automatically place contributors under a degree of scrutiny with regard to episodes of care. It is important that a clear message is conveyed to staff that audit/monitoring visits are not for personal scrutiny, but to review systems within the organization, which have a direct or indirect impact on patient care. Overcoming these barriers will assist in preventing failures during any form of audit, and those key factors should form part of the risk assessment, planning implementation program, and evaluation. As successful audits or monitoring visits are indicative (based on presented data and observations of practice) of the quality of care based on and above the set standards, careful consideration must be given to the following key strategies, which are inextricably linked, to avoid failures.

3.2.1 **Leadership**

Leadership comes with different styles, whether it is executed within or outside the acute or other healthcare settings [5]. Irrespective of the style engaged, undeniably, managers differ in characteristics from leaders in that; the latter has an impact on their followers and are concerned about leading, influencing, and giving direction, albeit with no delegated authority. In addition to leading by example so that others can emulate, good leaders demonstrate drive, passion, and challenging and proposing innovations [6]. This is evident in the cases reported in the Francis Report [7] and the Berwick Review [8] showing a clear nexus between a lack of good leadership and a negative impact on patient safety [8]. It is important that clinicians sit on leadership boards/equivalent to better evaluate the clinical component of the requirements and give a more realistic assessment of current compliance status, details on gaps and strategic insight, and rich contribution to improvement plans.

Some may argue that in cases where there is a financial incentive, healthcare leaders are passionate to flood their organizations with regular communications and pour out resources to achieve success in the particular initiative or program for the duration of the preparation time, leading up to the scheduled inspection date. Staff do not always view the drive as motivated by genuine care for embedding and maintaining, high-quality care, and patient safety. Leaders must have an enthusiasm that is commensurate with the compelling factors such as patient-focus elements under any form of quality assurance framework rather than seeking parity to justify the investment [9]. Purport that leadership is crucial and that leaders must be outward-facing and be prepared to learn from others [9].

Coherence of leadership is an important factor for the success of internal and external monitoring programs. It is understandable that depending on the size of the organization and the multiplicity of services offered to patients, there may be competing priorities, for example, in terms of allocating the resources to the various quality improvement initiatives. However, emphasis must be placed on the alignment of immediate, medium-, and long-term strategies with robust financial planning and achieving the end goal, quality assurance. The process for each organization must be saturated with quality controls agreed upon and followed through at all levels, and there must be a readiness to amend those to align with new evidence/evidence-based practice or other compelling factors such as national recommendations. This is poignant in the age of COVID-19 and the triangulation with infection, prevention, and control standards. A typical example is the shift in the advice on the use of personal protective equipment (PPE) that all clinical staff must now wear face masks at all times.

A key impetus for ensuring good leadership as integral to maintain a robust quality assurance is seen in the recently released NHS long-term plan, stressing on the importance of healthcare leaders being the inspiration behind the system-wide processes and connecting meaningfully with each part [10].

3.2.2 Creating a conducive culture

It is often said that the culture of the healthcare setting plays an important factor in the success of any quality assurance agenda. It must be a collaborative effort from the entire workforce and the underpinning messages must not be divorced from the embedded philosophy, visions, and values, usually manufactured and/or endorsed by the leaders. Quality assurance must also form a key performance indicator (KPI) [11]. In doing so, this remains live not only at meetings but remaining key to the daily business agenda.

Over the years, much has been written about the pull on resources, especially shortages of key workers such as nurses, midwives, and doctors in the National Health Service (NHS). Running alongside the absolute necessity of having the appropriate skill mix and appropriate care pathways, is the assurance required by Boards that compliance with required standards is achieved by givers of care.

A top-down approach, working in tandem with the bottom-up approach is required to permeate through the entire workforce so that staff are appreciated and it demands a regular sharing of information to staff through different, but user-friendly and easily accessible media and platforms. Any success requires staff to embrace, work with, and alongside the organization-wide strategy for improving quality. Equally, healthcare leaders must be visibly supportive and proactive toward any agreed system set up to enhance the quality assurance agenda by way of audit and monitoring standards [12]. Highlight the psychological dynamics such as omnipotence (leaders feeling entitled), cultural numbness (people playing along), and justified neglect (failing to speak up against ethical breaches to appease the powerful), which may be factors impacting success, but may be more deeply engrained in the organization, sitting as barriers to the success of any quality assurance agenda.

The organizational culture must be free from attitudes steeped in the beliefs that these different forms of monitoring lend themselves to a mere tick-box exercise and solely belong to roles of a much lower class. Rather, the organization must ensure that it has buy-in from each staff, whether clinical or nonclinical, and most importantly, it fosters proactivity rather than reactivity. By doing so, there is a constant appetite for necessary change toward improvement. De Jonge et al. [13] refer to this as moving toward the proactive with the end result being a generative culture [13]. Embedding such culture often takes time, effort, dedication, commitment, and active steps to identify and address all forms of hindrances.

Lessons learned from mistakes must form a core feature of the organization, whether it is through audits, monitoring visits, or other types of assessment measures. This requires active communication and dissemination, appropriate to the different groups of staff to achieve practical meaning. Placing an A4 sheet of paper highlighting all lessons learned on a display board in the manager's office will have no impact on a group of surgeons who barely have the time to take a break in between procedures. Similarly, sending key points of learning by email to clinical nurses will receive little appeal.

A culture that is deeply embedded within the quality assurance paradigm will drive staff to be passionate about showcasing their strengths and the improvement plans for their weaknesses. Buy-in for the quality agenda will result in a sort of pride for the type of care offered to their patients, especially if this is constantly measured through systems such as Friends and Family test. Such a staff response will be readily available and deliverable at any inspection and will impress upon others that a visit is not considered a chore but an opportunity to assure external stakeholders and well their patients and the public that the stake is high within this organization for quality assurance.

3.2.3 Adequate and appropriate resources

Resources must be appropriate to match the need and enable the success of quality assurance standards and programs. Patient care remains the focus of any recovery journey, but one which must be of the highest quality. To achieve this, the appropriate financial resources must be allocated to ensure the appropriate discharge of skills and interactions with staff on the shop floor and team players, including key leaders within the service.

Resources are critical to the planning and implementation of strategies for any preparation of audits and inspections. These resources are broad in nature; not least that of staffing. Clinical staff are usually heavily occupied with patient care and often not in a position to access and read emails, and little attention has been focused on addressing the futility of this medium. A proficient workforce is important from the recruitment stage and remains on a continuum toward the development and training of its staff [14]. Although adequate staffing is essential, the organization must ensure that those in strategic positions have the relevant expertise and the desired commitment to the cause, to achieve the commonly set goals.

Importantly, owing to the nature of audits, it requires the dedication of a designated member of staff with the requisite expertise, experience, and skills to lead the program. Although most organizations are moving towards having within its workforce, audit leads and/or Quality Assurance leads, it cannot be overstated that this role demands one with pristine knowledge and understanding of this area and is passionate about improving quality: use audit as a conduit or vehicle to achieve this objective. It can be safely argued that the advantage of administrative skills is in itself inadequate for this particular role, whether it is within the Research and Development team or other sections of the organization.

3.2.4 Review, monitoring, and evaluation

The constant review, monitoring, and evaluation of implemented programs should not be left to designated leads akin to a "one-man" show, as this can sometimes feel as *flogging a dead horse*. The quality assurance agenda is a matter for each limb of the organization and the drive for success requires total team engagement to meaningfully address the gaps to enable sustainable improvement in patient care.

Self-assessments are an open and direct way of monitoring each organization's status against the required standards. However, it requires genuine and stringent gap analyses, applying a holistic approach to the requirements and having a low threshold for incomplete compliance. A different approach void of targeted plans has the tendency to be laissez-faire, and tolerance for low standards may become routine and acceptable, thus defeating the entire objective of the organization-wide strategy for improving quality. Furthermore, a stringent approach toward an internal review process has the potential to recognize and address significant issues along the way before any formal audit or monitoring visit takes place. This process is of significant benefit to the organization, as it demonstrates a genuine commitment to quality improvement. This review process must include mini-inspections using an objective approach, such as a matron for theater conducting a mini-inspection of a surgical ward, away from the environment to which she has developed an attachment.

References

[1] Johnston G, Crombie IK, Davies HT, et al. Reviewing audit: barriers and facilitating factors for effective clinical audit. Qual Health Care 2000;9:23—36.

[2] Framework agreement between the Department of Health and the National Health Service Litigation Authority. NHS Litigation authority. NHS Litigation Authority framework agreement. 2017.

[3] Haslam D. What is the Healthcare Commission trying to achieve? J R Soc Med January 2007;100(1):15—8. https://doi.org/10.1177/014107680710000109. PMID: 17197681; PMCID: PMC1761661.

[4] Health and Social Care Act 2008. Available on: www.legislation.gov.uk. Accessed 6 August 2023.

[5] Kouzes JM, Posner BZ. Credibility: how leaders gain and lose it, why people demand it. John Wiley and Sons; 2011.

[6] Appleby J, Raleigh V, Frosini F, Bevan G, Gao H, Lyscom T. Variations in health care. The good, the bad and the inexplicable. London: The King's Fund; 2011.

[7] Francis R. Report of the mid Staffordshire NHS Foundation Trust public inquiry: executive summaryvol 947. The Stationery Office; 2013.

[8] Berwick D. On behalf of the national advisory group on the safety of patients in England. Improving the safety of patients in England: a promise to learn—a commitment to act. London: The Stationery Office; 2013.

[9] Fulop NJ, Ramsay AI. How organisations contribute to improving the quality of healthcare. Br Med J 2019;365.

[10] Safety culture: learning from best practice. Safety culture context within the NHS patient safety strategy. Available in: NHS England » Safety culture: learning from best practice. Accessed 6 August 2023.

[11] Jabbal J, Lewis M. Approaches to better value in the NHS: improving quality and cost. King's Fund; 2018.

[12] Wedell-Wedellsborg M. The psychology behind unethical behavior. Harv Bus Rev 2019;12:2–6.

[13] De Jonge V, Nicolaas JS, van Leerdam ME, Kuipers EJ. Overview of the quality assurance movement in health care. Best Pract Res Clin Gastroenterol 2011;25(3):337–47.

[14] Gandhi A, Luyckx K, Baetens I, Kiekens G, Sleuwaegen E, Berens A, Claes L. Age of onset of non-suicidal self-injury in Dutch-speaking adolescents and emerging adults: an event history analysis of pooled data. Compr Psychiatr 2018;80:170–8.

Inspections

4

Abstract

A regulatory inspection is a formal evaluation conducted by a regulatory authority to assess compliance with relevant laws, regulations, guidelines, and standards in a specific industry or field. These inspections are conducted by government agencies or other authorized entities and serve to ensure that organizations, institutions, or individuals are adhering to the established rules and requirements that govern their activities (Delanerolle et al., 2023). Regulatory inspections are common in various sectors, including healthcare, pharmaceuticals, biotechnology, medical devices, food and drug manufacturing, environmental protection, financial services, and more (Shetty et al., 2024). The specific focus of an inspection depends on the industry and the applicable regulations. The inspection process may involve reviewing documents, conducting interviews, and observing operations to verify compliance (UK Medical Research Council Clinical Trials Toolkit, 2006).

Keywords: Guidelines; Healthcare; Regulations; Regulatory inspections; Organizations.

Key messages

- Regulatory inspections are becoming more important within the research lifecycle.
- Regulations form the undercurrent for testing any intervention rigorously in animal models and humans.
- It is imperative that researchers understand the changing regulatory landscape.
- Nonprimate studies are highly important, especially if interventions are being licensed under the animal rule.
- Preparation for any inspection should cover three primary areas: Ensuring all pertinent documents are organized and filed as required, making staff required for the inspection available, and completing a mock inspection with the internal quality assurance team.

4.1 Introduction

A regulatory inspection is a formal evaluation conducted by a regulatory authority to assess compliance with relevant laws, regulations, guidelines, and standards in a specific industry or field. These inspections are conducted by government agencies or other authorized entities and serve to ensure that organizations, institutions, or

Quality Assurance Management. https://doi.org/10.1016/B978-0-12-822732-9.00006-0

individuals are adhering to the established rules and requirements that govern their activities [1]. Regulatory inspections are common in various sectors, including healthcare, pharmaceuticals, biotechnology, medical devices, food and drug manufacturing, environmental protection, financial services, and more [2]. The specific focus of an inspection depends on the industry and the applicable regulations. The inspection process may involve reviewing documents, conducting interviews, and observing operations to verify compliance [3].

Regulatory inspections in research are of paramount importance for several reasons. These inspections help ensure that research activities, particularly in fields like pharmaceuticals, biotechnology, medical devices, and clinical trials, are conducted ethically, safely, and in compliance with relevant laws, regulations, and guidelines. The most common reasons for regulatory inspections are as follows [4–7]:

- Protection of human subjects: There is an ethical and moral obligation to protect research participants, which is well defined by the Declaration of Helsinki and good clinical practice guidelines. In clinical research, regulatory inspections ensure the protection of human subjects involved in clinical trials. Inspections verify that informed consent processes are followed, participants' rights are respected, and potential risks are minimized. This safeguards the well-being and rights of research participants.
- Quality and integrity of data: Regulatory inspections verify the accuracy and integrity of research data. They ensure that data is collected, recorded, and maintained in accordance with good clinical practices or good laboratory practices, depending on the type of research. This is vital to ensuring the reliability and validity of research findings.
- Adherence to protocols and standards: Inspections ensure that research protocols are followed correctly, and standard operating procedures (SOPs) are adhered to. This helps maintain consistency in research procedures and data collection making research results more meaningful and reproducible.
- Compliance with regulatory requirements: Research in many fields is subject to strict regulations imposed by government agencies and international bodies. Regulatory inspections assess whether researchers and institutions are complying with these requirements. Noncompliance can lead to serious consequences, such as the suspension of research activities or the withdrawal of approvals.
- Ethical conduct of research: Inspections assess whether research is conducted ethically, with a focus on minimizing potential risks to participants and ensuring that benefits outweigh potential harms. Ethical research is essential for maintaining public trust in the scientific community.
- Drug and product safety: In pharmaceutical and biotechnology research, regulatory inspections assess the safety of drugs and products being developed. This helps protect public health by ensuring that only safe and effective treatments reach the market.

- Credibility and reputation: A positive outcome in regulatory inspections enhances the credibility and reputation of researchers, institutions, and the research itself. This, in turn, can attract funding, collaborations, and participation from both other researchers and the public.
- Continuous improvement: Inspections often provide feedback and recommendations for improvement. Researchers and institutions can use this feedback to enhance their research processes, implement best practices, and strengthen their overall research capabilities.
- Global collaboration: Many regulatory inspections are conducted in accordance with international standards, facilitating collaboration between researchers and institutions across borders. This helps accelerate the progress of research and the development of new treatments and technologies.

4.2 Key areas for regulatory inspections

There are a variety of components that are covered within a regulatory inspection. However, the fundamental components for inspection preparedness in the context of the following points are important [8,9].

1. Purpose: The primary purpose of a regulatory inspection is to evaluate whether the entity being inspected is operating in accordance with the laws, regulations, and standards that govern its activities. The aim is to ensure public safety, protect consumers, and maintain the integrity of the industry.
2. Regulatory authority: Inspections are carried out by government agencies or authorized bodies with the legal mandate to oversee a specific industry or sector. These regulatory authorities have the power to enforce compliance, issue warnings, impose fines, or even suspend operations if violations are found.
3. Scope: The scope of an inspection can vary based on the regulatory framework and the specific aspects of the industry being assessed. It may involve assessing compliance with safety standards, quality control procedures, record-keeping, ethical guidelines, environmental regulations, and more.
4. Frequency: The frequency of inspections can vary depending on the industry and the risk associated with the activities being regulated. Some industries may undergo routine inspections, while others may be inspected in response to specific incidents or complaints.
5. Inspection process: The inspection process typically involves a combination of document review, site visits, interviews with personnel, and direct observations of operations. Inspectors may request access to records, interview employees, and examine facilities and equipment.
6. Findings and follow-up: After the inspection, the regulatory authority provides the inspected entity with a report detailing their findings. This report may include any identified violations, recommendations for corrective actions, and timelines for compliance. The inspected entity is usually required to address any

issues found and report back to the regulatory authority with their corrective actions.

7. Consequences: Depending on the severity and frequency of violations, consequences for noncompliance can range from warnings and fines to license revocation, legal action, or other penalties.

Of the above, for those delivering an inspection, it is imperative to understand the process. The inspection process involves a systematic and structured evaluation of an organization, facility, or operation to assess its compliance with relevant laws, regulations, guidelines, and standards [1,2,4,5]. The specific steps and procedures may vary depending on the industry, the regulatory authority, and the scope of the inspection. However, the general inspection process typically includes the following key components [3,10–12].

1. Preinspection preparation: The regulatory authority informs the organization about the upcoming inspection and provides details regarding the purpose, scope, and objectives of the inspection. The organization prepares the relevant documents, records, and data required for the inspection. Internal preparation may involve conducting self-assessments to identify potential compliance issues.

2. Opening meeting: The inspection usually begins with an opening meeting, where the regulatory authority's representatives and the organization's key personnel participate. During the opening meeting, the objectives and expectations of the inspection are discussed, and the schedule and logistics are established.

3. Document review: Inspectors review relevant documents, records, and procedures to assess compliance with applicable regulations and standards. Documents may include SOPs, protocols, training records, quality control data, safety reports, and other relevant documentation.

4. On-site inspection: Inspectors conduct a physical examination of the organization's facilities, equipment, and operations. They may observe processes, practices, and behaviors to verify compliance with regulatory requirements. Inspectors may also interview personnel to gain insights into their knowledge of procedures and adherence to regulations.

5. Data and sample collection: Inspectors may collect samples of products, materials, or substances for further analysis and testing if applicable to the industry. In certain cases, data may be collected and analyzed to ensure data integrity and accuracy.

6. Identification of Noncompliance: During the inspection, any instances of noncompliance or deviations from regulations are documented. Noncompliance may range from minor issues with documentation to more significant violations affecting safety or quality.

7. Closing meeting: After the inspection activities are completed, a closing meeting is held between the regulatory authority and the organization's

representatives. Inspection findings are discussed, and any noncompliance issues are communicated.

8. Inspection report: The regulatory authority prepares an inspection report that includes detailed findings, observations, and any identified noncompliance. The report may also include recommendations for corrective actions and timelines for compliance.

9. Corrective action and follow-up: The organization is expected to address any noncompliance issues identified during the inspection. A corrective action plan is developed and implemented to rectify the identified deficiencies. In some cases, the regulatory authority may conduct follow-up inspections to ensure that corrective actions have been effectively implemented.

10. Regulatory decision: Based on the inspection findings and the organization's response to corrective actions, the regulatory authority makes decisions regarding further actions, such as follow-up inspections, sanctions, or enforcement measures.

4.3 Introduction to developing a specialist specific inspection plan and policy

Over the years, the drive to achieve hospital ratings through formal monitoring from external organizations such as the Care Quality Commission has sometimes been seen to be financially motivated rather than quality-driven, with patients being the ultimate beneficiaries [13,14]. The time and effort put into preparing for these visits do carry an element of exhaustion, complete engagement, and education. Contributing factors for the by-products of such preparations are often in the vein of disjointed and illogical planning, the absence of or inadequate subject-specific policies to assist with systematic preparations [15]. This, like audits, is a key component of clinical governance, which is considered the bedrock of healthcare and is wholly applicable to every specialty as part of a whole organization.

Clinical governance is "a system through which NHS organizations are accountable for continuously improving the quality of their services and safeguarding high standards of care by creating an environment in which excellence in clinical care will flourish [16]".

Policies must be strategically designed, sufficiently broad to enable staff members to understand the objectives, and narrowed to the point that staff gain a rich understanding of the specific requirements for each standard [1,17]. Policies created and agreed for this purpose must not only appear on the face of it to incorporate the key components to satisfy a particular format or expectation, but the document must also be easily accessible, user-friendly, and written in plain, clear language. Abbreviations and acronyms must be decoded to aid understanding of the document. It is advisable that a glossary be added where there is a large volume of abbreviations or unusual words.

Inspection plans must be specific to each specialty, whether it is imaging, oncology, maternity and gynecology, medicine, surgery, intensive and emergency care, or those that fall under the nonclinical umbrella [1,17,18]. Good planning is of utmost importance for success in audits and inspections, and challenges to noncompliance must be routine and tolerable as a safeguard to improve the quality of care. Further, accountability is paramount for preparation for and leading on the preparation for any inspection, avoiding the mistake of giving the responsibility of the process to all but, at the same time, to none.

Each specific specialist inspection plan must totally focus on two main factors: The specialization to be inspected and the specific specialist standard. Within these constructs should fall the crucial element of monitoring, which ensures risks are mitigated in the event of unplanned occurrences and gives reassurance that there is continuous review of the state of compliance and completion of tasks in readiness for the inspection [1,2,4,5]. For instance, if an acute specialist area such as maternity services is to be inspected by an external organization on its governance arrangements, it would be fatal to design an inspection plan and policy that covered the organization's general governance arrangements, although inevitably, the latter would be relied upon for triangulation as part of the inspection process.

Additionally, plans and policies must include quality measures that are realistic in terms of achievements. Therefore, it must be established that the key requirements can be converted into auditable standards that stand alone. It is advisable to avoid developing measures that, in reality, cannot be audited, just to satisfy an inspection program, but which have no meaning for the organization and its alignment with its patients, who are the beneficiaries of care. Assurance of team engagement is essential in preparing for any plan to support any succession planning, and the manner in which this is communicated must be consistent with the organization's strategic objective, which sits at a central point on the quality improvement agenda.

One extremely important point that is usually not mentioned in preparations for inspections is the need for total transparency across the services. An organization that prides itself on upholding the quality agenda at its core and central to its business should always be prepared to withstand scrutiny at unannounced and planned visits at any time. The measures and contingencies put in place to ensure safety for patients should rise above crises such as overcapacity or resource constraints [3,9–12]. During inspections, which are not limited to unannounced episodes, external reviewers sometimes find that there is some concealment of poor practices. This extends to ensuring only permanent staff and an overabundance of staff are on duty, and updated policies and data on the safety thermometer and audits are hidden out of sight for fear of discovery. This gives the impression that the organization is not entirely honest about some of its practices and the quality of its services, and this poses a threat to patients in that the outcome of inspections will not reflect its current status. This would be deemed as placing more risk on patients and a failure to desire to learn lessons to improve the quality of care.

4.3.1 **How to address major and critical findings?**

Inspections always culminate in an outcome that may be unfavorable for the organization. The unfavorable outcome does not only impact the team's morale but sometimes negatively on the financial pot, owing to monies spent in advance in the hope that a successful inspection will yield financial rewards beyond the specific expenditure [7,8]. Each inspection protocol dictates the timing of the release of the findings and may, in some instances, be placed in the public domain.

A systems' approach looks beyond the narrow margins and fosters a broad outlook, incorporating people and resources consistently at all levels. Critically, the objective is not to work toward passing an inspection each time it occurs but to make the attainment of high-quality care routine with the service structure recognized by all those working within it [1,2,4—7].

Individual inspection programs will have set frameworks with criteria assessments to determine the organization's compliance with the standards. These are usually based on national recommendations through organizations such as the National Institute of Clinical Health and Care Excellence (NICE) [19]. These expectations would have been made available to and well known to the healthcare organization that should be using this as a guide to planning and delivering care to users of their services. While none is perfect, the organization will be judged against the set standards for their level of compliance, and the methodology may be a mixture of observation of practice and document checks such as approved policies and minutes of meetings.

While some may regard the process as survival of the fittest and, to some degree, an appetite for competition, it is crucially important how the findings are viewed in light of quality improvement and assurance. An organization that is transparent and true to its strategic objectives would be astute in terms of its benchmarking status during self-assessments and during the period of actual formal inspection.

Findings of inspections must be read repeatedly, digested, and studied intently by the leaders of the organization, the accountable lead for the inspection, and all other relevant staff [16—19].

4.3.2 **Important factors**

- The findings must be made available to staff in the most user-friendly manner, easily accessible, and appropriate to the specific individuals or groups.
- A comparative exercise must be undertaken of the organization's most recent self-assessment prior to the inspection to identify the disparities. This is important as it may just highlight a number of issues, such as a failure to fully understand the requirements of the inspection standards or a misjudgment in terms of evidence matching.
- The positive points and strengths must first be extracted, as they not only demonstrate good practice but will also boost staff morale.

- Lessons must be learned, and this must be clearly demonstrated in practice in a consistent manner. This should be followed up with meaningful and measurable action plans that are regularly reviewed and communicated through the appropriate streams.
- The need for pragmatism is essential to ensuring sustainable progress.

Different methods for ensuring the gaps are addressed in a timely manner will be based on accurate assessments of the workforce and the type of resources available and set aside for remedial work postinspections. Good examples include the appointment of local champions, setting up subcommittees with clinical staff involvement, reporting to the leaders on progress, and robust follow-up on action plans.

4.3.3 Building a culture of resilience and adherence to quality assurance and management

Each organization must be prepared to embrace and embed quality assurance within the ethos of clinical governance, which is the backbone of all aspects of its services. While this may have a different meaning for various groups of staff, the principles will remain the same for all specialties, deeply rooted in clinical practice [19,20].

This culture of resilience moves away from a one-dimensional approach where quality assurance becomes only a project led by a designated person. It demands major factors such as dedicated, motivational, and supportive leadership, fostering a culture steeped in excellence as the gold standard for everyday practice in all services. The visibility and representation of leaders at key forums are key elements in building a conducive culture that promotes and supports adherence to quality assurance.

The terms resilience and adherence may connote a firm and stringent approach. This can be viewed as positive, as the organization can promote the workforce to be accountable to each other [20]. Where staff are fully conversant and appreciative of the set objectives as they work together individually and cooperatively, there will be this growing culture to challenge poor practice, partial or noncompliance with set standards. An attractive approach is also one that encourages praise for good work and provides support to enhance and improve on weak areas. For example, during hospital inspections, staff have praised their organizations for adopting a reward scheme in the form of *Star of the Month* for other programs to show true appreciation for compliance at a number of levels [20,21]. Conversely, to ensure consistency and avoid a drop in standards, it would be considered dangerous to ignore those who fail to adhere to principles of quality control and assurance. The organization must always work to assure its users and stakeholders of the delivery of high-quality care with a high degree of consistency and have in place a system whereby noncompliance can be managed effectively and in a timely manner. It is accepted that mistakes will be made, but it is the approach to them that will make the difference [22].

The staff recruitment process plays an important role in ensuring the appropriate culture is maintained within the organization. Excellence as a goal requires broad application, and pockets of the workforce with standards less than this will ultimately result in unwanted outcomes, which may reflect anomalies with the universal understanding, appreciation, application of, and approach to compliance with the principles set out in the quality agenda framework. A committed collective approach carries with it a desire to achieve the goals set both at local and national levels, which will include the incorporation of appropriate initiatives toward achieving improvement.

One may ask what other types of initiatives can be used when clinical staff, in particular, are overworked and exhausted trying to deliver basic care to patients. One must bear in mind that since patients are the end users of the delivery of care, they would have valuable contributions on what excellent looks like for them. This then invites the suggestion of patient involvement and feedback on services. It may seem at the initial stage that the Friends and Family Test was a good indicator of how trusts are performing by way of perception of care. As clearly indicated in their report, NHS England (2014) outlines one key ambition: The provision of data that can be compared to hold trusts to account includes an element of reward for better-performing trusts [23].

Communication is a key component of embedding a desirable culture within the framework of quality assurance. A thorough assessment of the workforce is paramount to assessing the suitability of different types of communication. It is absurd to forward electronic mails on plans and actions required of staff to those who work in acute clinical areas such as the maternity delivery suite or the operation theater, as the unpredictable nature of their acuity would not routinely lend itself to opportunities for downtime for access [23]. The method of communication must be carefully selected for maximum benefit, including the opening of opportunities for staff to make contributions. Equally, the language must be titrated to encourage inclusiveness and make a positive impact [1,2,4–6]. As pertaining to inclusiveness, it is well known that within the health service, there is little opportunity for staff on the shop floor to attend important meetings owing to the failure to ensure protection for this purpose. Nurses and midwives are usually the most affected groups, and feedback is rather rare. There is little commitment to ensuring the entire workforce is fully represented in all of the organization's key business, including essential meetings that provide face-to-face updates and a real-time opportunity to provide information, receive feedback, and make suggestions for improvement.

Staff training is an important factor for success; in that sense, the area of quality assurance can be seen as complex to some. While it is agreed that quality assurance is not usually presented as a package to the workforce but translated into parts that relate to specialisms, groups, and departments, the requirements are not always easily understood and appreciated by them. This also demands a training analysis approach so that staff are conversant, clear, and well-guided so that all aim toward a common goal.

References

[1] Delanerolle G, Cavalini H, Taylor J, Hinchliff S, Talaulikar V, Zingela Z, Toh T-H, Wong X-S, Lee K-Y, Lee JS-Y, Pati S, Rathnayake N, Sundarappeuma T, Mudalige T, Dasanayake L, Dasanayake D, Pathiraja V, Herath P, Kurmi O, Shetty A, Irfan M, Kareem R, Kemp H, Palo SK, Eleje GU, Vwalika B, Zhao W, Shi JQ, Phiri P. An exploration of the mental health impact among menopausal women: The MARIE project protocol (International Arm). medRxiv 2023;11(26):23299012. https://doi.org/10.1101/2023.11.26.23299012.

[2] Shetty A, Delanerolle G, Cavalini H, et al. A systematic review and network meta-analysis of pharmaceutical interventions used to manage chronic pain. Sci Rep 2024; 14:1621. https://doi.org/10.1038/s41598-023-49761-3.

[3] UK Medical Research Council Clinical Trials Toolkit. How to prepare for an inspection for good clinical practice by the medicines and healthcare products regulatory agency (MHRA): a guide for NHS organisations that sponsor or host clinical trials of medicinal products. 2006.

[4] Introduction to regulatory affairs in clinical research https://careers.iconplc.com/blogs/2024-1/the-role-of-regulatory-affairs-in-clinical-research. accessed on 26th of January 2024.

[5] Good clinical practice regulatory authority inspections. Good clinical practice regulatory authority inspections booklet | research quality association | RQA. therqa.com. accessed on 26th of January 2024.

[6] OECD regulatory enforcement and inspections toolkit. https://www.oecd.org/gov/regulatory-policy. accessed on 26th of January 2024.

[7] Regulatory inspection 101. Regulatory inspection 101 | research in action | advancing health ubc.ca. accessed on 26th of January 2024.

[8] McGowan I. 1-U01-AI068633-01 DAIDS protocol#. 2007.

[9] Inuwa M, Rahim SBA. Lean readiness factors and organizational readiness for change in manufacturing SMEs: the role of organizational culture. J Crit Rev 2020;7(5):56–67.

[10] Franck LS, et al. Quality assurance for clinical research: challenges in implementing research governance in UK hospitals. Int J Health Care Qual Assur 2004;17(5):239–48.

[11] Holford S. Keeping an eye on the incubators. PharmaFocus; 2003. July [Online]. Available from: http://www.inpharm.com/news/keeping-eye-incubators.

[12] Kurdziel TJ. Regulatory authority inspections – lessons learned. In: New Zealand clinical research conference, August, Auckland, New Zealand; 2008.

[13] Valania M. 'Quality control and assurance in clinical research – a system of checks and examinations that helps ensure the quality of clinical trials', Applied Clinical Trials. 2006.

[14] Akinleye DD, McNutt LA, Lazariu V, McLaughlin CC. Correlation between hospital finances and quality and safety of patient care. PLoS One 2019;14(8):e0219124.

[15] Dubas-Jakóbczyk K, Kocot E, Tambor M, et al. The association between hospital financial performance and the quality of care—a scoping review protocol. Syst Rev 2021;10: 221. https://doi.org/10.1186/s13643-021-01778-3.

[16] Scally G, Donaldson LJ. Clinical governance and the drive for quality improvement in the. New NHS England BMJ 1998;317:61. https://doi.org/10.1136/bmj.317.7150.61.

[17] Delanerolle G, Phiri P, Cavalini H, Benfield D, Shetty A, Bouchareb Y, et al. Synthetic data & the future of women's health: a synergistic relationship. May 24, 2023. Available at: SSRN 4441808.

[18] Delanerolle G, McCauley M, Hirsch M, Zeng Y, Cong X, Cavalini H, Phiri P. The prevalence of mental ill-health in women during pregnancy and after childbirth during the Covid-19 pandemic: a systematic review and Meta-analysis. BMC Pregn Childbirth 2023;23(1):1−40.

[19] National Institute for Health and Care Excellence. Fever in under 5s: assessment and initial management [NICE Guideline No. 143]. 2019. https://www.nice.org.uk/guidance/ng143.

[20] Davis MV, Mahanna E, Joly B, Zelek M, Riley W, Verma P, et al. Creating quality improvement culture in public health agencies. Am J Public Health 2014;104(1): e98−104.

[21] Reward in the NHS report. Available on: https://www.nhsemployers.org/publications/reward-nhs-report. accessed on 26th of January 2024.

[22] Kohn LT, Corrigan JM, Donaldson MS. Why do errors happen? In: To err is human: building a safer health system. National Academies Press (US; 2000).

[23] Friends and family test - maternity - 2014−15. Available on: https://data.england.nhs.uk/dataset/friends-and-family-test-maternity-2014-15. accessed on 26th of January 2024.

Quality assurance management in pain medicine

5

Abstract

Quality assurance is process-oriented and relies on systematic measurement of programs and treatment and their specific outcome measures. Feedback loops incorporated in the process prevent error generation. Quality assurance management in a symptom-based specialty such as pain medicine is often a challenge. Pain Medicine, like other specialties, has undergone a revolution in its scope in medical practice. The specialty is in its infancy compared to the other more established fields. New treatment modalities have to pass a more rigorous approval process than historically used ones.

Keywords: Acute pain; Analgesic; Chronic pain; End-of-life care; Feedback loops; Opioids; Pain management; Palliative care; Quality assurance.

Key messages

- There are a variety of quality control steps before quality assurance of any pain medicine treatment is provided
- Clinical research studies conducted in pain medicine are complex and challenging to complete due to the nature of the disease
- Novel interventions developed within pain medicine should be assessed for quality throughout the testing life cycle
- Quality assurance is closely linked to pain management and therefore becomes complex to assess in a simple manner

5.1 Introduction

Quality assurance is process-oriented and relies on systematic measurement of programs and treatment and their specific outcome measures. Feedback loops incorporated in the process prevent error generation. Quality assurance management in a symptom-based specialty such as pain medicine is often a challenge. Pain Medicine, like other specialties, has undergone a revolution in its scope in medical practice. The specialty is in its infancy compared to the other more established fields. New treatment modalities have to pass a more rigorous approval process than historically used ones.

Quality Assurance Management. https://doi.org/10.1016/B978-0-12-822732-9.00001-1

In medicine, quality assurance drives improvement within the defined program or treatment, resulting in better patient outcomes in clinical efficacy and safety. But what does this mean in Pain Medicine, and how can we replicate quality care in a specialty which is so subjective in its main outcome measures: experience of pain and patient satisfaction. Quality of care could be measured in terms of the elimination of pain. But, being "pain-free" does not correlate fully with patient satisfaction. Comley and DeMeyer [1] showed improved patient satisfaction following pain management treatment despite most patients reporting ongoing pain and ineffective treatment [1]. It highlights the difficulty pain medicine faces where pain management is often imperfect. Thus, we should consider other factors within the specialty when evaluating the quality of pain interventions. Cost-effectiveness is essential when considering new interventions and services. Secondary benefits could include early discharge following surgery, functional recovery, or return to work. Within the specialty, different areas need different strategies to measure quality. The focus of outcomes is on recovery and return to functional baseline in acute pain management compared with an emphasis on quality-of-life indicators in chronic pain management. In the end of life care and cancer pain, comfort is the leading indicator of quality care.

Providing pain relief is a central theme in medical care. Lobbying for providing high-quality pain relief is essential in the present-day health care environment. Pain, unless adequately assessed, remains in the background, and patients continue to suffer. The underlying framework across acute pain, cancer pain, and noncancer pain for ensuring high quality include comprehensive assessment, appropriate, cost-effective treatment strategy, reassessment to treatment, interdisciplinary approach, and access to specialty care when required [2].

Given the scope of Pain Medicine, it is unlikely that there will be a one-size-fits-all approach to maintaining quality throughout the system. It is already widely recognized that healthcare provision has significant variability [3]. Within Pain Medicine, differences in treatment decisions and follow-up of treatments will vary among physicians based on their training and experience. Approaches to reduce variation include nationalized guidelines intended to standardize patient care and pathways to promote quality patient care and safety [4]. Individual physicians alone might fail to impact the system and implement changes widely. This is circumvented by encouraging collaborations of physicians and formations of institutions to create guidelines and publish research and innovations. A scientific approach to assessing the current clinical practice is critical. Keeping quality goals such as a safe, patient-centered, productive, timely, equitable, and efficient treatment plan will aid in this process [5]. Merely improving pain assessment and documentation and using unimodal treatment strategies will not improve the quality. Evidence-based clinical management tailored to the patient is essential. An interdisciplinary approach should be used, increasing the quality experienced by the patient perceptibly. Quality assurance should also be applied to research and training/education to guide future practice among clinicians.

5.2 **Rationale for quality assurance in pain medicine**

Pain is universal. It is one of the most common reasons for patients seeking medical advice [6]. It can affect a patient's physical and mental well-being and, when not effectively managed, can negatively impact the quality of life [7]. Chronic pain syndromes can have complex etiologies associated with multiple pathologies and psychosocial disorders. Chronic pain affects about one-third of people in the United Kingdom, increasing incidence in an aging population [8]. Pain management practices vary across the United Kingdom, and the provision of pain services is highly variable in different regions [9]. Pain management services are delivered by various health care professionals, including but not limited to physicians, psychiatrists, psychologists, specialist nurses, physiotherapists, and occupational therapists. In the United Kingdom, training in Pain Medicine is currently limited to trainees in anesthesiology. All clinicians will be responsible for managing pain to some degree, which further leads to variance in prescribing and management, which can impact the patient's experience of pain.

Given the large spread of healthcare professionals (HCPs) involved in diagnosing and managing pain, structures and pathways for maintaining quality are paramount. One of the critical areas within pain medicine that are monitored is the responsible use of drugs. This has been acknowledged as a crucial component in achieving quality care for patients [10]. The responsible use of drugs is a global concern, with reports suggesting that 50% of medications are prescribed or dispensed without the need [10]. This should be of particular concern to clinicians working in pain medicine. Recent NICE guidance suggested that most treatments commonly prescribed for patients with chronic pain did more harm than good [11].

The biopsychosocial complexity of pain makes it challenging to determine what treatments will work best for an individual. Pain lacks prominent clinical biomarkers to identify a common etiology or response to treatment. Individuals respond differently to different interventions even when they share a common cause for their pain, which makes defining outcomes and standardizing research difficult in pain medicine. The quality of data available in this cohort of patients is limited, and large-scale RCTs providing good quality data are lacking, with available trials often underpowered [12]. Recruitment for large clinical trials in pain medicine is difficult given the range of comorbidities and complexity, which means confounders are challenging to remove, leading to small study populations. Outcome data for extensive trials in pain medicine is also reliant on patient-reported outcome measures and thus is at risk of bias in situations where patients and clinicians are unblended [13]. Research in pain medicine is also affected due to the lack of suitable translational studies. It is difficult for animal models to mimic complex biopsychosocial pain syndromes or give any practical outcome on subjective pain experience. Due to these difficulties, pharmaceutical companies have tended to shy away from traditional analgesic research and development [14].

Medicine is undergoing a technological revolution, and pain medicine is no different. That means that new technologies and medical devices are now available to both clinicians and patients within the field of practice. Web-based applications, mobile devices, and wearable technologies are now available to help diagnose, track, and potentially treat chronic pain syndromes. HCPs practicing pain medicine should utilize these technologies in patient care and research. This requires legislation and good data collection so that the quality of care can be assured and maintained for patients.

5.2.1 Pain classification and varying quality management approaches

5.2.1.1 Acute pain

Anesthetic departments have traditionally led acute pain services. Although postoperative pain remains a core element of their work, it has expanded as the scope and background of hospital inpatients have changed. It has resulted in most quality assurance projects focusing on postsurgical pain relief, recovery, and return to function. Postsurgical pain is usually predictable, lasts less time, and can be managed with a range of treatments compared to chronic pain syndromes. However, poor postsurgical pain management can result in reduced patient satisfaction, increased time in the hospital, and increased cardiovascular and pulmonary complications [15]. Inadequate pain management in the acute setting has also been associated with an increased incidence of chronic pain [17]. Management of acute pain is a significant issue, and variances between services lead to different patient experiences. It is essential to focus on what to measure, which can lead to quality improvements.

Measuring quality in acute pain medicine is difficult given the complexity of the issue. Many factors influence the outcome and determine the quality. Identifying quality measures is essential as they allow a careful evaluation of services, comparison of services, and guide future care directed at patients. The goal of quality indicators is to distinguish good from poor quality care. Meissner et al. [20] considered the different ways of monitoring quality when considering an acute pain management program [15]. They highlighted three areas where the acute pain services could be monitored for quality:

1. Structural—(an indication of the resources available when care occurs). Meissner et al. [20] identified several areas with significant discrepancies across pain services in health care settings: acute pain services; appropriate numbers of trained staff; the presence of standard operating procedures/protocols; access to technical equipment, including patient-controlled analgesic devices.
2. Process—(an indication of the care provided and the extent of how well it has been performed). Monitoring is focused on patients being treated according to guidelines and how that care is recorded. For example, there is significant variance in how pain is recorded in the acute setting. One European study showed less than half of postoperative patients had their pain documented in the bedside chart [18].

3. Outcome—(indicates the best clinical outcome for the patient). In practice, this would seem to be practical and straightforward. Complete pain relief in the acute setting would seem to be the best clinical outcome for the patient and thus determine the quality of care. However, using pain relief as the outcome to measure quality must be taken in its clinical context. For example, it is increasingly recognized that pain relief alone is not an indicator of an excellent postoperative outcome and does not correlate with the length of stay or recovery [19]. Pain is subjective, and direct reproducible measurements are not possible. Patient scales (Numeric Rating Scale 0—10 (NRS); visual analog scale (VAS)) are used to quantify pain. Given that patient interpretations of pain differ from subject to subject, they cannot on their own be used to determine treatment, for example. NRS scales have only been shown to add fair value to identifying clinically meaningful pain syndromes in primary care [20]. NRS scores are more likely to be of value in monitoring a patient's response to treatment. This helps the clinician understand the patient's perspective and monitor changes over time.

The PAIN OUT Study, funded by the European Union, pulled together a series of outcome measures to improve the quality of postoperative pain management [21]. Patient satisfaction was closely correlated with patient involvement in the decision making and subsequent degree of pain reduction. The type of analgesic, delivery method, and intensity of pain were poor correlates with patient satisfaction in this study, suggesting that patient satisfaction is more closely linked with the perception of improvement and suitability of care. Thus when considering quality assurance outcomes in acute pain services, results should focus on patient experience. Various guidelines have been published concerning acute pain management, allowing for gold-standard comparison and standardization of services [22].

5.2.1.2 Chronic pain

The struggle for quality assurance in chronic pain lies in the variance in the patient background, presentation, and contributing factors. Guidelines in the acute setting can be clear about presenting causes and give stepwise management plans. Medications can be introduced in a stepwise and escalating manner. Outcomes, even though pain relief as described above may not be the most accurate, can focus on secondary goals, including length of stay and function return. Chronic pain is harder to characterize, where patients have had persistent pain over months and years with the associated secondary effects on both physical and mental health. Establishing clear outcome measures in this context is a challenge. In chronic pain, it is already accepted that pain relief (where the pain is 0) is not a meaningful outcome and may contribute to clinicians chasing the wrong treatments. Ballantyne and Sullivan [54] argue that clinicians' desire to treat and relieve pain in patients with chronic pain in the United States has likely contributed to the epidemic of prescription opioid abuse with no associated improvement in the incidence of chronic pain [23]. In this sense, chasing outcomes to demonstrate quality should be taken with caution and emphasize the importance of evidence-based practice when considering quality indicators. Opioids have good efficacy when used acutely, but little evidence supporting their long-term use. Yet despite this, NRS scales were used as the principal outcome measure when considering opioids in chronic pain patients [23]. One reason why this falls as a reliable measure is that the intensity of pain in patients with persistent pain does not correlate with the severity of the original injury or process or give any reliable indication as to the potential tissue damage. This is due to pain being an experience rather than a true reflection of active nociception.

Therefore, evaluating the quality of pain service requires a broader understanding of the patient's experience and outcome measures that focused on quality of life and functional goals—pain management programs in general focus on "living with" persistent pain rather than cure. The IMMPACT trial recommended six core outcome measures when considering chronic pain services: (1) pain; (2) physical functioning; (3) emotional functioning; (4) patient rating of satisfaction and improvement; (5) symptoms and adverse events; (6) participant disposition [24]. There are several patient-validated questionnaires with which this information can be collated [25]. However, the challenge lies in adequate data collection. The variance and range of data needed to demonstrate the quality of care are vast and unpredictable. This makes it difficult for chronic pain programs to demonstrate improved patient outcomes in terms of satisfaction and physical benefit and provide a cost-effective service. Given the rarity of chronic pain programs, the long-term follow-up data are also scarce compared with acute pain services, which are smaller, more local, and have more definable outcome measures.

Technology may be one answer for measuring patient outcomes and satisfaction in the longer term. Increasing web-based applications and handheld devices means data collection is improving. For larger cohorts of patients, guidelines and standards of care can be based on reliable well-collected evidence. Guidelines to set standards of care do exist [4]. However, the scope for guidelines is significant given the scale of chronic pain and its lack of definability outside of the presentation. This makes it hard for single clinicians or services to maintain quality standards. A few examples of commonly available pain medication include the following:

- Paracetamol: The efficacy of paracetamol (acetaminophen) in addressing chronic pain varies depending on the specific type of pain. High-quality evidence suggests that paracetamol is ineffective in reducing pain and disability or enhancing the quality of life in patients with low back pain. Furthermore, its benefits are only marginal and not clinically significant for pain and disability reduction in patients with hip or knee osteoarthritis. A combination therapy involving paracetamol at a dosage of 1000–4000 mg daily, along with ibuprofen 400 mg, has demonstrated superiority over paracetamol alone in patients with hip or knee osteoarthritis. However, it is essential to note that this combination therapy is associated with an increased risk of gastrointestinal bleeding. Additionally, when prescribing paracetamol, the dosage should be adjusted appropriately for patients weighing less than 50 kg. These considerations highlight the nuanced approach required in prescribing paracetamol for chronic pain, taking into account the specific type of pain, potential combination therapies, and individual patient characteristics to optimize effectiveness while minimizing associated risks

- NSAIDs: Nonsteroidal antiinflammatory drugs (NSAIDs) have an established role in the treatment of conditions such as rheumatoid arthritis and gout, and they provide some benefits in managing chronic low back pain and certain forms of osteoarthritis. It is important to note that NSAIDs are associated with cardiovascular and gastrointestinal risk factors. In prescribing NSAIDs, a cautious approach is recommended. Lower-risk agents should be the first-line choice, prescribed at the lowest effective dose and for the shortest duration necessary to control symptoms. For example, ibuprofen in doses up to 1.2 g daily or naproxen at 0.5−1 g daily have not been associated with significant thrombotic or cardiovascular risks. If one NSAID proves ineffective, consideration can be given to switching to a different NSAID, as individual responses to these medications may vary. It is crucial to exercise extra caution when using NSAIDs in frail patients, where there is an increased risk of acute kidney injury, particularly in the presence of dehydrating illnesses. For more detailed guidance in such cases, clinicians are advised to refer to specific polypharmacy considerations. This approach underscores the importance of tailoring NSAID therapy to individual patient needs, considering both the potential benefits and associated risks.

- Topical NSAID: Topical NSAIDs are deemed safe, potentially effective, and should be considered as a treatment option for patients experiencing chronic pain from musculoskeletal conditions. This is particularly relevant for individuals who may have difficulty tolerating oral NSAIDs. Additionally, topical rubefacients are considered safe and may be effective in managing pain associated with musculoskeletal conditions. These products can be purchased over the counter, aligning with self-management goals for individuals seeking relief. The use of topical treatments provides an alternative and localized approach to pain management, potentially minimizing systemic side effects associated with oral medications. The accessibility of over-the-counter rubefacients further supports self-care strategies for individuals dealing with musculoskeletal pain.

Despite the potential safety improvement of prescribing single-component dihydrocodeine or codeine in situations where patients may be overusing the medicine, local formularies and guidance should be consulted, especially in areas where prescription diversion is a concern. Initiating opioids with a "Starting low" and "Going slow" strategy is advisable to minimize side effects [4−7]. Combining low-dose codeine or dihydrocodeine with paracetamol (e.g., Co-codamol) is a therapeutic option for all patients, particularly those susceptible to opioid side effects. This approach allows for the development of tolerance before titrating up to therapeutic doses. It is essential to acknowledge the lack of evidence for the long-term efficacy of opioids in treating chronic pain, coupled with significant risks such as increased risk of overdose, fractures, abuse, or dependence. Clinicians should explicitly discuss these risks with patients. Recent Cochrane reviews have indicated an elevated risk of adverse events with opioids compared to placebo and nonopioid active comparators. The authors highlight the need for a clear demonstration of clinically relevant benefits before considering long-term opioid use in individuals with chronic noncancer pain. Despite limited evidence for the use of co-codamol 8/500 mg, it may be appropriate for a small percentage of patients who cannot tolerate stronger opioids [5,6]. However, there are associated risks such as addiction and constipation, so a trial with a step-down to paracetamol alone should be considered. Patients coprescribed to two opioids for mild-to-moderate pain should undergo regular review.

Strong opioids, including Tramadol, Morphine, Oxycodone, Fentanyl, and Tapentadol, are recommended for prescription instead of, not in conjunction with, lower-strength opioids. The optimal approach is to use them in combination with nonopioid analgesic medications to minimize dosing and side effects. Dose equivalence calculators and tapering guides are available to facilitate the transition or discontinuation of opioids. It is crucial to note that equivalent analgesic dose conversions are estimates, and patients may exhibit varying sensitivity to the new opioid, potentially leading to unexpected outcomes such as life-threatening oversedation or respiratory suppression. When switching opioids, it is important to reduce the dose on the new agent to ensure patient safety. The use of a tapering tool, as demonstrated in the provided screenshot, can be a valuable resource in the process of transitioning or discontinuing opioids. This tool aids in the gradual reduction of opioid doses, promoting a safer and more manageable adjustment for patients [4,5].

In the United Kingdom, Tramadol is classified as a strong opioid according to the National Therapeutic Indicators. The recommended dose range is 50−100 mg every 4−6 hours, with a maximum of 400 mg in 24 hours. Tramadol shares a similar adverse effect profile with codeine and dihydrocodeine but has a higher potential for drug interactions. It is not advisable to combine Tramadol with other opioids for mild-to-moderate pain [4]. When converting to or from Tramadol and another opioid, clinicians should be mindful of the wide morphine equivalence range. Additionally, caution is warranted when prescribing Tramadol with an SSRI, as it may lead to potentially serious side effects like serotonin syndrome. It is important to acknowledge that opioids are not universally effective in every patient, and this should be discussed before initiating treatment [5]. Opioids are not routinely recommended for managing acute or chronic lower back pain. If opioids are deemed appropriate, a realistic goal should be a minimum of a 30% improvement in pain and/or a significant enhancement in functional ability. Complete pain relief is rarely achieved with opioids. A 1 to 2-week trial approach is recommended to assess efficacy, tolerability, and suitability, with a patient review within 4 weeks of initiating opioid treatment. Evidence suggests that a majority of patients taking opioids for moderate to severe pain will develop opioid-induced constipation, and tolerance does not develop to this side effect [7]. Local formularies should be consulted for guidance on specific agents for opioid-induced constipation. Once a stable regimen is established, with substantial relief of symptoms reported by the patient and no significant concerns dictating otherwise, opioids should be reviewed at least every 6 months. Continuing opioids is advised only after confirming clinically meaningful improvements in pain and function without significant risks or harm. Various thresholds are quoted where the risk of harm outweighs the benefits, and careful consideration is recommended when increasing the dosage. The US Department of Health suggests reconsidering the benefits and risks when increasing dosage to ≥ 50 Morphine Equivalent Dose (MED)/day, avoiding increasing dosage to ≥ 90 MED/day or justifying a decision to titrate dosage to ≥ 90 MED/day [4−7]. The risk of harm substantially increases at doses of ≥ 120 mg MED/day with no increase in benefit. Regular and careful monitoring is crucial to ensure the safe and effective use of opioids in the management of pain. A few case studies demonstrating quality management with prescribing include the following.

5.2.1.2.1 Case study—NHS Forth Valley

A patient with a diagnosis of Fibromyalgia, experiencing widespread body pain and low back pain, was referred to the pharmacist-led pain management clinic in NHS Forth Valley. At the time of referral, the patient was prescribed eight medications: MST 50 mg twice daily, regular Oramorph, amitriptyline 50 mg, pregabalin 150 mg twice daily, mirtazapine 30 mg, cetirizine, lansoprazole, and letrozole. The primary concern for the patient was waking up at night with restless legs. Following a comprehensive review, the pharmacist recommended the reduction or cessation of one medication, mirtazapine. After a 6-week period, the medicine was successfully stopped, and the restless leg issue was resolved. Subsequent reviews allowed for the cessation of another medication (Oramorph) and the reduction of another (MST). As a result of these adjustments, the patient experienced significant improvement, enabling a return to work. This case highlights the valuable role of pharmacist-led pain management clinics in conducting thorough medication reviews, identifying opportunities for optimization, and collaborating with patients to achieve positive outcomes in managing chronic pain.

General Practitioners (GPs) in NHS Fife conducted an audit of 10 patients who were newly initiated on opioids, aligning with the criteria outlined in the practice prescribing policy recommended by NHS Fife. The audit aimed to ensure compliance with five established standards and was repeated within the year to assess improvements.

The audit standards were as follows:

- Indication document: Ensure that 90% of patients newly initiated on an opioid have an indication document.
- No-pharmacological advice: Ensure that 90% of newly initiated patients receive nonpharmacological advice on managing their pain and are provided information on the side effects of opioids.
- Acute prescription: Ensure that 90% of all newly initiated opioids are issued on acute prescriptions, indicating a single-use prescription rather than a repeat

- Daily limit: Ensure that 90% of patients newly initiated on opioids are prescribed no more than a 30 days supply for initial and subsequent prescriptions.
- Prescription review: Ensure that 90% of all newly initiated prescriptions for an opioid undergo a review before the next supply, within a maximum of 8 weeks.

Comparison between baseline and follow-up data revealed improvements across all standards, indicating the successful implementation of the audit and the positive impact on opioid prescribing practices within the NHS Fife setting. This case study highlights the commitment to quality improvement and patient safety through regular audits and adherence to prescribing guidelines.

NHS Scotland colleagues have adapted a resource originally developed in New Zealand, which consolidates various elements of care into a tool for quality improvement. This tool is designed to aid in the audit and review of patients who have been prescribed opioids. The bundle incorporates several principles that align with the tools utilized in NHS Fife, demonstrating a collaborative effort to enhance the quality of care and prescribing practices related to opioids within the healthcare system. This adaptation reflects a commitment to incorporating best practices from diverse sources to optimize patient outcomes and safety.

5.2.1.2.2 Neuropathic pain

There are significant risks of addiction and abuse associated with gabapentin and pregabalin, prompting considerations for reclassification as controlled drugs due to a reported increase in related deaths [21,22]. The number of drug-related deaths involving gabapentin and pregabalin rose from 2 in 2009 to 225 in 2016. Clinicians are advised to conduct annual reviews for patients prescribed these medications. Tools are provided alongside this document to assist in identifying this patient cohort and optimizing their care. Additionally, the prescribing of lidocaine should be reviewed. Currently, there is no evidence from high-quality randomized controlled studies supporting the use of topical lidocaine for treating neuropathic pain. However, some low-quality individual studies suggest that it may have a role in pain relief. Clinicians are encouraged to critically evaluate the evidence and exercise caution when considering lidocaine prescriptions for neuropathic pain.

It is crucial to assess whether there are elements of neuropathic pain, defined by the International Association for the Study of Pain as pain caused by a lesion or disease of the somatosensory nervous system. According to SIGN 136 guidelines, first-line pharmacological treatments for neuropathic pain include amitriptyline or gabapentin. The choice between these two drugs primarily depends on clinical preference and patient factors. If the response to the first agent is insufficient, the other may be used as a replacement or in combination. Pregabalin is considered an alternative for patients who have not benefited from or tolerated amitriptyline or gabapentin. A recent meta-analysis on the pharmacotherapy for neuropathic pain in adults revealed relatively modest outcomes. The trials included treatments lasting longer than 3 weeks, achieving 50% pain relief, with corresponding numbers needed to treat (NNT) and numbers needed to harm (NNH). The information in the following table is based on the meta-analysis conducted by Finnerup et al.[16]

Drug	NNT for 50% pain relief	NNH for harmful effects
Amitriptyline	4.4	8.3
Duloxetine	6.5	12.5
Pregabalin	6.7	9.2
Gabapentin	7.7	11.4
Oxycodone	8.3	5.0
Tramadol	11.1	8.3

The quality of the evidence identified could be summarized as follows:

Drug	Number needed to treat	Number needed to harm	Quality of final evidence
Tricyclic antidepressants	3.6 (95% CI 3.0–4.4)	13.4 (9.3–24.4)	Moderate
Serotonin-noradrenaline reuptake inhibitor (SNRI) antidepressants, duloxetine and venlafaxine	6.4 (95% CI 5.2–8.4)	11.8 (9.5–15.2)	High
Pregabalin	7.7 (95% CI 6.5–9.4)	13.9 (11/5–17.4)	High
Gabapentin	7.2 (95% CI 5.0–8.3)	25.6 (15.3–78.6) and 31.9 for ER preps	High
Tramadol	4.7 (3.6–6.7)	12.6 (8.4–25.3)	Moderate
Morphine/oxycodone	4.3 (3.4–5.8)	11.7 (8.4–19.3)	Moderate
Topical lidocaine	No information	No information	Low
Capsaicin 8%	10.6 (7.4–19)	No information	High

The results of the meta-analysis indicate that the efficacy of systemic drug treatments for neuropathic pain is generally not dependent on the underlying disorder's etiology. Despite the low NNTs for tramadol and opioids, the quality of evidence is considered moderate.

There is currently no evidence from high-quality randomized controlled studies supporting the use of topical lidocaine for treating neuropathic pain. However, some individual studies of low quality suggest its potential effectiveness in pain relief. Lidocaine 5% medicated plaster is licensed for use in postherpetic neuralgia (PHN). It may be considered in patients with very localized neuropathic pain who are intolerant of first-line therapies or for whom these therapies have proven ineffective [26].

5.2.1.2.3 Improving quality of prescribing

NHS Fife, in collaboration with a community pharmacy, initiated a project to enhance the role of community pharmacist prescribers in the management of patients on high-risk pain medications [26–29]. Through the NHS Education for Scotland (NES) Teach and Treat process, community pharmacist prescribers were up-skilled, allowing them to review patients on high-risk pain medications and offer an exit strategy for those transitioning from the pain service. Specific funding from NES facilitated the training and up-skilling of community pharmacist prescribers, with a coordinator appointed to drive the training one session per week. Collaboration and support from the multidisciplinary team in the pain service were crucial for shadowing and training, and the local lead pharmacist played a key role in developing community pharmacy services and prescribing clinics. Additional funding from the Scottish Government supported prescribing clinics in community pharmacies. Initial project protocols were developed to target specific patient groups, and patients received 30—45 minutes initial appointments for comprehensive engagement, pain medication history, and discussions about self-management. The benefits of the initiative were significant. Patients could receive care closer to home, with ample time during appointments to discuss fears and beliefs hindering safe and effective analgesic use. Follow-up appointments facilitated the implementation of plans, including adjustments to pain medication and regular reviews to achieve the optimum combination. Patient feedback was very positive, highlighting the benefits of having dedicated time for discussions and medication reviews. Patients who did not regularly attend their GP or specialist services could have their pain medication reviewed, contributing to improved medication management. Patient surveys confirmed these benefits, emphasizing the success of the initiative in enhancing patient care and medication management for chronic pain.

5.2.1.2.4 NHS Greater Glasgow and Clyde implemented a comprehensive whole-system approach that delivered significant benefits

NHS Greater Glasgow and Clyde (GGC) initiated a pilot program with the objective of fostering self-management of chronic pain and enhancing overall quality of life. This collaborative effort involved a diverse group of healthcare professionals, including pharmacists, physiotherapists, GPs, a pain consultant, a psychologist, health improvement experts, and patient representatives [29]. The project, conducted in partnership with the local Health and Social Care Partnership (HSCP), the Chronic Pain Managed Clinical Network, and the community pharmacy development team, aimed to optimize primary care pathways for chronic pain by April 2016. Key components included pharmacist-led pain clinics, enhanced services by up-skilled Musculoskeletal physiotherapists, early intervention through patient education sessions, a community pharmacist pilot for chronic pain medication review, and professional education sessions for healthcare practitioners involved in the project. The benefits were notable for patients, GPs, and healthcare boards, including improved access to information, reduced pain severity scores, streamlined chronic pain management pathways, decreased GP consultations on chronic pain, enhanced professional satisfaction for GPs, and positive impacts on analgesic utilization and drug expenditure reduction for healthcare boards. This multifaceted approach demonstrated the potential for collaborative efforts to positively influence chronic pain management across different stakeholders.

5.2.1.3 Cancer pain and palliative care

Recognition, diagnosis, and treatment of patients with cancer pain remain a significant problem. For these patients who have cancer, pain is one of the symptoms in a spectrum that includes respiratory distress, nausea, confusion, and other psychological conditions. The World Health Organization (WHO) began efforts in the 1980s to improve the quality of pain care worldwide. The guideline highlighting the analgesic ladder remains the most important quality improvement step for cancer pain. The logical approach highlighted in the guideline has improved pain education across the globe and, in the process, improved the quality of palliative care.

Seow et al. introduced a framework to assess the quality of care in cancer patients at the end of life [26]. The five steps of this framework can be used to develop and evaluate quality indicators for end-of-life care. It is done by defining:

- Population of focus
- Broad quality domains
- Specific target areas
- Steps of the care process
- Evaluation criteria for quality indicators

Clinicians can use this framework to provide better care by measuring their practice effectively. Researchers, policymakers, and developers of quality indicators also benefit from them. The economic, policy-related, and institutional barriers and inadequate training and education of HCPs have caused the scarcity of access to palliative and cancer pain treatment. In addition to obstacles to delivering adequate care, there are practical barriers to implementing quality indicators. Identifying the population of patients requiring end-of-life care is difficult owing to the unpredictability of this period. Documentation remains inadequate, leading to limitations in data collection, affecting quality indicators that rely on accuracy in documentation. Many indicators are still dependent on the abstract inference of medical records. Electronic medical records offer a solution to this barrier but lack the universal nature in availability. Indicators designed for one system may not work in others due to differences in demographics. Future research needs to develop indicators specific to the setting and population and answer scientific questions to refine the quality of end-of-life/cancer care. A few case studies that demonstrate quality improvement are as follows.

5.2.1.3.1 NHS Lanarkshire achieved noteworthy enhancements in the prescription of lidocaine

Lidocaine 5% medicated plasters are recommended for alleviating neuropathic pain associated with prior herpes zoster infection (postherpetic neuralgia, PHN) in adults. However, there is limited available data comparing the clinical effectiveness of lidocaine plasters. Despite their restricted role in therapy, the prescription of lidocaine plasters has been on the rise. NHS Lanarkshire has been evaluating lidocaine patch prescribing for several years, with limited success. In the 2015−16 period, a new incentive scheme for General Practitioners (GPs) was introduced. Patients using lidocaine patches were invited for a face-to-face review with their GP to ensure the appropriateness and effectiveness of the therapy. Patients undergoing regular treatment were encouraged to undergo a plaster-free trial in accordance with guidelines. The scheme particularly targeted prescribing outside the licensed indications. A review cycle was deemed successful if at least 50% of patients reviewed had their therapy discontinued. The aim of the scheme was to encourage prescribing for neuropathic pain in accordance with NHS Lanarkshire formulary guidelines and to reduce inappropriate use of lidocaine 5% medicated plasters without compromising patient safety or care. This was achieved by implementing:

- GP face-to-face reviews of patients prescribed lidocaine patches
- Each practice agreeing and implementing a policy of prescribing formulary first-line choices for neuropathic pain

Benefits of this include patients being provided with the chance to undergo a face-to-face review with their GP regarding their lidocaine therapy. This resulted in a more suitable utilization of lidocaine patches, fostering an improved understanding of the indications and evidence supporting their use. The initiative also led to enhanced adherence to formulary guidelines and, consequently, a decrease in the utilization of lidocaine patches, contributing to a reduction in overall drug expenditure.

5.2.1.3.2 NHS Fife initiated efforts to enhance the interface between primary and secondary care

Collaborating across the primary/secondary care interface, NHS Fife prioritized morphine as the first-line choice for strong opioids in their formulary. Concerns were raised by GPs regarding patients being discharged on oxycodone without clear review guidance, leading to potential long-term prescriptions. To address this issue, a primary care pharmacist collaborated with a senior hospital-based pharmacist to review a month's worth of discharge letters. This collaborative effort identified a specific directorate with higher oxycodone usage. The primary care pharmacist then met with the Lead Clinician of the service to understand the prescribing rationale and explore the potential use of morphine. Through education, intervention, and regular on-site presence, the Acute Based Pain Nurse and Clinical Pharmacist influenced change within the highlighted directorate. This resulted in a decreased use of oxycodone, increased utilization of morphine as the first-line choice, and the establishment of clear review plans for all patients discharged on strong opioids from this service. This successful collaboration underscores the positive outcomes achievable when primary and secondary care clinicians work together to enhance prescribing practices. Ongoing efforts are being made to further comprehend and address oxycodone use in other directorates.

5.3 Patient-centered outcomes

Patient satisfaction is closely linked with pain relief [27]. This leads to medical care being rated by the patient based on the quality of analgesia provided. The delicate balance between achieving the patient's desired outcome and the clinician's concern about the adverse effects of treatment should be appreciated. The use of opioids in this context has been most concerning in the recent past. Opioids are potent depressants of respiratory drive and are lethal. The demand from patients to have absolute autonomy over opioid medications keeping in line with the control they enjoy in other aspects of health care led to increased use and later abuse of these drugs [28,29]. Patient choice needs to be appreciated. However, clinicians need to respect the drawbacks and cooperatively educate the patients. Patients want their pain recognized, evaluated thoroughly, and treated safely [30,31]. They need to feel that they are not isolated and have some control over their treatment. The ethical dilemma occurs when the clinician and the patient disagree over the course of the treatment. Despite their primary duty toward the patient, can clinicians neglect the broader impact on society, seen as an increase in abuse and deaths? Can the clinician ignore the scientific evidence that does not support the long-term use of opioids? Targeting patient-centered outcomes, applicable in other areas of medicine, should be approached with trepidation in pain management and is a subject of ethical debate.

5.4 Interventional pain management

Interventional pain management (IPM) is a field with a history of 3 decades. Zhou et al. [59] published the first research study on quality assurance in this field [32]. The degree of immediate pain relief, patient satisfaction, and incidence of adverse events were the three criteria they highlighted. This study was done in a university pain clinic, and the authors concluded that quality assurance could be achieved in IPM. These criteria can form the backbone for training fellows and residents to high quality. The authors highlight the importance of attaining good immediate pain relief. As most IPM procedures deliver local anesthetic, frequently with a corticosteroid to the diagnosed pain generator (for example nerve root injections), immediate pain relief will confirm the accuracy of diagnosis and the needle placement on the target. This makes immediate pain relief a good quality indicator and a good predictor of long-term relief. Patient safety is at the core of IPM philosophy. Achieving a low rate of complications is vital for improving quality. Guidelines developed by international and national pain bodies for peri-procedural and procedure-specific management have been instrumental in bringing down the rate of complications [33]. Overall quality of health care has a positive relationship with patient satisfaction [34]. Decreased pain postprocedure leads to satisfied patients. The skillful execution of the procedure with clear communication in the peri-procedural period is crucial for improving satisfaction. When the study was done for quality assurance in IPM procedures in private practice, the criteria remained similar [35]. These studies highlighted the possibility of using a quality assurance program in IPM and the promise that the quality of IPM can be improved.

5.4.1 **Polypharmacy and the impact in pain care**

Medication stands out as the most prevalent form of medical intervention, with approximately 300,000 prescriptions issued daily in Scotland. The term "polypharmacy" itself simply refers to the use of many medications and is commonly defined as occurring when a patient takes five or more medications. It is essential to emphasize that polypharmacy is not inherently negative; it can be both rational and necessary [28,29]. The critical distinction lies in differentiating appropriate polypharmacy from inappropriate polypharmacy. Inappropriate polypharmacy occurs when one or more drugs are prescribed that are unnecessary or no longer needed, or when there are hazardous interactions between medications. The Scottish Government initially published Polypharmacy Guidance in 2012, followed by a revised version in 2015. Notably, it has become more common for patients in Scotland to have two or more long-term conditions rather than just one. The chart below illustrates the relative coprevalence of various conditions. Chronic pain emerges as one of the most frequent comorbidities associated with other long-term conditions, including heart and respiratory disease, cancer, and diabetes. This shift in the healthcare landscape underscores the importance of managing polypharmacy effectively, particularly in the context of coexisting chronic pain and other long-term conditions. The goal is to ensure that medication regimens are rational, necessary, and free from potential risks associated with inappropriate drug combinations or unnecessary prescriptions. The ongoing guidance and initiatives from the Scottish Government play a crucial role in navigating the complexities of polypharmacy and optimizing patient care in the presence of multiple health conditions. The prescribing practices for individuals dealing with chronic pain are explicitly outlined in SIGN 136 (Scottish Intercollegiate Guidelines Network 136). Although NICE (National Institute for Health and Care Excellence) has also generated guidelines on chronic pain management, clinicians within NHS Scotland are directed to consult SIGN as their primary reference. SIGN is regarded as the sole comprehensive, evidence-based guideline for managing chronic pain in nonspecialist healthcare settings. These principles serve as a guide for clinicians, ensuring a standardized and evidence-based approach to prescribing in the context of chronic pain. The emphasis on evidence-based guidelines reflects a commitment to optimizing patient care and outcomes in the management of chronic pain within the NHS Scotland healthcare system.

The seven steps provided serve as a comprehensive guide for structuring the medication review process. Commencing with Step 1, the focus is on discerning the patient's priorities and objectives for drug therapy, necessitating an understanding of patient demographics, medical history, and social context. Moving to Step 2, the review categorizes current medications into essential and potentially stoppable, emphasizing the importance of expert guidance for discontinuing essential drugs. Step 3 involves scrutinizing the necessity of remaining drugs based on therapeutic objectives and updated evidence. Subsequent steps address the effectiveness of current drugs, identification of adverse drug reactions (ADRs), consideration of cost-effectiveness, and exploration of patient adherence. The final step, Step 7, emphasizes the importance of optimizing the drug regimen to enhance adherence by involving patients in decision-making about treatment goals and balancing effectiveness with safety and symptom control [29]. Together, these steps form a comprehensive framework for a thorough and patient-centric medication review [29].

5.5 Quality assurance in pain management—challenges and confounders

The goal of Pain Medicine, in reality, is simple—to prevent and control pain. The complexity is derived from the individual's experience of pain and the complex mix of medical and psychological comorbidities that might exist in the studied population. To date, no clinical tool exists that objectively captures all the dimensions of pain, and thus outcomes are dependent on subjective measures. Therefore, ensuring that patient-reported outcome data is of high quality is vital for the specialty of pain medicine in providing quality care.

This makes research into best practices difficult. Guidance has been developed by the British Pain Society for clinicians conducting research into pain medicine on the best use of outcome measures [36]. The rationale for this was to try and standardize practice across the United Kingdom, having noted the variance between services. Having reliable outcome measures is one way in which quality can be maintained. One of the issues for pain medicine is that the outcome measures may simplify and trivialize complex presentations. For example, the NRS and VAS are tools that have been validated for use in adults to monitor pain response [37]. These scores are quick and easy to use for clinicians and patients and may be particularly helpful, especially in monitoring change. The challenge in pain medicine is its simplicity. This may be a reasonable choice when conducting research in acute pain, where intervention and effect may be easier to capture with fewer confounders.

Other areas within Pain Management where outcome measures have been sought include pain interference, emotional distress and functioning, and quality of life questionnaires [36]. Some of these more in-depth scales, for example, the Oswestry Low Back Pain Disability Questionnaire, have only been validated for specific pain presentations. This limits their use in more generalized pain research. Quality of life measures, such as the EQ-5D, have emerged as potential outcome measures in Pain Research [38]. Within chronic pain, these tools likely offer the most reliable data outcomes for monitoring services and interventions, given the scope of the questionnaires and the many impacts of chronic pain. However, they can be time-consuming to complete and create multiple data points. These tools have been shown to have value in pain research and can signpost meaningful changes after the intervention. However, were not developed with pain as their primary measure.

Within pain medicine, experts have worked to try and create specific multimodal outcome measures to monitor chronic pain [39]. This research is time-consuming and requires consensus among many HCPs, with different experiences and ideas on what demonstrates a good outcome. One recent study identified as many as eight domains when considering chronic pain outcomes [40]:

(1) Pain intensity
(2) Pain frequency
(3) Emotional well-being
(4) Satisfaction with social roles and activity
(5) Productivity
(6) health-related quality of life
(7) Physical activity
(8) Patient's perception of treatment goal achievement

Not only does this highlight the complexity of chronic pain and its effects on an individual beyond the pain itself, but it also reinforces how difficult this area is to research and validate.

Randomized control trials remain the gold standard for providing evidence, but constructing a trial for this cohort has challenges. In addition to the difficulty of accepting outcome measures, identifying the correct eligibility criteria for patients is also challenging in this cohort. Chronic pain presentations vary and do not follow a standard disease course making traditional study designs difficult. RCTs within this group are likely to be of small size and lack generalizability as a result of complex patients' selection and suitable outcome measures. As this is the usual measure for creating evidence-based guidelines to influence quality care, it follows that this is lacking within the existing structures of pain medicine. RCTs in chronic pain patients may also suffer from two other biases: selection bias and loss to follow-up. There is likely to be a higher number of participants who have not responded to conventional treatments and would consider participating in an RCT. Second, loss to follow-up is likely to be high in this cohort of patients who may seek alternative treatments if they perceive the trial is not effective. Real-world evidence (RWE) is described as "information related to healthcare derived from various sources outside conventional clinical research settings." This field has witnessed rapid growth, thanks to technological advancements over the past decades, particularly the widespread availability of extensive databases and computational tools facilitating secondary research use of data not originally collected for this purpose. Some have even proposed that, in specific contexts, RWE studies could complement randomized controlled trials (RCTs). However, the potential advantages of utilizing routine data are tempered by challenges such as the absence [23] of randomization, frequently limited data quality and quality control issues (e.g., incomplete or incorrect data), and the potential for significant confounding effects [24−27]. This underscores the crucial importance of deriving valid RWE from well-designed, meticulously conducted studies that use carefully curated data and address data quality concerns [26]. As part of an initiative by ACTTION (Analgesic, Aesthetic, and Addiction Clinical Trial Translations, Innovations, Opportunities, and Networks) IMMPACT (Initiative on Methods, Measurement, and Pain Assessment in Clinical

Trials), this qualitative systematic review aims to identify the approaches employed in assessing the effectiveness of pain treatments in RWE studies [28–30]. Additionally, it seeks to provide an overview of the methods employed thus far in designing, conducting, and analyzing RWE studies in pain research. Importantly, this review focuses on the methodology employed in studies using retrospective data to compare two or more groups [31,32]. The emphasis is on the challenging aspects of retrospective design and how valid causal inferences about interventions can be drawn in the absence of randomization, despite noncomparability issues. It is worth noting that this discussion excludes two significant categories of potential RWE studies: prospective trials, which were previously addressed in our work on "pragmatic trials," and single-arm cohort studies, as they contribute to a distinct trail of evidence [33]. A notable revelation from this review is the infrequent use of terms like "real-world data" and "real-world evidence" in reports. Specifically, fewer than six articles mentioned "real-world data" as a phrase, only one article used the term "real-world evidence," and merely two studies incorporated "real-world" in their titles [33,34]. Paradoxically, the term "real-world" is commonly employed to characterize investigations, such as pragmatic trials, which may not necessarily fall under the classification of "real-world evidence" studies. This practice is often a way of distinguishing them from laboratory settings [34,35]. The lack of consensus on the appropriate usage of the term RWE adds complexity to the matter. This issue is significant because for RWE studies to serve as an alternative to conventional RCT data in treatment decisions, the studies must be accessible and robust for evidence synthesis through systematic reviews and meta-analyses [38–40]. The problem for RCTs when considering patients with pain is this: are the results demonstrated generalizable enough to dictate decision making at a population level? In general, it seems that this is not the case, and this has led to difficulties when creating guidelines and standardizing care throughout the profession [41]. In contrast to clinical trials that adhere to clearly defined terms like "randomized," "placebo-controlled," and "double-blind," thanks to initiatives like CONSORT, RWE studies lack such standardized language. For instance, these defining terms will be present in the title of all randomized, placebo-controlled, double-blind clinical trials. This standardized approach is absent in the realm of RWE studies. A search for sensitivity, such as using PubMed for "pain AND (real-world OR real world)," yields thousands of results, escalating the workload for systematic reviews with very low specificity. Furthermore, the term "real world" may not be used by many relevant studies, suggesting that even such a search string might not be entirely sensitive. Consequently, the search conducted here is likely not exhaustive and can only offer a partial understanding of real-world studies [37,38]. Therefore, achieving consensus on standard terminology and the quality of methods and assessments is crucial for the field. This consensus is essential to build a body of work that can effectively contribute to evidence synthesis in the field of medicine.

This reflects large databases becoming publicly available recently, improved search methods and data base indexing, and growing awareness of using routinely collected health data for research purposes. Although some sources have been created specifically for future research, like the Spine Tango Registry and the Collaborative Health Outcomes Information Registry (CHOIR), in other cases, large data sets of national health bodies were made accessible to enable research [41,42]. These often include naturally large unified systems, like the US Department of Veterans Affairs or the United Kingdom's National Health Service, a single-payer system, under which UK residents have single identification numbers under which multiple records across multiple health services are identifiable. Such secondary use of data should certainly be welcomed because it can increase research value without additional burden on patients [43,44]. More than 90% of the studies included in our analysis used propensity scores to account for potential confounding, making it by far the dominant method. This may partly be the result of our search string (which included "propensity score" as a term) [45,46]. However, other statistical methods in our string were not picked up at all. Propensity score matching or adjustment is an appropriate method for reducing confounding effects. However, these methods depend on the measurement and inclusion of all important confounders. Vollert et al. study showed the wide use of propensity matching over other uses of propensity scores, such as stratification or inverse probability weighting, especially in large databases [47]. The absence of more modern methods, such as marginal structural models, was conspicuous, possibly because of the relative simplicity of implementing propensity score-based methods [48]. The use of appropriate statistical methods for drawing valid causal inferences is a crucial element for the success of RWE studies, and the potential of emerging methods has been shown [48]. The fast-emerging field of causal inference develops methods designated to drawing high degrees of evidence from nonexperimental data and can be especially used in RWE studies. Over 90% of the studies included in our analysis relied heavily on propensity scores as the predominant method for addressing potential confounding, indicating its widespread use. It is worth noting that this prevalence may be influenced, at least in part, by our search string, which specifically included "propensity score" as a term. However, it is noteworthy that other statistical methods specified in our search string were not identified at all. The utilization of propensity score matching or adjustment is recognized as an appropriate approach for mitigating confounding effects. Nonetheless, the effectiveness of these methods hinges on the accurate measurement and inclusion of all relevant confounders. What struck us as particularly surprising was the extensive use of propensity matching in comparison to other applications of propensity scores, such as stratification or inverse probability weighting, especially in the context of large databases. The noticeable absence of more contemporary methods, like marginal structural models, stands out, possibly attributed to the perceived simplicity of implementing propensity score-based approaches. Recognizing the pivotal role of employing appropriate statistical methods for drawing valid causal inferences, the potential of emerging methods has been demonstrated in previous research. The rapidly evolving field of causal inference is actively developing methods specifically designed to extract high-quality evidence from nonexperimental data. These advancements hold particular promise for the realm of real-world evidence (RWE) studies, emphasizing the importance of staying abreast of and incorporating innovative approaches in the ongoing pursuit of robust causal inference.

5.5.1 Quality assurance in pain management—a potential solution?

The need for data to drive quality is evident. But if the usual routes for collecting this don't apply, pain medicine may need to look beyond conventional methods. One area which could prove fruitful is the creation of patient registries. A patient registry is a structured system using observational study methods to collect data, both clinical and nonclinical, in a systematic way [42]. The benefit of this is it allows the study of a population defined by a disease or condition and allows the user to assess specific outcomes. It will enable comparing epidemiological differences that may otherwise be difficult to account for in smaller studies. Data are collected in a way that fits the clinical narrative based on the decisions of the physician and patient rather than as a result of the designs and protocols of the study [42]. Data derived from studies is likely to mirror actual clinical practice closely, and although they may resemble sizable observational cohort studies, they have the potential to adapt and prioritize new ideas over time. This makes them a valuable tool in studying populations over long periods.

As the healthcare industry grapples with the ever-expanding volume of patient-related data, the curation and management of these vast data sources pose a challenge for an overwhelmed health workforce. The integration of artificial intelligence (AI), with its automation and rapid processing capabilities for large-scale data, is met with mixed reactions among clinicians. Although some embrace the potential benefits, others express concerns about the potential consequences. One of the logistical challenges in assessing the impact of AI on clinical care revolves around the ability to evaluate and monitor its effects. Operationalizing AI for decision support entails a comprehensive process, including design, development, selection, use, and ongoing surveillance. In the field of pain medicine, the primary intersection with AI occurs through advancements in adjacent clinical domains and the application of clinical decision support (CDS). Notably, CDS related to opioid prescribing has been designated as a medical device, requiring approval from the US Food and Drug Administration (FDA) if the system lacks algorithmic transparency or employs a closed-loop process, as seen in some prescription drug monitoring programs (PDMPs) calculating opioid risk scores. Although CDS has a substantial body of literature supporting its benefits, concerns about associated alarm fatigue have also been raised. As the integration of AI into clinical settings is evaluated, it is crucial to consider both its strengths and weaknesses. The FDA has, to date, approved at least 29 AI health devices and algorithms for patient care. However, a major challenge lies in recognizing that these algorithms are constructed by humans, introducing inherent biases and blind spots that can potentially be amplified and encoded into clinical care, exacerbating issues related to access and health equity.

An illustrative example comes from anesthesiology, where the development of pulse oximetry in Japan, influenced by melanin levels, posed risks for undertreated oxygenation issues, particularly impactful during the COVID-19 pandemic. Ultimately, the overarching goal for physicians caring for patients with pain is to provide the safest and most effective care. The escalating volume of digital health data poses a significant burden. Although clinicians may triage the most critical data points, AI holds the promise of performing this task more efficiently and presumably with fewer critical omissions. Additionally, AI could enhance the effectiveness of querying scientific databases for real-time answers to clinical questions. This examination aims to explore both the strengths and limitations of integrating AI and automated technologies in the clinical care sphere for pain medicine.

Pain medicine could benefit significantly from the creation and maintenance of patient registries. They are already used successfully within cancer populations, for example, to drive change in diagnosis, prevention, treatment, and end-of-life care [43]. In essence, the creation of patient registries can provide a level of surveillance to a nonspecific population that presents with pain. Registries can be used at a local level, a national level, or even an international level [42]. A further advantage to creating patient registries at all of these levels is that through real-time feedback, data quality improvement can be at the forefront of data collection. For a specialty such as Pain medicine, where this process is complex, the creation of patient registries may provide an answer to its problems.

Several large-scale registries for Pain Medicine have been created to try and address this problem. The PAIN OUT registry is an international patient registry focusing on acute perioperative pain [21]. It has enrolled nearly 50,000 subjects and aims to use "real life" data to identify best practices and aid decision making by both patients and physicians. Further registries have now been created specifically with interventional procedures [44] and chronic pain in mind [45].

Digital medicine is likely to play a crucial role in developing patient registries in Pain Medicine and could allow for better data collection, patient participation, outcome measurement, and analysis. Electronic health records are one tool that could be used to contribute to and maintain specific patient registries [46]. Mobile applications, increasing accessible with increasing ownership of smart devices, have the potential to capture real-time data from the patient [49]. Within Pain Medicine, this could allow clinicians to chart the effects of interventions more accurately and give patients more ownership over their disease. Recognition of pain is one of the most critical[50–53 aspects for patients when they consider the effectiveness of their treatment. Patient satisfaction is an important marker of quality care [54,55]. Thus, it makes sense that incorporating available and potential technologies that promote autonomy will lead to improvements in the quality of care, particularly in a specialty such as pain management [56,57].

Although AI has demonstrated quantitative benefits in specific healthcare settings, its success is often contingent on the availability of large amounts of reliable discrete data, particularly in clinical areas such as radiology [58,59]. However, AI has not reached a level of development where it can operate independently without physician oversight [60−65]. This is evident in radiology, where standalone AI is outperformed by radiologists. Although AI may identify suspicious lesions overlooked by radiologists, it also increases the workload by augmenting the number of scans for review [65]. Moreover, in scenarios where AI flags a potential issue, but a physician overrides the AI classification, the physician assumes increased liability if the patient later develops a health concern [66,67]. AI's applicability in imaging-related tasks is more acceptable when dealing with numerous and relatively homogenous data, such as breast mammograms or brachial plexus ultrasounds [68−73]. However, in complex clinical situations like determining the cause of low back pain, AI is likely to underperform compared to a clinician, as demonstrated in the multifaceted environment of the emergency department [74]. Beyond diagnosis, AI struggles to construct treatment plans, even within a limited algorithmic scope [75−79]. For instance, ML using genetic profiling couldn't predict opioid doses for cancer patients, raising doubts about its efficacy in formulating complex analgesic regimens for chronic noncancer pain [80,81]. Similarly, a digital tool for managing low back pain was deemed "noninferior" to clinician time but failed to match patient satisfaction levels, with some feeling that clinician involvement would have been superior. Other concerns pertain to breaches of patient confidentiality and diminished agency associated with AI technologies. For instance, using large insurance databases to predict morbidity and mortality in patients with opioid use disorder for harm reduction initiatives raises privacy concerns [82−86]. Additionally, AI has the potential to exacerbate biases and reduce patient agency, particularly in complex clinical scenarios, potentially diminishing the individual's role in their own care. As healthcare systems prioritize efficiency and cost savings, there is a risk that AI implementation could decrease access to care for patients with state-funded insurance or complex diagnoses [83,84]. Current models often lack consideration of social determinants of health (SDH), and there is a concern that factors considered high risk for poor outcomes may be excluded from consideration, resulting in inequity for pharmaceutical or interventional candidates [84,85]. Certainly, if AI is effectively harnessed to provide genuine support, the benefits could be substantial for frontline clinicians. For instance, a Prescription Drug Monitoring Program (PDMP) guided by intelligent AI that directs clinicians toward safer opioid prescribing practices could significantly improve patient morbidity. Similarly, the application of machine learning (ML) to predict patient responses to spinal cord stimulation shows promise, with early studies suggesting transformative outcomes. EHRs are already presenting crucial data in real time as clinicians order medications, such as displaying creatinine values when renally cleared medications are prescribed [46,84,86]. Enhancing this capability to alleviate the cognitive burden on pain providers, who are already stretched to maximum efficiency, has the potential to improve patient outcomes. Moreover, utilizing AI to predict the duration of care, optimizing healthcare resource utilization, can contribute to cost containment. The opportunity to enhance patient access by streamlining efficiency, reducing mundane tasks, and precisely selecting therapeutics could be truly transformative.

References

[1] Comley AL, DeMeyer E. Assessing patient satisfaction with pain management through a continuous quality improvement effort. J Pain Symptom Manag 2001;21(1):27–40. https://doi.org/10.1016/s0885-3924(00)00229-3.

[2] Gordon DB, Pellino TA, Miaskowski C, et al. A 10-year review of quality improvement monitoring in pain management: recommendations for standardized outcome measures. Pain Manag Nurs 2002;3(4):116–30. https://doi.org/10.1053/jpmn.2002.127570.

[3] Swensen SJ, Meyer GS, Nelson EC, et al. Cottage industry to postindustrial care–the revolution in health care delivery. N Engl J Med 2010;362(5):e12. https://doi.org/10.1056/NEJMp0911199.

[4] Nice low back pain and sciatica in over 16s. 2016. p. 29. SIGN 136 – Management of Chronic Pain, https://www.nice.org.uk/guidance/ng193.

[5] A structured approach to opioid prescribing. Faculty of Pain Medicine https://fpm.ac.uk/opioids-aware/structured-approach-opioid-prescribing

[6] US Dept of Health – Centres for Disease Control and Prevention. Checklist for prescribing opioids for chronic pain. 2016.

[7] CKS Scenario: constipation in adults. NICE. Available on: https://cks.nice.org.uk/topics/constipation/management/adults/. accessed in 25th of November 2023.

[8] Garimella V, Cellini C. Postoperative pain control. Clin Colon Rectal Surg September, 2013;26(3):191–6. https://doi.org/10.1055/s-0033-1351138. PMID: 24436674; PMCID: PMC3747287.

[9] Institute of Medicine (US) Committee on Quality of Health Care in America. Crossing the quality chasm: a new health system for the 21st century. Washington (DC): National Academies Press (US); 2001. Faculty of Pain Medicine.

[10] St Sauver JL, Warner DO, Yawn BP, et al. Why patients visit their doctors: assessing the most prevalent conditions in a defined American population. Mayo Clin Proc 2013; 88(1):56–67. https://doi.org/10.1016/j.mayocp.2012.08.020.

[11] Katz N. The impact of pain management on quality of life. J Pain Symptom Manag 2002;24(Suppl. l):S38–47. https://doi.org/10.1016/s0885-3924(02)00411-6.

[12] Fayaz A, Croft P, Langford RM, Donaldson LJ, Jones GT. Prevalence of chronic pain in the UK: a systematic review and meta-analysis of population studies. BMJ Open 2016; 6(6):e010364. https://doi.org/10.1136/bmjopen-2015-010364. Published 2016 Jun 20.

[13] Rockett M, Vanstone R, Chand J, Waeland D. A survey of acute pain services in the UK. Anaesthesia 2017;72(10):1237–42. https://doi.org/10.1111/anae.14007.

[14] Fujita K, Moles RJ, Chen TF. Quality indicators for responsible use of medicines: a systematic review. BMJ Open 2018;8(7):e020437. https://doi.org/10.1136/bmjopen-2017-020437. Published 2018 Jul 16.

[15] National Institute for Health and Care Excellence (NICE). Chronic pain (primary and secondary) in over 16s: assessment of all chronic pain and management of chronic primary pain. NICE guideline [NG193]. Published: 7 April 2021. Available from: https://www.nice.org.uk/guidance/ng193.

[16] Finnerup NB, Kirsten F-F, Johnsen E, Jensen TS. Screening for motor neuron involvement in patients with pure lower motor neuron disease: a clinical, neurophysiological and neuropathological study. Eur J Neurol 2015;22(2):218–26. https://doi.org/10.1111/ene.12579.

[17] Poply K, Mehta V. The dilemma of interventional pain trials: thinking beyond the box. Br J Anaesth 2017;119(4):718–9. https://doi.org/10.1093/bja/aex301.

[18] Hróbjartsson A, Emanuelsson F, Skou Thomsen AS, Hilden J, Brorson S. Bias due to lack of patient blinding in clinical trials. A systematic review of trials randomizing patients to blind and nonblind sub-studies. Int J Epidemiol 2014;43(4):1272−83. https://doi.org/10.1093/ije/dyu115.

[19] Mao J. Current challenges in translational pain research. Trend Pharmacol Sci 2012; 33(11):568−73. https://doi.org/10.1016/j.tips.2012.08.001.

[20] Meissner W, Huygen F, Neugebauer EAM, Osterbrink J, Benhamou D, Betteridge N, Coluzzi F, De Andres J, Fawcett W, Fletcher D, Kalso E, Kehlet H, Morlion B, Montes Pérez A, Pergolizzi J, Schäfer M. Management of acute pain in the postoperative setting: the importance of quality indicators. Curr Med Res Opin 2018;34(1): 187−96. https://doi.org/10.1080/03007995.2017.1391081. Epub 2017 Nov 15. PMID: 29019421.

[21] Derry S, Wiffen PJ, Moore RA, Quinlan J. Topical lidocaine for neuropathic pain in adults. Cochrane Database Syst Rev 2014;(7).

[22] Kehlet H, Jensen TS, Woolf CJ. Persistent postsurgical pain: risk factors and prevention. Lancet 2006;367(9522):1618−25. https://doi.org/10.1016/S0140-6736(06)68700-X.

[23] Goh GS, Zeng GJ, Tay DK, Lo NN, Yeo SJ, Liow MHL. Does obesity lead to lower rates of clinically meaningful improvement or satisfaction after total hip arthroplasty? A propensity score-matched study. Hip Int 2020;32(5):610−9.

[24] Hah JM, Sturgeon JA, Zocca J, Sharifzadeh Y, Mackey SC. Factors associated with prescription opioid misuse in a cross-sectional cohort of patients with chronic non-cancer pain. J Pain Res 2017;10:979−87.

[25] Han DG, Koh W, Shin JS, Lee J, Lee YJ, Kim MR, et al. Cervical surgery rate in neck pain patients with and without acupuncture treatment: a retrospective cohort study. Acupunct Med 2019;37:268−76.

[26] Han L, Goulet JL, Skanderson M, Bathulapalli H, Luther SL, Kerns RD, Brandt CA. Evaluation of complementary and integrative health approaches among US veterans with musculoskeletal pain using propensity score methods. Pain Med 2019;20(1):90-102.

[27] Harrold LR, Shan Y, Rebello S, Kramer N, Connolly SE, Alemao E, Kelly S, Kremer JM, Rosenstein ED. Disease activity and patient-reported outcomes in patients with rheumatoid arthritis and Sjögren's syndrome enrolled in a large observational US registry. Rheumatol Int 2020;40(8):1239-1248.

[28] Benhamou D, Berti M, Brodner G, et al. Postoperative Analgesic THerapy Observa- tional Survey (PATHOS): a practice pattern study in 7 central/southern European countries. Pain 2008;136(1−2):134−41. https://doi.org/10.1016/j.pain.2007.06.028.

[29] Helwig U, Mross M, Schubert S, Hartmann H, Brandes A, Stein D, et al. Real-world clinical effectiveness and safety of vedolizumab and anti-tumor necrosis factor alpha treatment in ulcerative colitis and Crohn's disease patients: a German retrospective chart review. BMC Gastroenterol 2020;20:211.

[30] Herman PM, Yuan AH, Cefalu MS, Chu K, Zeng Q, Marshall N, et al. The use of complementary and integrative health approaches for chronic musculoskeletal pain in younger US veterans: an economic evaluation. PLoS One 2019;14:e0217831.

[31] Hermansen E, Romild UK, Austevoll IM, Solberg T, Storheim K, Brox JI, et al. Does surgical technique influence clinical outcome after lumbar spinal stenosis decompression? A comparative effectiveness study from the Norwegian Registry for Spine Surgery. Eur Spine J 2017;26:420−7.

[32] Hirsch BP, Khechen B, Patel DV, Cardinal KL, Guntin JA, Singh K. Safety and efficacy of revision minimally invasive lumbar decompression in the ambulatory setting. Spine 2019;44:E494−e499.

[33] Ho M, van der Laan M, Lee H, Chen J, Lee K, Fang Y, et al. The current landscape in biostatistics of real-world data and evidence: causal inference frameworks for study design and analysis. Stat Biopharm Res 2021:1–14.

[34] Hohenschurz-Schmidt D, Kleykamp BA, Draper-Rodi J, Vollert J, Chan J, Ferguson M, et al. Pragmatic trials of pain therapies: a systematic review of methods. Pain 2022;163: 21–46.

[35] Aasvang EK, Luna IE, Kehlet H. Challenges in postdischarge function and recovery: the case of fast-track hip and knee arthroplasty. Br J Anaesth 2015;115(6):861–6. https:// doi.org/10.1093/bja/aev257.

[36] Hu CG, Zheng K, Liu GH, Li ZL, Zhao YL, Lian JH, et al. Effectiveness and postoperative pain level of single-port versus two-port thoracoscopic lobectomy for lung cancer: a retrospective cohort study. Gen Thorac Cardiovasc Surg 2021;69:318–25.

[37] Il Kim J, Kim YT, Jung HJ, Lee JK. Does adding corticosteroids to periarticular injection affect the postoperative acute phase response after total knee arthroplasty? Knee 2020;27:493–9.

[38] Jeong HJ, Kim HS, Rhee SM, Oh JH. Risk factors for and prognosis of folded rotator cuff tears: a comparative study using propensity score matching. J Shoulder Elbow Surg 2021;30:826–35.

[39] a Jung H, Lee KH, Jeong Y, Yoon S, Kim WH, Lee HJ. Effect of fentanyl-based intravenous patient-controlled analgesia with and without basal infusion on postoperative opioid consumption and opioid-related side effects: a retrospective cohort study. J Pain Res 2020;13:3095–106.
      b Kockerling F, Bittner R, Kofler M, Mayer F, Adolf D, Kuthe A, Weyhe D. Lichtenstein versus total extraperitoneal patch plasty versus transabdominal patch plasty technique for primary unilateral inguinal hernia repair: a registry-based, propensity score-matched comparison of 57, 906 patients. Ann Surg 2019;269:351–7.

[40] Krebs EE, Carey TS, Weinberger M. Accuracy of the pain numeric rating scale as a screening test in primary care. J Gen Intern Med 2007;22(10):1453–8. https:// doi.org/10.1007/s11606-007-0321-2.

[41] Kockerling F, Koch A, Adolf D, Keller T, Lorenz R, Fortelny RH, et al. Has shouldice repair in a selected group of patients with inguinal hernia comparable results to lichtenstein, TEP and TAPP techniques? World J Surg 2018;42:2001–10.

[42] Kockerling F, Simon T, Adolf D, Kockerling D, Mayer F, Reinpold W, et al. Laparoscopic IPOM versus open sublay technique for elective incisional hernia repair: a registry-based, propensity score-matched comparison of 9907 patients. Surg Endosc 2019;33:3361–9.

[43] Derry S, Wiffen PJ, Moore RA, Quinlan J. Topical lidocaine for neuropathic pain in adults. Cochrane Database Syst Rev 2014;7.

[44] Zaslansky R, Rothaug J, Chapman CR, et al. Pain out: the making of an international acute pain registry. Eur J Pain 2015;19(4):490–502. https://doi.org/10.1002/ejp.571.

[45] Kim MK, Kang H, Choi GJ, Kang KH. Robotic thyroidectomy decreases postoperative pain compared with conventional thyroidectomy. Surg Laparosc Endosc Percutaneous Tech 2019;29:255–60.

[46] Kim MK, Yi MS, Kang H, Choi GJ. Effects of remifentanil versus nitrous oxide on postoperative nausea, vomiting, and pain in patients receiving thyroidectomy: propensity score matching analysis. Medicine 2016;95:e5135.

[47] Krauss I, Mueller G, Haupt G, Steinhilber B, Janssen P, Jentner N, et al. Effectiveness and efficiency of an 11-week exercise intervention for patients with hip or knee

osteoarthritis: a protocol for a controlled study in the context of health services research. BMC Publ Health 2016;16:367.

[48] Lee H-J, Wong JB, Jia B, Qi X, DeLong ER. Empirical use of causal inference methods to evaluate survival differences in a real-world registry vs those found in randomized clinical trials. Stat Med 2020;39:3003—21.

[49] Chou R, Gordon DB, de Leon-Casasola OA, et al. Management of postoperative pain: a clinical practice guideline from the American pain society, the American society of regional anesthesia and pain medicine, and the American society of anesthesiologists committee on regional anesthesia, executive committee, and administrative council. J Pain 2016;17(2):131—510. https://doi.org/10.1016/j.jpain.2015.12.008.

[50] Quality prescribing for chronic pain — an introduction. Available on: https://www.therapeutics.scot.nhs.uk/wp-content/uploads/2018/03/Strategy-Chronic-Pain-Quality-Prescribing-for-Chronic-Pain-2018.pdf. Accessed in 25th of November 2023.

[51] Kerr NL. Harking: hypothesizing after the results are known. Personal Soc Psychol Rev official J Soc Personal Soc Psychol Inc 1998;2:196—217.

[52] Khan JS, Hah JM, Mackey SC. Effects of smoking on patients with chronic pain: a propensity-weighted analysis on the Collaborative Health Outcomes Information Registry. Pain 2019;160:2374—9.

[53] Kim MK, Kang H, Choi GJ, Kang KH. Robotic thyroidectomy decreases postoperative pain compared with conventional thyroidectomy. Surg Laparosc Endosc Percutaneous Tech 2019;29:255—60.

[54] Ballantyne JC, Sullivan MD. Intensity of chronic pain–the wrong metric? N Engl J Med 2015;373(22):2098—9. https://doi.org/10.1056/NEJMp1507136.

[55] Turk DC, Dworkin RH, Allen RR, et al. Core outcome domains for chronic pain clinical trials: IMMPACT recommendations. Pain 2003;106(3):337—45. https://doi.org/10.1016/j.pain.2003.08.001.

[56] APM Council on Ethics. Ethics charter from American academy of pain medicine. Pain Med May, 2005;6(3):203—12. https://doi.org/10.1111/j.1526-4637.2005.05040.x.

[57] Dubois MY. The birth of an ethics charter for pain medicine. Pain Med 2005;6(3):201—2.

[58] McNeill JA, Sherwood GD, Starck PL, et al. Assessing clinical outcomes: patient satisfaction with pain management. J Pain Symptom Manag 1998;16(1):29—40.

[59] Zhou Y, Furgang FA, Zhang Y. Quality assurance for interventional pain management procedures. Pain Phys 2006;9:107—14.

[60] Vila Jr H, Smith RA, Augustyniak MJ, Nagi PA, Soto RG, Ross TW, et al. The efficacy and safety of pain management beforeand after implementation of hospitalwide pain management standards: is patient safety compromised by treatment based solely on numerical painratings? Anesth Analg 2005;101:474—80.

[61] Gonzalez N, Quintana JM, Bilbao A, Escobar A, Aizpuru F, Thompson A, et al. Development and validation of an inpatient satisfaction questionnaire. Int J Qual Health Care 2005;17:465—72.

[62] Zhou Y, Thompson S. Quality assurance for interventional pain management procedures in private practice. Pain Physic 2008;11(1):43—55. PMID: 18196169.

[63] Mao J. Current challenges in translational pain research. Trend Pharmacol Sci 2012;33(11):568—73. https://doi.org/10.1016/j.tips.2012.08.001.

[64] Joos E, Peretz A, Beguin S, Famaey JP. Reliability and reproducibility of visual analogue scale and numeric rating scale for therapeutic evaluation of pain in rheumatic patients. J Rheumatol 1991;18(8):1269—70.

[65] Obradovic M, Lal A, Liedgens H. Validity and responsiveness of EuroQol-5 dimension (EQ-5D) versus Short Form-6 dimension (SF-6D) questionnaire in chronic pain. Health Qual Life Outcome 2013;11:110. https://doi.org/10.1186/1477-7525-11-110. Published 2013 Jul 1.

[66] Kaiser U, Kopkow C, Deckert S, et al. Developing a core outcome domain set to assessing effectiveness of interdisciplinary multimodal pain therapy: the VAPAIN consensus statement on core outcome domains. Pain 2018;159(4):673−83. https://doi.org/10.1097/j.pain.0000000000001129.

[67] Gordon DB, de Leon-Casasola OA, Wu CL, Sluka KA, Brennan TJ, Chou R. Research gaps in practice guidelines for acute postoperative pain management in adults: findings from a review of the evidence for an American pain society clinical practice guideline. J Pain 2016;17(2):158−66. https://doi.org/10.1016/j.jpain.2015.10.023.

[68] Gliklich RE, Dreyer NA, Leavy MB, editors. Registries for evaluating patient outcomes: a user's guide. 3rd ed. Rockville (MD): Agency for Healthcare Research and Quality (US); 2014 Patient Registries. Available from: https://www.ncbi.nlm.nih.gov/books/NBK208643/.

[69] Parkin DM. The role of cancer registries in cancer control. Int J Clin Oncol 2008;13(2):102−11. https://doi.org/10.1007/s10147-008-0762-6.

[70] Licciardone JC, Gatchel RJ, Phillips N, Aryal S. The Pain Registry for Epidemiological, Clinical, and Interventional Studies and Innovation (PRECISION): registry overview and protocol for a propensity score-matched study of opioid prescribing in patients with low back pain. J Pain Res 2018;11:1751−60. https://doi.org/10.2147/JPR.S169275. Published 2018 Sep. 6.

[71] Langley PC. A practice based chronic pain management registry (CPMR): structure and content of proposed patient and patient/provider platforms. Innov Pharm 2019;10(1). https://doi.org/10.24926/iip.v10i1.1628. Published 2019 Aug 31. doi:10.24926/iip.v10i1.1628.

[72] Ehrenstein V, Kharrazi H, Lehmann H, et al. Obtaining data from electronic health records. In: Gliklich RE, Leavy MB, Dreyer NA, editors. Tools and technologies for registry interoperability, registries for evaluating patient outcomes: a user's guide. 3rd ed. Rockville (MD): Agency for Healthcare Research and Quality (US); October, 2019. Addendum 2 [Internet].

[73] Ventola CL. Mobile devices and apps for health care professionals: uses and benefits. P T 2014;39(5):356−64.

[74] Magrabi F, Ammenwerth E, McNair JB, et al. Artificial intelligence in clinical decision support: challenges for evaluating AI and practical implications. Yearb Med Inform 2019;28:128−34. https://doi.org/10.1055/s-0039-1677903. https://rapm.bmj.com/lookup/google-scholar?link_type=googlescholar&gs_type=article&author%5B0%5D=F+Magrabi&author%5B1%5D=E+Ammenwerth&author%5B2%5D=JB+McNair&title=Artificial+intelligence+in+clinical+decision+support:+challenges+for+evaluating+AI+and+practical+implications&publication_year=2019&journal=Yearb+Med+Inform&volume=28&pages=128-34"GoogleScholar.

[75] Clinical decision support software: guidance for industry and food and drug administration staff [U.S. Food and Drug Administration]. Available: https://www.fda.gov/regulatory-information/search-fda-guidance-documents/clinical-decision-support-software [Accessed 11 April 2023].

[76] Your clinical decision support software, is it a medical device? U.S. Food and Drug Administration Available: https://www.fda.gov/medical-devices/software-medical-device-samd/your-clinical-decision-support-software-it-medical-device [Accessed 11 Apr 2023].

[77] Hussain MI, Nelson AM, Yeung BG, et al. How the presentation of patient information and decision-support advisories influences opioid prescribing behavior: a simulation study. J Am Med Inf Assoc 2020;27:613−20.

[78] Thomas LB, Mastorides SM, Viswanadhan NA, et al. Artificial intelligence: review of current and future applications in medicine. Fed Pract 2021;38:527−38.

[79] Cabanas AM, Fuentes-Guajardo M, Latorre K, et al. Skin pigmentation influence on pulse oximetry accuracy: a systematic review and bibliometric analysis. Sensors 2022;22:3402.

[80] Patterson BK, Guevara-Coto J, Yogendra R, et al. Immune-based prediction of covid-19 severity and chronicity decoded using machine learning. Front Immunol 2021;12: 700782.

[81] Rozova V, Witt K, Robinson J, et al. Detection of self-harm and suicidal ideation in emergency department triage notes. J Am Med Inf Assoc 2022;29:472−80.

[82] Hornung AL, Hornung CM, Mallow GM, et al. Artificial intelligence in spine care: current applications and future utility. Eur Spine J 2022;31:2057−81. https://doi.org/10.1007/s00586-022-07176-0.

[83] Yagi M, Michikawa T, Yamamoto T, et al. Development and validation of machine learning-based predictive model for clinical outcome of decompression surgery for lumbar spinal canal stenosis. Spine J 2022;22:1768−77. https://doi.org/10.1016/j.spinee.2022.06.008.

[84] Ngiam KY, Khor IW. Big data and machine learning algorithms for health-care delivery. Lancet Oncol 2019;20:e262−73. https://doi.org/10.1016/S1470-2045(19)30149-4 [published correction appears in Lancet oncol. 2019 Jun; 20 (6):293].

[85] Gabriel RA, Harjai B, Prasad RS, et al. Machine learning approach to predicting persistent opioid use following lower extremity joint arthroplasty. Reg Anesth Pain Med 2022;47: 313−9. https://doi.org/10.1136/rapm-2021-103299. Abstract/FREE Full TextHYPERLINK, https://rapm.bmj.com/lookup/google-scholar?link_type=googlescholar&gs_type=article&author%5B0%5D=RA+Gabriel&author%5B1%5D=B+Harjai&author%5B2%5D=RS+Prasad&title=Machine+learning+approach+to+predicting+persistent+opioid+use+following+lower+extremity+joint+arthroplasty&publication_year=2022&journal=Reg+Anesth+Pain+Med&volume=47&pages=313-9"GoogleScholar.

[86] Zhong H, Poeran J, Gu A, et al. Machine learning approaches in predicting ambulatory same day discharge patients after total hip arthroplasty. Reg Anesth Pain Med 2021;46: 779−83. https://doi.org/10.1136/rapm-2021-102715.

Further reading

[1] Quality Prescribing for Chronic Pain - A guide for Improvement. Available on: https://www.therapeutics.scot.nhs.uk/wp-content/uploads/2018/03/Strategy-Chronic-Pain-Quality-Prescribing-for-Chronic-Pain-2018.pdf. [Accessed 25th November 2023].

[2] Gupta A, et al. Quality assurance and assessment in pain management. Anesthesiol Clin 2011;29:123—33. https://doi.org/10.1016/j.anclin.2010.11.008.

[3] Seow H, Snyder CF, Mularski RA, et al. A framework for assessing quality indicators for cancer care at the end of life. J Pain Symptom Manag 2009;38(6):903—12.

[4] Comley AL, DeMeyer E. Assessing patient satisfaction with pain management through a continuous quality improvement effort. J Pain Symptom Manag 2001;21(1):27—40.

[5] McCracken LM, Klock PA, Mingay DJ, et al. Assessment of satisfaction with treatment for chronic pain. J Pain Symptom Manag 1997;14(5):292—9.

[6] Kaiser U, Kopkow C, Deckert S, Sabatowski R, Schmitt J. Validation and application of a core set of patient-relevant outcome domains to assess the effectiveness of multimodal pain therapy (VAPAIN): a study protocol. BMJ Open 2015;5(11):e008146. https://doi.org/10.1136/bmjopen-2015-008146. Published 2015 Nov 6.

Quality assurance management in maternity care

6

Abstract

Maternity care is nuanced because pregnancy is not deemed an illness that requires treatment. Furthermore, unlike other areas of healthcare, maternity has the added complexity of care episodes being targeted to both mother and baby/unborn at any given time. This demands an approach underpinned by constant risk assessments, surveillance, and application of policies and guidelines.

Keywords: Clinical epidemiology; Episiotomy; Maternity care; Pregnancy; Quality assurance; Quality management.

Key messages

- Quality assurance is vital to operate a high-quality maternity service given the significant volume of births
- Obstetric services are unique as it involves two patients that could lead to unanticipated adverse new-born and maternal outcomes such as maternal mortality or postpartum hemorrhage
- Using evidence-based practices is vital and beneficial to improving safety and patient outcomes
- Conducting quality management activities such as seminars, workshops, and regular team meetings as well as training events alongside regular assessment of quality indicators are important to continue to operate a safe healthcare service
- There are variations in quality standards across a variety of clinical settings

6.1 Introduction

Maternity care is nuanced because pregnancy is not deemed an illness that requires treatment. Furthermore, unlike other areas of healthcare, maternity has the added complexity of care episodes being targeted to both mother and baby/unborn at any given time. This demands an approach underpinned by constant risk assessments, surveillance, and application of policies and guidelines.

Over many years and in the wake of several inquiries, discussions on risk and safety have been ubiquitous, as the underpinning factors toward plans for improvement. Arulkumaran [1] purports that safety is the core pillar of quality that dictates

Quality Assurance Management. https://doi.org/10.1016/B978-0-12-822732-9.00002-3

the setting of appropriate standards. Improvement of quality requires a multipronged approach involving key stakeholders such as women, their families, midwives, obstetricians, and other care givers and policy makers [2]. The Changing Childbirth document [2] was inspired by the government's response to a previous review of maternity services [3] and focused on women's choice and involvement in and promoting continuity of care.

The Morecambe Bay investigation [4] highlighted a catalog of issues from failure to identify abnormalities, to missed opportunities that resulted in harm and in some cases death. In the Ockendon Report [3], recommendations were made, which point to addressing appropriate risk assessments and escalation of risks, as well as introducing senior roles to focus on fetal outcomes. Maternity services have seen a plethora of national policies and recommendations directly targeting pregnancy and childbirth. Better Births was then published in 2016 [5], setting out plans for safe delivery of maternity services, focusing on women as well as staff. Dame Cumberlege asserted the problem of different adaptations of quality, disparities in data collection systems, and poor team work across the different disciplines [5]. The report highlighted things go wrong too frequently and with that comes the consequential pay-outs.

Maternity care is also influenced by guidance issued by the National Institute for care and Health Excellence (NICE) [6] on various aspects of care in pregnancy and childbirth. Although these are regarded as guidance, they are often integrated into local policies and guidelines to inform care, and outcomes are usually judged by the level of compliance.

The NHS (National Health Service) Patient Safety Strategy [7] has patient safety at the heart of its objectives. Its underpinning safety principles are embedded in quality through key facets such as staffing, learning from incidents, exploration of women's experiences of care, inequalities in care, and a culture based on positive learning.

The care quality commission (CQC) continues to closely monitor standards in maternity care, and its recent report expressed concern that improvements were not at a rapid rate [8]. In essence, maternity care is governed by a plethora of standards by which obstetricians, midwives, and other team members function in practice in delivering woman-centered care, which is safe. Drawing on the recommendations of recent inquiries into poor care within maternity services, it is safe to say that factors such as those affecting the culture and dynamics of the teams do have an impact on outcomes. Midwives are trained to be leaders of normality (natural/usual), and it can be argued that the current medical model of care seems to interfere with the execution of their role and threaten the normality discourse [9], especially working in such a risk-averse environment. Within maternity care, standards and quality are determined by factors such as policies, training and competence, culture, leadership, women's experiences and involvement, national guidance, inadequate risk assessments, and team dynamics.

It follows then, that in terms of quality assurance in maternity care, the issues arising are as follows:

- Arrangements for effective audit programs: although maternity services tend to have an audit program, it is usually taken up by doctors in training to satisfy the requirement for progression or by specialist midwives to meet a particular expectation, for example, under the umbrella of a quality improvement program.
- Data collection systems: the area of informatics is a growing trend in maternity, aimed at improving the way in which vital information on care and services are collated as part of systems and frameworks. It can be argued that the focus on having a universally recognized informatics system in place is underpinned and influenced by financial gain. Maternity services work closely with commissioners and one way of assuring them of standard setting is to provide certain data in an effective way, but accurately reflecting events. It is ubiquitous in maternity to retrospectively amend birth details soon after the event, following quality checks by the specialist midwives for informatics. Any form of alacrity or avoidance of checks will negatively impact the mother, her family, and the organization. Health records have been seen to be an area for improvement in maternity services. It is compounded by the weak management of paper records or the debacle arising through the use of two different health record systems—paper and electronics. Health records must be managed appropriately as these may be required to respond to complaints or for litigation.
- Innovation and research: maternity staff are rarely involved in research and indulging in new ideas. In many maternity units, this is often left to a small research team who are usually only facilitating the information giving and consent taking from women for a study or trial. Better Births [5] encouraged support for staff in the promotion of innovations.
- Poor working relationships: highlighted in several maternity inquiries undoubtedly creates a challenge for achieving objectives under the auspices of quality assurance.

6.2 Association of quality management and clinical epidemiology

Epidemiological data play a vital role in quality management, with maternity and perinatal services. Within the United Kingdom, the national maternity and perinatal audit (NMPA) [10] program is led by the Royal College of Obstetricians and Gynecologists (RCOG) [11] in partnership with the Royal College of Paediatricians and Child Health (RCPCH) [12], the London School of Hygiene and Tropical Medicine (LSHTM), and the Royal College of Midwives. The NMPA uses data and information from maternity services in the United Kingdom to better understand both maternity care including hospital admissions and the journey undertaken by its service users. The report comprised birth data by way of NHS Digital's maternity services data and hospital episode statistics records based on over half a million birthing people and women as well as their babies born between April 1, 2018, and March 31, 2019, within Wales and England. A key finding was that a third of women and birthing people who were at singleton pregnancies at term had induced labor, while 1 in 20 women who experienced instrumental birth by forceps had no episiotomy. Of these birthing people and women, 31% had a third- or fourth-degree tear. Women and birthing people that opted for a vaginal birth following a prior cesarean birth were recorded as 61%, which was 10% lower than the proportions reported as part of national guidance (72%–75%). The report also showed that postnatal readmission rates were higher postcesarean birth in comparison with vaginal birth in Wales (4.7% vs. 3.3%) and England (4.3% vs. 2.9%). Approximately 23% of women and birthing people had an instrumental birth while 44% had an episiotomy during their vaginal birth. The report also showed that around 50% of the babies born after their due date were small for their gestational age, which was also in contrast to the national guidelines. The guidelines recommend early induction should be considered if there are concerns around gestational age. A key quality assurance point that was highlighted in the NMPA was the lack of data completeness linked to quality indicators such as augmentation, anesthesia, episiotomy, body mass index, smoking status at birth, labor onset, and maternal ethnicity. The NMPA report was unable to indicate the pain relief received by a birthing person or woman during labor. Underreporting of preconception conditions such as high blood pressure was another key issue the NMPA report indicated.

Improving the availability of the information is as important as the quality of the data gathered about possible interventions during labor and birth. This would aid maternal health services to improve the care offered and individualize evidence-based approaches such as the availability of multiple language formats to help decision making and consent tools. These quality indicators are vital to start engaging in discussions with healthcare professionals to resolve the problems, starting with amending data fields when gathering data, especially about timelines of epidural anesthesia, intrapartum analgesia by type, and the type of anesthesia used, at a granular level. There are also differences in the data captured even between the divulged nations within the United Kingdom, where postnatal variables differ within maternity datasets with regard to skin-to-skin measures or breast milk use for example. There is recognition that the current postnatal variables do not capture the experience of women, birthing people, and their babies. Therefore, adding processes to address these problems and introducing better quality control steps as well as using core characteristics (Table 6.1) should be considered as a priority to optimize outcomes for maternity services.

Maternity record book (MRB) has been another quality assurance approach that has been used in some low-middle-income countries (LMICs). Galadanci and colleagues [13] conducted a research study using a structured MRB approach for midwives and nurses to record information in rural settings. In the initial stages of the study, five hospitals in the northern region of Nigeria were used as sites, followed by nine sites in the south and south-western regions of Nigeria. The study team

Table 6.1 Characteristics that can be used as variables to better report maternity service outcomes along with key quality control steps that can be introduced to manage quality assurance.

Characteristics	Quality control approach	Quality assurance
Age <20, 20−24, 25−29, 30−34, 35−39 and 40+ Index of multiple deprivation BMI <18.5, 18.5−24.9, 25−29.9, and ≥30 Ethnicity and race: White, South Asian, Black, Mixed, Hispanic, and others Obstetric history including parity, primiparous, multiparous, and prior cesarean birth Preexisting comorbidities such as hypertension, diabetes, endometriosis, and mental illness Multiplicity: singleton, twins, triplets, or more Gestation at birth; $0-23^{+6}$, $24-33^{+6}$, $34-36^{+6}$, $37-41^{+6}$ and 42+ weeks Modes of birth: unassisted vaginal birth, assisted vaginal birth, elective cesarean birth, or emergency cesarean birth	Introduce a process within electronic systems to prevent the submission of the patient care record for the visit if the age details are not entered Introduce a verification step as part of an existing checklist on paper healthcare records to be completed before a patient is released from the hospital Introduce a checklist for all home health visitors that support home births to complete as part of their record-keeping process Use of a digital dashboard to report the overall outcomes of each patient within hospital environments, which indicates real-time data	Periodic auditing of the services Introduce an audit program for the services Introduce awareness days for healthcare staff that work to promote a *lessons-learned* approach Introduce digital dashboards to ward areas that would show how teams are performing

trained midwives to collate the data and the notes were supervised by local hospital-based obstetricians. The data showed Eclampsia and Preeclampsia were the two most common and challenging diseases within the population during pregnancy and labor. Although MRBs are a cost-effective way to gather longitudinal data and understand trends that can be used as quality indicators, it can be challenging to keep these notes long-term as these can be misplaced [14]. Although these are potential and known risks, using the MRB update has been a useful tool for healthcare staff working in rural regions.

Another aspect that needs considering is the multimorbidity status as this is becoming more common in pregnant women. Pregnant women with multimorbidity have a high risk of an adverse outcome for mother and child although maternal morbidity in this cohort is rare. The MuM-PreDiCT group indicated [15−17] that multimorbidity is distributed across the United Kingdom and the common combinations of health conditions such as depression and anxiety were highly prevalent in pregnant women. Mental health conditions attributed to approximately 70% of multimorbidity among pregnant women while psychiatric comorbidities were a leading cause of maternal death. These results were clinically and socially vital for integrating mental health and maternal services as well as access to perinatal mental health services to improve safety and overall care provided. This could also act as a quality control step to improve quality assurance management across maternity care offered in the United Kingdom. This would aid with quantifying the impact of multimorbidity on maternal and child outcomes for the current and future populations. The development of comprehensive quality indicators could further aid in understanding and categorizing high-risk pregnancies using evidence-based approaches that could optimize clinical practice.

The COVID-19 pandemic originated in Wuhan [18], China, in December 2019, caused by the novel virus SARS-CoV-2. It quickly spread globally, leading to millions of confirmed cases and significant morbidity and mortality [18,19]. Pregnant individuals were of particular concern due to physiological and immunological changes, potentially increasing the risk of severe respiratory morbidity, akin to SARS-CoV-1 and MERS-CoV [20]. Efforts to control the virus were initially hindered by factors such as asymptomatic carriers, limited testing, and a lack of knowledge about the novel virus. The United States faced challenges in implementing effective quarantines due to these issues. Other countries, including Taiwan, Singapore, and South Korea, implemented more robust testing, tracking, and quarantine measures, resulting in lower infection rates and better outcomes [20,21]. The review article aims to cover the general epidemiology of the COVID-19 pandemic, including its geographic spread, symptomatology, transmission, and current gaps in knowledge, with a specific focus on the obstetric population. Testing for antibodies (IgM and IgG) to SARS-CoV-2 is mentioned as a tool for identifying past exposures although the validation of many assays remains unclear [22]. The article aims to provide an overview of the pandemic's impact and challenges, particularly in the context of pregnancy. As of the publication date, there were approximately 8.6 million confirmed COVID-19 cases worldwide, with over 450,000 deaths. The United States had the highest case count, with 2,218,457 confirmed cases and 119,061 deaths as of June 19, 2020. The Chinese government first acknowledged cases of the disease on December 31, 2019, reporting dozens of pneumonia cases of unknown cause, initially presumed to be a zoonotic illness from a wet market in Wuhan. By January 21, cases had been reported in several countries, including Japan, South Korea, Thailand, and the United States. The city of Wuhan, with a population of over 11 million, was locked down on January 23, with travel restrictions implemented both within the city and for major transportation modes leaving the city. One week later, after thousands of cases had been reported in China, the World Health Organization (WHO) declared a global health emergency. This timeline highlights the rapid spread of the virus, leading to significant global impacts and public health responses, including lockdowns and travel restrictions. The WHO's declaration of a global health emergency underscored the severity and urgency of the situation. The weeks following the lockdown in Wuhan saw the emergence of COVID-19 cases worldwide [23–25]. Countries responded differently to the outbreak, applying lessons from China to their unique populations and health infrastructures. Italy experienced a major outbreak, becoming the first country outside China to record a high death rate. Italy's first cases were reported on January 31st, and a state of emergency was declared on the same day [26,27]. Clusters of cases emerged, particularly in Northern Italy, overwhelming the healthcare system with demands for critical care. In contrast, Japan experienced relatively low mortality, with 17,658 cases and 951 deaths as of June 19, 2020. Japan employed a cluster-based testing approach, traced infections to single sources, and emphasized the "three C method" to avoid closed spaces, crowded spaces, and close contact. The cultural practice of wearing masks in public and different social customs for greetings may have contributed to lower rates of community transmission.

As of early May 2020, efforts to contain the spread of COVID-19 highlighted several high-risk populations for uncontrolled transmission. Cruise ships became notable hotspots, with 40 ships confirming COVID-19 cases on board. The Diamond Princess, quarantined off the coast of Yokohama, Japan, saw over 500 passengers testing positive, resulting in a rate of 19.2% out of 3711 people [23,26,27]. Cruise ships, with confined and closely quartered populations, posed challenges for controlling infectious diseases, especially given the high average age of passengers and potential issues with air circulation Nursing homes also faced significant challenges, with a long-term care center in King County, Washington, being the site of the first COVID-19 outbreak in the United States [28–30]. The outbreak resulted in 34 deaths among residents, highlighting the vulnerability of elderly populations in such settings. Nursing homes across the country implemented measures ranging from strict visitation restrictions to complete lockdowns, doorstep meal deliveries, and the cancellation of group activities. Pregnant women were initially considered a high-risk population for severe morbidity and mortality due to COVID-19. Previous experiences with related viruses (SARS-CoV-1 and MERS-CoV) had shown high rates of ICU admission. However, a moderate-sized series of COVID-19 cases among pregnant women did not suggest high rates of ICU admission, although severe complications and deaths were reported. Similar to the general population, a significant proportion of pregnant women infected with SARS-CoV-2 are asymptomatic. Delanerolle et al. in a systematic review, found that substantiate the ubiquity of depressive, anxious, posttraumatic stress disorder (PTSD), stress-related, and sleep-related symptoms during both the gestational phase and the postpartum period amid the COVID-19 pandemic. Noteworthy is the prevalence, with approximately 24.9% of women disclosing manifestations of depression, 32.8% experiencing anxiety, 29.44% reporting stress-related symptoms, 27.93% indicating PTSD symptoms, and 24.38% exhibiting sleep disorders [31]. In one study conducted at two New York City hospitals, 88% of women who screened positive upon admission for delivery were without symptoms. In a systematic review of 538 pregnancies complicated by COVID-19, common symptoms included fever (48%), cough (46%), myalgias (17%), dyspnea (16%), fatigue (15%), and headache (9%)

[31]. Severe complications have been reported among pregnant patients, including cardiomyopathy, the need for extracorporeal membrane oxygenation, and death. In the systematic review, 1.4% of women were admitted to an intensive care unit [32]. Estimates of critical illness in obstetric patients with COVID-19 are imprecise due to the rare nature of such events. In a series of 158 pregnant patients with COVID-19 in New York City, 11 women experienced symptomatic hypoxia requiring oxygen, with 9 requiring ICU or step-down level care. There were no cases of stroke, thromboembolism, or cardiomyopathy in that series. Symptomatic presentation may be indicative of prognosis; for example, in the New York series, women who were initially asymptomatic had a lower likelihood of developing moderate or severe symptoms compared to those with mild symptoms on presentation. Women with underlying medical conditions, such as asthma, were more likely to develop moderate or severe symptoms.

6.3 Governance implications on issues with maternity care

Assurance of quality demands appropriate staff training and competencies. In addition to competencies gained at their formal training, healthcare professionals should acquire the requisite competence to provide care of the highest standard. Statutory and mandatory training should be completed following an organizational agreement and decision on what constitutes an appropriate training needs analysis (TNA). Embedded in the training should be learning from incidents, claims, and complaints, so that staff are able to improve their practice and professionally challenge colleagues. Some units have what seems like plausible education and training programs with desirable targets. However, when putting these to a rigorous test, there are major weaknesses in that, there is no safeguard or fail safe to ensure staff who fail to attend training have done so in a timely manner. This means that staff are not always up to date with their skills, knowledge, and personal development and are likely to give suboptimal care, creating risks for patients.

Good leadership is a pivotal aspect of good governance, specifically leading on a drive for quality improvements and safety. Leadership visibility should form one of the underpinning factors, providing staff of all grades with confidence that the top listens, is concerned about their well-being, and promotes open dialogue. Weak leadership from the Board level down to shop floor staff creates a culture that does not uphold transparency and openness. It is important that leaders are concerned for patients, support the risk management structures, create opportunities for learning, development, and research, and foster good relationships and ease of using risk management systems.

Most maternity units now use the Datix system for reporting incidents. Staff must be conversant with the process for reporting incidents, including what triggers a report. It is helpful to provide guidance by way of an incident trigger list and supporting policy. Reporting incidents should not be a platform for blaming individuals when things go wrong but should drive learning to improve care. Equally, investigations into moderate-to-serious incidents must be timely, incorporating women and families, focused on systems failure rather than individuals, and sharing learning through various accessible platforms.

Mobile Health (mHealth) constitutes a vital component of electronic health (eHealth) systems [33,34], specifically referring to health services delivered through smartphones [35]. In the dynamic landscape of health services, the optimal functioning of mHealth is crucial as it facilitates the accessibility of health services through communication technology [33]. The WHO defines mHealth as the utilization of mobile devices, particularly smartphones, as monitoring tools for health services [33,35]. The prevalence of smartphones has ushered in advanced communication and health systems, meeting the escalating demands in the field. Smartphones are recognized for their role in simplifying health information searches and enhancing health information systems. The integration of mHealth systems not only enhances the quality of health and patient life but also fosters communication between healthcare providers and patients [36−39]. However, the effective implementation of mHealth in the community is not without challenges [40,41]. The transformative impact of information and communication technologies, notably the internet, has reshaped how individuals seek health information and make health-related decisions. Within the spectrum of information and communication technologies encompassing mHealth in eHealth, health practices are supported by communication tools such as smartphones, patient monitoring tools, and various wireless devices [42,43]. The evolution of mHealth technology has been particularly notable in lower-middle-income countries [44]. mHealth resources offer secure and accessible access to care-related information, encompassing surveillance, health education, training, and diverse research initiatives [45]. The services provided through mHealth applications extend to communication between users and healthcare systems, including call centers, appointment scheduling, and timely maintenance reminders [33,46]. The health of pregnant women stands as a critical indicator of a nation's health status, influencing developmental and quality-of-life indices [47]. Recognizing the global need for comprehensive health services, the WHO initiated an international program to address the health needs of at least 400 million people lacking access to essential health services [48,49]. The health status of pregnant women is intricately linked to adequate prenatal care, safeguarding against complications and mortality during childbirth, as well as ensuring fetal growth and health [50,51]. To enhance health services, it is essential to identify and address factors related to maternal and child health, thereby contributing to the reduction of maternal mortality (MMR) and infant mortality (IMR) [35,52]. mHealth applications play a pivotal role in recording information about the health of pregnant women. These applications empower pregnant women by providing information on antenatal care, enabling health workers to manage examination data efficiently, and offering consultation services. These applications prove instrumental in aiding pregnant women in overcoming challenges experienced during pregnancy [53,54]. Moreover, geographical constraints and distance limitations that impede equal access to health services can be mitigated through long-distance health services, often referred to as telehealth, telemedicine, and telenursing [37,53]. Telemedicine has demonstrated economic advantages, reducing health costs and enhancing diagnostics in women with high-risk pregnancies [37]. Pregnant women increasingly utilize their smartphones to access information about birth preparation, share experiences, and provide comprehensive support to others on social media platforms [54]. Although numerous articles have explored the use of mHealth in pregnancy care, there remains a gap in the literature concerning a comparative analysis of pregnancy care using mHealth and conventional approaches in developing countries.

The widespread adoption of electronic health records (EHRs) among obstetrician–gynecologists has been driven by the recognition of their potential benefits and government programs incentivizing their use. Health information technology (IT) brings various advantages, including efficient data storage and retrieval, rapid communication of patient information in a legible format, improved medication safety through enhanced legibility, and ease of information retrieval. The potential for enhancing patient safety through health IT is substantial, incorporating features such as medication alerts, clinical flags and reminders, improved tracking and reporting of consultations and diagnostic testing, clinical decision support, and comprehensive patient data availability. Health IT data can be leveraged to assess therapeutic interventions' efficacy, leading to improvements in medical practice. Alerts play a crucial role in optimizing adherence to guidelines and evidence-based care, while record uniformity reduces practice variations and facilitates systematic audits for quality assurance. Moreover, health IT promotes patient engagement by providing consumers access to their medical records, fostering greater knowledge about their conditions, and encouraging active participation in shared decision making. Beyond the patient encounter, health IT improves follow-up for missed appointments, consultations, and diagnostic testing, enhancing overall healthcare delivery. However, challenges and hazards are associated with health IT. Alert fatigue, arising from the sheer volume of alerts, poses a significant concern, necessitating the development of systems to manage alerts effectively. Computerized physician order entry has improved legibility but raises concerns about increased order placement times and disruptions to healthcare provider workflows. Patient engagement tools, while enhancing involvement, introduce concerns regarding data reliability and privacy invasion when using unprotected portable devices. Patient data mismatches and inaccuracies may occur with electronic charting, highlighting the importance of thorough review and editing of automated templates and copied notes to ensure accuracy. Achieving robust interoperability, allowing seamless data exchange across healthcare settings and providers, remains a challenge due to proprietary code use by vendors. Automated templates, intended to save time, may inadvertently compromise the accuracy of medical records, requiring careful review and editing. Barriers to addressing patient safety concerns in health IT systems include the absence of mandatory reporting for related medical errors, concerns about violating nondisclosure clauses, and vendors' intellectual property rights. Although health IT brings significant benefits to healthcare, ongoing efforts are essential to address challenges and ensure the safe and effective implementation of these technologies in medical practice.

Remote monitoring has the potential to transform prenatal care by enabling more frequent contact with less inconvenience for expectant mothers [55]. A study conducted by Marko et al. demonstrated a 43% reduction in clinic visits, increased satisfaction, enhanced engagement, and no change in perinatal outcomes with remote monitoring [56,57]. In this study, 100 low-risk, first-trimester patients were divided into two groups, with one receiving remote monitoring and reduced clinic visits (8 vs. 14) and the other receiving standard care. The remote monitoring group generated significantly more data points for weight and blood pressure measurements per patient [55,57]. Ochsner Health has developed a similar system called Connected Maternity Online Monitoring—Connected MOM, providing expectant mothers with a tote bag containing a wireless scale, a wireless blood pressure cuff, and an at-home urine protein kit [58]. Patient data points recorded at home are securely uploaded to a system where physicians can access the information, fostering communication between physicians and patients without the need for clinic visits or phone calls [59]. Various adaptations of this model support the notion that mobile monitoring leads to better care and higher patient satisfaction compared to standard care although more objective data on significant outcomes are needed [58]. In addition to home monitoring, telemedicine has been seamlessly integrated into the care of pregnant patients. Since 1997, studies, such as that by Nores et al., have shown that the interpretation of first-trimester obstetric ultrasonography using video review is equivalent to live video telemedicine [59]. At Ochsner Health, maternal—fetal medicine ultrasounds are often recorded by skilled technicians and later evaluated by physicians, contributing to increased efficiency without compromising quality. Furthermore, electronic fetal monitoring, aimed at reducing cerebral palsy, neonatal seizures, or intrapartum fetal death by monitoring a fetus's heart rate, can be conducted remotely. Ochsner Health's TeleStork system centralizes live, beat-to-beat monitoring of fetal heart tracings from laboring patients across the system. Trained registered nurses monitor the system, promptly notifying in-house physicians if an abnormal fetal heart tracing is detected. Despite the subjectivity and interpretative challenges of electronic fetal monitoring, it remains the most commonly used method for intrapartum surveillance during labor.

6.4 **Advice for improvement**

Meaningful investments should be made if audits are undertaken using a multiprofessional approach so that learning can occur together, and joint working would drive a more workable way of addressing areas for improvement. Types of audits to be undertaken must be influenced and driven by themes from claims, complaints and incidents, patient experiences and where relevant-national platforms. All audits are required to include measurable action plans with set timescales and a mechanism for monitoring progress toward agreed goals. Conducting clinical audits should be for the main purpose of learning and improving standards. Identifying gaps in compliance with standards should lead to plans for setting workable and manageable objectives [60]. This will not only give assurance and confidence to maternity or Trust Boards but to women and their families about the quality of care and strategies for continuous improvements.

Unlike audit, research is focused on producing and enhancing new knowledge. The involvement of staff is important and should be encouraged for improving the quality of care. Society is changing, women are having babies at a later age, diseases are increasing, and research must be on par with these societal developments.

A robust system of informatics/maternity information systems with appropriate and specialist oversight is important to improve the quality of information produced about care and services. Information systems must be fit for purpose and be able to withstand scrutiny. This should be embedded within the maternity care services and reflect a close-knit method of working with the audit and quality improvement teams. The development or purchase of a health record system requires a robust risk assessment by those with the appropriate expertise. The decision making must not be in isolation, but integrated into the centrality of risk management and clinical governance systems within the service. Review and evaluation of current systems are essential, and this should include users of the systems.

The meaningful use of dashboards (scorecards) is pivotal, not as an academic exercise, but for use as a transparent method and a form of self-assessment and judging standards, using set benchmarks or key performance indicators. Such a mechanism can be used as a sounding board on performance in key areas of delivery of care and services. In a number of inspections by the CQC, maternity services have been unable to convict inspectors of the validity of claims made about targets and benchmarking on certain outcomes. Often, weak and unreliable systems are in place, which are disjointed and unsustainable at a number of levels. It must be borne in mind that in the midst of cultivating a sense of readiness for external audits and accreditations, pregnant women must feel safe throughout their journey.

Pregnant women are at the core of maternity care. They rely on health professionals who are experts in care, to give them the confidence that all are working toward achieving safe outcomes for both mother and their baby. If a culture of fractions between teams exists, there are potential adverse implications for women because of the impact on communication. For example, in the event of an emergency, the lack of teamwork will be reflected in the management of the event and can have devastating consequences. Ways to improve teamwork include regular joint meetings, staff listening clinics, appropriate staff training on conflict and well-being, and structured simulations in the workplace with formal feedback, giving participants the opportunity to voice their perceptions on the management process.

It is important to have in place stringent processes to support the quality agenda. Although this may be prescriptive in nature in some instances, they should be sufficiently flexible to embrace the expertise of all appropriate stakeholders. The Health Foundation [61] asserts that it is the manner in which providers and givers of care function as a team that will determine the quality of care. In addition to strong leadership, this process demands taking time to identify and review the issues and causes and enlist the engagement of all grades of staff. Monitoring the efficacy of processes is paramount through a combination of appropriate tools such as pilot studies, periodic reviews, and even audits to avoid repeating past mistakes.

Robust measures taken toward achieving quality assurance, if approached systematically, would aim to improve fundamental aspects of practice and models of care. The legal requirements provided that Supervisors of Midwives serve a particular purpose, to protect pregnant women by ensuring midwives practiced safely [62]. Following the Nursing and Midwifery Council's review of the failings highlighted in the Morecambe Bay [4] and other inquiries, it decided that the arrangements were not addressing public protection and removed statutory supervision. This is one typical example of assuring quality from a staff perspective to ensure patients are receiving a high standard of care. The replacement system through Professional Midwifery Advocates (PMAs) employs several mechanisms including listening clinics for women and midwives separately. The learning is then disseminated to staff and used to inform changes to practice. It can be argued that in the absence of a legal footing, there is not yet a review to ascertain its effectiveness within maternity services.

Case reviews are a grounded practice in maternity services. Within maternity service, the delivery suite is one area of high acuity and often, owing to the rapid turn of events, there may be several emergency situations that require a multiprofessional approach (midwives, obstetricians, theater staff, anesthetists, and neonatologist/pediatrician). Case reviews are a platform for learning why and how things go wrong and are the drivers for change in practice and better models of care. In some cases, case review sessions are rarely attended by staff members such as midwives. Doctors tend to get protected time for these sessions, and therefore, other staff members are not able to reap the benefits of attendance and engagement with the process. Quality assurance provides the confidence of a competent workforce and one where the culture is steeped in constant learning and improvement.

Change management demands effective planning and adequate and appropriate resources. This will require, as a first step, a comprehensive risk assessment to identify risks and agree on a plan for mitigation and evaluation of implemented actions.

The reported incidence of failed tracheal intubation during cesarean sections has persisted between 1:238 and 1:808, showing limited improvement despite advancements in airway equipment, training programs, and the publication of difficult airway algorithms. Most instances of failed intubations in obstetric cases occur after regular working hours and often involve trainee anesthetists. This situation is associated with a mortality rate of 1 in 90. Over the last 30 years, there has been a decrease in the use of general anesthesia for obstetric cases, primarily due to the increased popularity of neuraxial anesthesia [63]. This shift is influenced by changing public expectations for a positive birthing experience, improved postoperative analgesia, and the desire to avoid airway complications associated with general anesthesia, including the risk of aspiration and subsequent litigation. Managing a difficult airway in obstetric cases is a critical skill, but the decline in general aesthetic rates, coupled with training restrictions, has reduced opportunities for trainees to practice this skill. The current curriculum for novice trainees includes didactic teaching, work-based exposure, and assessments. Simulation training has been recommended to provide a safe environment for exposure and practice, but it can be resource-intensive. Virtual reality (VR) has emerged as a promising tool in medical education, offering advantages such as enhanced realism, repeatability, adaptability, and the ability to provide varied scenarios. However, most existing VR tools rely on computer graphics, which may compromise environmental realism. In this context, there is a need to explore the potential of VR in training novice trainees to manage difficult airways in obstetric cases. VR has demonstrated effectiveness in surgical training, endoscopy, crisis scenario preparation, and pediatric airway management. Leveraging the advantages of VR, such as improved environmental realism, could address the limitations of existing simulation curricula and better prepare trainees for critical events in a safe and controlled setting.

Chan and colleagues [63a] developed a VR tool inspired by Kolb's experiential learning theory, which posits that knowledge is generated through the transformation of experiences. Kolb's learning cycle is iterative, commencing with an experience that triggers reflection, followed by abstract conceptualization, experimentation, and application. The learning process involves a continuous cycle where new information, depending on the scenarios presented, guides learners through the stages of redefining preexisting knowledge structures and mental models. This experiential learning approach, as implemented in the VR tool, provides a dynamic and immersive environment for learners to engage with scenarios, reflect on their experiences, and actively participate in the learning process. The utilization of high-fidelity VR simulation in anesthesia crisis scenarios has not been investigated in our local context. Additionally, there is a lack of exploration into the perceptions of novice learners regarding VR simulation. Therefore, our objectives were twofold: firstly, to assess the learning needs of our novice junior residents when confronted with the management of a difficult obstetric airway; and secondly, to understand how these junior residents perceived VR as a learning tool for enhancing decision-making skills in crisis scenarios related to obstetric difficult airways. To address these objectives, specific research questions were formulated to investigate the learner's perspective on: (1) their readiness in managing an obstetric difficult airway crisis; and (2) the effectiveness of a VR game in facilitating the acquisition of decision-making skills in the context of a obstetric difficult airway crisis [64]. This study was conducted at KK Women's and Children's Hospital in Singapore from August 10, 2018, to October 31, 2022 [64–66]. Ethical approval for the study was obtained from the SingHealth Centralised Institutional Review Board (Singhealth CIRB 2018/2610). The participants in this study were novice junior residents in their second year of training who were undergoing the obstetric anesthesia training module. All residents included in the study provided informed consent before participating [67]. The study took place after the completion of multiple-choice question (MCQ) and short answer question (SAQ) examinations, as well as the objective structured clinical examination (OSCE), all of which are part of the standard curriculum [64]. The recruitment for this study faced delays due to restrictions on the rotations of residents imposed during the COVID-19 pandemic. Clinical reasoning is a complex process involving both formal and informal strategies to analyze patient information and evaluate its validity. This multidimensional approach is recursive and plays a crucial role in making diagnostic decisions [68]. One widely accepted model of clinical reasoning is the dual-process theory, which encompasses two independent systems [69]. System 1 is automatic, intuitive, nonanalytical, and prone to errors, while System 2 is slower, analytical, and conscious. Both systems work simultaneously in most clinical scenarios, contributing to improved diagnostic outcomes [70,71]. Decision making is considered both a component and an outcome of clinical reasoning. Various teaching methods for clinical reasoning have been reviewed, with the dual-process theory providing valuable insights [72,73]. However, the field still requires more research and evidence to recommend effective approaches for teaching clinical reasoning. Teaching clinical decision making is particularly challenging for medical educators, especially in complex clinical situations such as the obstetric difficult airway crisis [74]. Although didactic settings can impart knowledge on managing obstetric difficult airways, and task trainers can help develop technical skills like tracheal intubation, simulation training emerges as a crucial tool for teaching communication, situational awareness, and the intricate clinical decision-making processes involved in these complex scenarios [75]. VR emerges as a valuable modality for teaching clinical decision making, offering advantages such as repetitive practice, adjustable difficulty levels, built-in performance feedback, and cognitive interactivity [76,77]. In contrast to current teaching methods, VR provides an immersive, realistic experience that replicates the stress levels encountered in actual crisis scenarios [77,78]. However, this study uncovered gaps in the existing curriculum for equipping novice junior residents with the skills needed to manage an obstetric difficult airway crisis [77]. With novice learners primarily focusing on theoretical knowledge in the early years and limited training opportunities for managing obstetric difficult airways, more frequent simulation training becomes essential, posing challenges in terms of time, staffing, and resource constraints [79]. Although technology alone does not guarantee educational improvement, its appropriate application can enhance learning effectively. The study implemented a VR simulation program specifically targeting clinical decision making in obstetric difficult airway scenarios [80,81]. Learners provided positive feedback on the portable VR program, citing its immersive, realistic, and interactive experience within a safe environment [82]. However, several areas for improvement were identified for future work [83–85]. Several limitations were acknowledged, including varied perceptions from novice learners, the potential influence of power dynamics on interview responses, and limitations in physical and equipment fidelity with VR, particularly regarding haptic feedback for technical procedures [86,87]. The study's methodology incorporated data triangulation, comparison with existing studies, and external feedback to enhance research quality and objectivity. The focus on decision making, rather than task performance, was considered when addressing limitations related to physical and equipment fidelity in the VR scenario design.

6.5 Digital technology for quality management

The use of digital technologies could help with maternity transformation programs that are adjunct to quality assuring the services provided. The use of EHRs, smartphones, dashboards, or other software can assist clinicians and service users alike. In the United Kingdom, the Maternity Transformation Program included a work stream aimed at harnessing digital technologies with a special focus on digital maternity interoperability, digital toolsets, and women's digital care records [88–92]. The digital maternity interoperability project in particular focuses on enabling the exchange of maternity records between women and healthcare professionals irrespective of their location or clinical system [93–96]. This approach enhances the ability of healthcare professionals in a primary, secondary, or tertiary setting to become aware of a woman's medical history and any ongoing care. The digital tools in particular are vital to improve the personalization of the care offered to women by way of providing evidence-based advice and specific information that will allow them to make informed choices.

Digital tools can also be used to manage complications such as pregnancy-induced hypertension, which complicates approximately 6%–10% of pregnancies. This could also lead to the likes of preeclampsia, cerebrovascular hemorrhage, intrauterine growth restriction, prematurity placental abruption, renal and liver failure, and fetal death. In the United Kingdom, the National Institute for Health and Care Excellence (NICE) guidelines recommend weekly monitoring for those with mild hypertension and twice weekly for those with moderate hypertension. Increases in the number of visits to a maternity service can be burdensome to the patients and stretch clinical services, equally. A possible solution could be the use of home-based monitoring systems with telehealth technology where both the patient and the maternity service healthcare professionals could monitor the blood pressure. Telehealth has shown much promise in a variety of clinical disciplines. Therefore, a number of telehealth systems have been developed and are being tested with the objective to demonstrate its applicability and viability to help reduce face-to-face consultations at a healthcare service for blood pressure monitoring but still objectively obtain the required information to make informed decisions. A study conducted by Fazal and colleagues [53] indicated that this approach using a system called FLORENCE was safe and effective and could be used as a QA tool to improve pregnancy-related outcomes and reduce potential complications. FLORENCE is now used in clinical practice, in some healthcare organization in the United Kingdom. The tool also showed its value during the COVID-19 pandemic as it enabled healthcare professionals to support pregnancies in a safe and convenient manner.

The sensation of pain during labor is recognized as the most intense form of pain, persisting throughout the three stages of labor: dilation of the uterus, delivery of the fetus, and delivery of the placenta [97]. Although it is a natural occurrence, excessive pain during labor can result in adverse physiological effects, including heightened neuroendocrine stress, maternal academia, and prolonged labor. Hence, it is imperative to reasonably mitigate pain intensity and duration while ensuring safety.

Although epidural analgesia, the predominant method of pain relief during labor, is proven to be effective, it is associated with prolonged labor and increased surgical interventions [98]. Opioids, like pethidine, alleviate labor pain but bring about side effects such as maternal drowsiness, nausea, vomiting, and respiratory depression [99,100]. Moreover, pharmacological interventions do not address the cognitive and emotional aspects influencing pain and anxiety. Consequently, the World Health Organization advocates for nonpharmaceutical approaches to pain relief. Various nonpharmacological methods, including music and aromatherapy, aim to reduce reliance on analgesic drugs but face challenges related to inconvenience and a steep learning curve [101,102]. Distraction, a common strategy in medical procedures, effectively reduces pain and anxiety [103]. VR, an integrated distraction technology utilizing computer technology to create immersive 3D environments, offers potential by diverting attention from external stimuli and promoting positive thinking [104]. By engaging users in a realistic 3D environment, VR stimulates multiple perceptions, influencing complex physiological pain modulation systems and reducing attention to pain [104,105]. Growing evidence supports VR as a safe and effective distraction intervention for various pain conditions in adults and children, including burns and acute pain [15−18]. However, labor pain, characterized by strong emotions and changing intensity, differs from other types of pain, necessitating a cautious interpretation of findings from general pain studies. Despite the promising potential of VR, limitations in equipment and variations in experimental design have resulted in small-scale clinical trials with controversial findings. Thus, a systematic review specifically focusing on the effectiveness of VR in maternal delivery becomes essential, as, to our knowledge, none have been conducted to date. Recent contributions from Chinese scholars in this field also warrant attention. The evidence aimed to assess the effectiveness and safety of VR as a method for alleviating maternal anxiety and pain, with the intention of providing insights for clinical practice and justifying investments in maternity hospital equipment. The impact of VR applications on maternal pain during childbirth was evaluated across four studies involving 405 patients [24,30,31,106]. Upon analysis using mean difference (MD), a substantial level of heterogeneity was observed among the studies (chi-square $P < .001$; I2 $= 88\%$). To address this heterogeneity, we categorized the studies into two groups for subgroup analysis: a continuity VR group, where VR was applied continuously from the first stage of labor until its conclusion [24,106], and an intermittent VR group, where interruptions occurred in the VR application [30,31]. A notably high level of heterogeneity was found between these two groups (chi-square $P < .001$; I2 $= 95.9\%$). However, within the intermittent VR group, there was no significant heterogeneity (chi-square $P = .76$; I2 $= 0\%$), and similarly, within the continuity VR group, no significant heterogeneity was observed (chi-square $P = .71$; I2 $= 0\%$). Consequently, we employed a fixed-effects model for the analysis to account for the observed heterogeneity showed a statistically significant ($P < .001$).

VR serves as a technological distraction therapy, capturing the user's attention and immersing them in a virtual environment [107]. This distraction is achieved by blending elements of fiction, reality, and imagination, providing a comprehensive virtual experience that engages visual, tactile, and kinesthetic perception [108]. Both clinical and experimental studies have demonstrated the efficacy of this user-friendly and noninvasive method as a safe and effective strategy during normal labor [109–112]. The outcomes of these studies consistently reveal positive effects, indicating that presenting nature, sea, and landscape images through VR during labor contributes to the reduction of pain and anxiety, regulation of blood pressure, shortening of labor stages, and an increase in childbirth satisfaction [109–113]. Drawing on the collective evidence from these studies, our aim is to conduct a systematic review and meta-analysis of randomized controlled trials, exploring the effects of VR methods on maternal health during normal delivery. Ensuring group homogeneity has proven challenging in studies examining the impact of VR on labor pain. To address this, the design of more rigorously controlled studies becomes imperative, aiming to maintain consistency in factors such as prior pain experience, coping skills, the most suitable VR experience, and the intended duration and frequency of VR use. Enhanced control over these variables may yield clearer and more conclusive results regarding the effectiveness of VR intervention on labor pain. This study also reveals a significant reduction in labor anxiety through VR intervention (SMD = −1.08, 95% CI [−1.75, 0.41], $P < .001$). Akin et al. [114] specifically noted significantly lower anxiety levels among women in the VR intervention group compared to the control group [114]. Anxiety in the context of labor can be characterized as a transient emotional state arising from the anticipation of potential harm, even when the likelihood of harm is low or uncertain [115,116]. Expectant individuals undergoing labor often grapple with fear and anxiety due to the anticipated pain, discomfort, and associated childbirth risks [117]. The fear and anxiety experienced by pregnant women during labor contribute to pelvic muscle tension, resulting in resistance to uterine contractions. This resistance can lead to prolonged labor, increased overall fatigue, heightened pain perception, and reduced pain-coping abilities [118]. Nonpharmacological methods are commonly employed alongside pharmacological approaches to alleviate anxiety and provide comfort during labor [117,119]. Notably, the study by Momenyan et al. [111] found that individuals using VR during labor reported lower anxiety levels, underscoring the efficacy of VR in reducing both pain and anxiety during labor [111]. Consistent with these findings, Wong and Gregory [120] reported that VR interventions were effective in reducing anxiety and pain during labor for the majority of women [120]. Further support is found in other studies demonstrating that VR interventions significantly decrease anxiety levels during labor [114,121,122].

Employing low-cost, nonpharmacologic interventions devoid of side effects, such as VR, during normal labor presents a promising avenue for reducing pain, anxiety, and the duration of labor, while simultaneously enhancing childbirth satisfaction. These positive outcomes not only have the potential to increase patient satisfaction but also contribute to an overall improvement in the quality of care provided. The strength of this meta-analysis lies in its inclusion of randomized controlled trials (RCTs), a robust methodological approach that adds credibility to the findings. However, it is essential to acknowledge the limitations of this study, particularly the analysis of a restricted number of studies meeting the inclusion criteria. The limited pool of eligible studies may impact the generalizability and comprehensive understanding of the effects of VR on maternal health during normal delivery. To address this limitation, future RCTs with larger sample sizes should be undertaken across multiple centers. This approach will not only serve to corroborate the present findings but also provide more robust evidence, contributing to a deeper understanding of the potential benefits and applications of VR in the context of normal labor.

Leung and colleagues [123] in their systematic review showed the potential of VR in alleviating pain during childbirth. Despite the notable heterogeneity among the included studies, a subgroup analysis was conducted, revealing that the interruption of VR had an impact on pain reduction. It is postulated that frequent interruptions may diminish the immersive and distracting effects of VR, potentially reducing its efficacy in pain relief. Additionally, the study suggests that prolonged exposure to VR might diminish the novelty of the technology, potentially decreasing maternal interest and, consequently, its pain-relieving effects. These results emphasize the importance of employing VR at an appropriate frequency for optimal effectiveness. In the context of the active phase of labor, a meta-analysis of three studies demonstrated that VR effectively reduced pain levels, consistent with findings from other reviews exploring the use of VR for pain relief [27,28]. Notably, one study specifically investigated VR in conjunction with epidural analgesia during labor, revealing a more pronounced pain relief effect in women using VR ($P < .001$) [25]. Given the growing population of women undergoing epidural procedures during labor, further studies are warranted to explore the combined effects of epidural anesthesia and VR, assessing whether a synergistic effect can be achieved. The VR interventions across the included studies employed varied contents and devices, with differences in intervention frequency. A study highlighted that the effectiveness of interventions was impacted by the content of VR; for instance, natural landscapes overlaid with positive thinking interventions, while video contents combining visual and auditory stimuli increased distraction levels. However, no conclusive evidence was presented regarding which type of content was more effective. Notably, the review did not identify studies employing multidimensional tools to measure pain intensity during labor. Moreover, information on pain levels in the second and third stages of labor was unavailable, possibly due to challenges in obtaining accurate information under extreme conditions. As a result, future studies should delve into the timing and duration of VR use during delivery, exploring the impact of different VR content on maternal delivery pain to optimize intervention results.

Although countries such as the United Kingdom could provide the required investment to improve the quality of care, many other parts of the world may find it challenging to use some of these options. Providing funding streams, web-based tools, and more portable devices could be useful alternatives to improve quality. In rural settings, in particular, adequate oversight and training to improve diagnostic accuracy or other quality assurance activities can be cumbersome. Advancing care

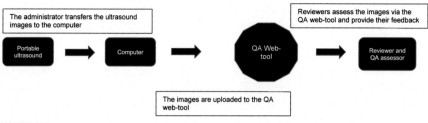

FIGURE 6.1

Step-by-step feedback mechanism for obtaining an evaluation of ultrasound scans using portable units in rural parts.

within these regions should include increasing internet capacity that could support digital technology use. Medical imaging is a key utensil that can advance centralized remote quality assurance by way of performing ultrasound examinations within rural sites. Clinical trials have been conducted to assess the use of portable ultrasounds and other web-based tools to improve pregnancy outcomes in countries such as the Democratic Republic of the Congo, Kenya, Zambia, Pakistan, and Guatemala [107]. The pilot phases including 3800 examinations followed by 5000 examinations in the clinical trial phase were evaluated by off-site QA reviewers who were radiologists based in the United States. The QA system used was a web-based tool (Fig. 6.1) from the Global Network Ultrasound website (GNUW) that allowed a rapid feedback loop to field sonographers working within remote regions. The GNUW acted as a central image reviewer and QS hub that also allowed country-specific sonographers to train other healthcare staff. This web-based QA prototype was developed by RTI International's Data Coordinating and Analysis Center as part of the Nulliparous Pregnancy Outcomes Study aimed to monitor mothers to be in the United States. The original study in the United States included 10,000 women to facilitate uterine artery Doppler assessments, fetal adrenal gland measurements, and cervical length measurements. This QA tool has the potential to be used globally and to act as a quality control step in the clinician decision-making process as well.

References

[1] Arulkumaran S. Clinical governance and standards in UK maternity care to improve quality and safety. Midwifery 2010;26(2010):485–7.

[2] DOH (Department of Health). Report of the expert maternity group: changing childbirth (Cumberlege report). London: HMSO; 1993.

[3] Ockendon D. Emerging findings and recommendations from the independent review of the maternity services at the Shrewsbury and Teleford Hospital NHS Trust. 2020. Available at: https://www.gov.uk/government/publications/ockenden-review-of-maternity-services-at-shrewsbury-and-telford-hospital-nhs-trust.

[4] Kirkup B. The report of the Morecambe Bay investigation. United Kingdom. The Stationery Office; 2015.

[5] Cumberlege J. BETTER BIRTHS -Improving outcomes of maternity services in England -A Five Year Forward View for maternity care. Available at: https://www.england.nhs.uk/publication/better-births-improving-outcomes-of-maternity-services-in-england-a-five-year-forward-view-for-maternity-care//; 2016.

[6] National Institute for Health and Care Excellence. Supporting adult carers (NICE guideline NG150). 2020. https://www.nice.org.uk/guidance/ng150/resources/supporting-adult-carers-pdf-66141833564869.

[7] England NHS, Improvement NHS. The NHS patient safety strategy. Safer culture, safer systems, safer patients. 2019.

[8] CQC (Care Quality Commission). Getting safer faster: key areas for improvement in maternity services. 2020. Available at: https://www.cqc.org.uk/publications/themed-work/getting-safer-faster-key-areas-improvement-maternity-services.

[9] Scamell M. The swan effect in midwifery talk and practice: a tension between the language of risk. Social Health Illn 2011;33(7):987−1001.

[10] NMPA Project Team. National Maternity and Perinatal Audit: clinical report 2022. https://maternityaudit.org.uk/FilesUploaded/Ref%20336%20NMPA%20Clinical%20Report_2022.pdf. Accessed 29 March 2023.

[11] Royal College of Obstetricians and Gynaecologists. Developing a green-top guideline. London: RCOG; 2020.

[12] Skinner R, Davies EG, Cant AI, Finn A, Foot A. Royal College of Paediatrics and Child Health (RCPCH) best practice statement on Immunisation in the immunocompromised child. Int J Infect Dis 2002;6:S58−9.

[13] Galadanci H, Künzel W, Zinser R, Shittu O, Adams S, Gruhl M. Experiences of 6 years quality assurance in obstetrics in Nigeria—a critical review of results and obstacles. J Perinat Med April 2016;44(3):301−8. https://doi.org/10.1515/jpm-2014-0302.

[14] Caruana EJ, Roman M, Hernández-Sánchez J, Solli P. Longitudinal studies. J Thorac Dis November 2015;7(11):E537−40. https://doi.org/10.3978/j.issn.2072-1439.2015.10.63.

[15] Admon LK, Winkelman TNA, Heisler M, Dalton VK. Obstetric out- comes and delivery-related health care utilization and costs among pregnant women with multiple chronic conditions. Prev Chronic Dis 2018;15:E21.

[16] D'Arcy R, Knight M, Mackillop L. A retrospective audit of the socio- demographic characteristics and pregnancy outcomes for all women with multiple medical problems giving birth at a tertiary hospital in the UK in 2016. BJOG An Int J Obstet Gynaecol 2019;126:128.

[17] Lee SI, Azcoaga-Lorenzo A, Agrawal U, et al. Epidemiology of pre-existing multimorbidity in pregnant women in the UK in 2018: a population-based cross-sectional study. BMC Pregnancy Childbirth 2022;22:120. https://doi.org/10.1186/s12884-022-04442-3.

[18] Wang CJ, Ng CY, Brook RH. Response to COVID-19 in Taiwan: big data analytics, new technology, and proactive testing. JAMA 2020;323(14):1341−2.

[19] Young BE, Ong SWX, Kalimuddin S, et al. Epidemiologic features and clinical course of patients infected with SARS-CoV-2 in Singapore. JAMA 2020;323:1488.

[20] Young BE, Ong SWX, Kalimuddin S, Low JG, Tan SY, Loh J, Singapore 2019 Novel Coronavirus Outbreak Research Team. Epidemiologic features and clinical course of patients infected with SARS-CoV-2 in Singapore. JAMA 2020;323(15):1488−94.

[21] Thompson D. What's behind South Korea's COVID-19 exceptionalism. Atlantic 2020;6.

[22] R. Castro, P.M. Luz, M.D. Wakimoto, V.G. Veloso, B. Grinsztejn, H Perazzo. COVID-19: a meta-analysis of diagnostic test accuracy of commercial assays registered in Brazil Braz J Infect Dis 24:180

[23] Johns Hopkins University & Medicine. Coronavirus Resource Center. Available at: coronavirus.jhu.edu/map.html. Accessed 19 June 2020.

[24] Wee SL, Wang V. China grapples with mystery pneumonia-like illness. New York Times; 2020.

[25] WHO. Origin of SARS-CoV-2. March 26, 2020. Available at: apps.who.int/iris/bitstream/handle/10665/332197/WHO-2019-nCoV-FAQ-Virus_origin-2020.1-eng.pdf. Google Scholar. Accessed 19 June 2020.

[26] Wuhan lockdown 'unprecedented', shows commitment to contain virus: WHO representative in China. Reuters, 23; 2020. Archived from the original on 24 January 2020. Retrieved 23 January 2020.

[27] NPR. WHO declares coronavirus outbreak A global health emergency. January 30, 2020. Available at: http://www.npr.org/sections/goatsandsoda/2020/01/30/798894428/who-declares-coronavirus-outbreak-a-global-health-emergency.GoogleScholar. Accessed 20 June 2020.

[28] Zheng L, Chen Q, Xu J, Wu F. Evaluation of intervention measures for respiratory disease transmission on cruise ships. Indoor Built Environ 2016;25(8):1267−78.

[29] McMichael TM, Currie DW, Clark S, Pogosjans S, Kay M, Schwartz NG, Duchin JS. Epidemiology of COVID-19 in a long-term care facility in King County, Washington. N Engl J Med 2020;382(21):2005−11.

[30] Sutton D, Bertozzi-Villa C, Lasky J, Fuchs K, Friedman A. Outcomes and epidemiology of COVID-19 infection in the obstetric population. Semin Perinatol November 2020;44(7):151283. WB Saunders.

[31] Delanerolle G, McCauley M, Hirsch M, Zeng Y, Cong X, Cavalini H, et al. The prevalence of mental ill-health in women during pregnancy and after childbirth during the Covid-19 pandemic: a systematic review and Meta-analysis. BMC Pregnancy Childbirth January 28, 2023;23(1):76. https://doi.org/10.1186/s12884-022-05243-4.

[32] The New York Times. Coronavirus Stalls Milan, Italy's economic engine. Available at: www.nytimes.com/2020/02/24/world/europe/24coronavirus-milan-italy.html. Accessed 19 June 2020.

[33] Kayyali R, Peletidi A, Ismail M, Hashim Z, Bandeira P, Bonnah J. Awareness and use of mHealth apps: a study from England. Pharmacy 2017;5:33. https://doi.org/10.3390/pharmacy5020033.

[34] Fahim M, Cebe HI, Rasheed J, Kiani F. mHealth: Blood donation application using android smartphone. In: Proceedings of the 2016 6th international conference on digital information and communication technology and its applications (DICTAP); Konya, Turkey. 21−23 July 2016; 2016. p. 35−8.

[35] Overdijkink SB, Velu AV, Rosman AN, van Beukering MDM, Kok M, Steegers-Theunissen RPM. The usability and effectiveness of mobile health technology−based lifestyle and medical intervention apps supporting health care during pregnancy: systematic review. JMIR mHealth uHealth 2018;6:e8834. https://doi.org/10.2196/mhealth.8834.

[36] Ghahramani F, Wang J. Impact of smartphones on quality of life: a health information behavior perspective. Inf Syst Front 2020;22:1275−90. https://doi.org/10.1007/s10796-019-09931-z.

[37] Zapata BC, Fernández-Alemán JL, Idri A, Toval A. Empirical studies on usability of mHealth apps: a systematic literature review. J Med Syst 2015;39:1—19. https://doi.org/10.1007/s10916-014-0182-2.

[38] Lee JH. Future of the smartphone for patients and healthcare providers. Healthc Inform Res 2016;22:1—2. https://doi.org/10.4258/hir.2016.22.1.1.

[39] Murthy N, Chandrasekharan S, Prakash MP, Kaonga NN, Peter J, Ganju A, et al. The impact of an mHealth voice message service (mMitra) on infant care knowledge, and practices among low-income women in India: findings from a pseudo-randomized controlled trial. Matern Child Health J 2019;23:1658—69. https://doi.org/10.1007/s10995-019-02805-.

[40] Shuwandy ML, Zaidan BB, Zaidan AA, Albahri AS. Sensor-based mHealth authentication for real-time remote healthcare monitoring system: a multilayer systematic review. J Med Syst 2019;43:33. https://doi.org/10.1007/s10916-018-1149-5.

[41] Gurupur VP, Wan TTH. Challenges in implementing mHealth interventions: a technical perspective. mHealth 2017;3:32. https://doi.org/10.21037/mhealth.2017.07.05.

[42] Arnaert A, Ponzoni N, Debe Z, Meda MM, Nana NG, Arnaert S. Experiences of women receiving mHealth-supported antenatal care in the village from community health workers in rural Burkina Faso, Africa. Digit Health 2019;5: 2055207619892756. https://doi.org/10.1177/2055207619892756.

[43] da Silva RM, Brasil CCP, Bezerra IC, de Sousa Nunes Queiroz FF. . Mobile health technology for gestational care: evaluation of the GestAção's app. Rev Bras Enferm 2019;72(Suppl. 3):266—73. https://doi.org/10.1590/0034-7167-2018-0641.

[44] Agarwal S, Perry HB, Long LA, Labrique AB. Evidence on feasibility and effective use of mHealth strategies by frontline health workers in developing countries: systematic review. Trop Med Int Health 2015;20:1003—14. https://doi.org/10.1111/tmi.12525.

[45] Sumarmi S. Model Sosio Ekologi Perilaku Kesehatan dan Pendekatan Continuum of care Untuk Menurunkan Angka Kematian. Ibu. Indones J Public Health 2017;12: 129. https://doi.org/10.20473/ijph.v12i1.2017.129-141.

[46] Ghebreyesus TA. All roads lead to universal health coverage. Lancet Glob Health 2017;5:e839—40. https://doi.org/10.1016/S2214-109X(17)30295-4.

[47] Kruk ME, Leslie HH, Verguet S, Mbaruku GM, Adanu RMK, Langer A. Quality of basic maternal care functions in health facilities of five African countries: an analysis of national health system surveys. Lancet Glob Health 2016;4:e845—55. https://doi.org/10.1016/S2214-109X(16)30180-2.

[48] Sklavos N. In: Zeadally S, Badra M, editors. Privacy in a digital, networked world: technologies, implications and solutions. Basel, Switzerland: Springer International Publishing; 2017. p. 418.

[49] Purbaningsih E, Hariyanti TS. Pemanfaatan Sistem telehealth Berbasis web Pada Ibu Hamil: Kajian Literatur. J Ilm Ilmu Keperawatan Indones 2020;10:163—71. https://doi.org/10.33221/jiiki.v10i04.683.

[50] Coleman J, Eriksen J, Black V, Thorson A, Hatcher A. The mobile alliance for maternal action text message—based mHealth intervention for maternal care in South Africa: qualitative user study. JMIR Hum Factors 2020;7:e14078. https://doi.org/10.2196/14078.

[51] Early J, Gonzalez C, Gordon-Dseagu V, Robles-Calderon L. Use of mobile health (mHealth) technologies and interventions among community health workers globally: a scoping review. Health Promot Pract 2019;20:805—17. https://doi.org/10.1177/1524839919855391.

[52] Zhu XH, Tao J, Jiang LY, Zhang ZF. Role of usual healthcare combined with telemedicine in the management of high-risk pregnancy in Hangzhou, China. J Healthc Eng 2019;2019:3815857. https://doi.org/10.1155/2019/3815857.

[53] Fazal N, Webb A, Bangoura J, et al. Telehealth: improving maternity services by modern technology BMJ Open. Quality 2020;9:e000895. https://doi.org/10.1136/bmjoq-2019-000895.

[54] Edwards KJ, Bradwell HL, Jones RB, Andrade J, Shawe JA. How do women with a history of gestational diabetes mellitus use mHealth during and after pregnancy? Qualitative exploration of women's views and experiences. Midwifery 2021;98:102995. https://doi.org/10.1016/j.midw.2021.102995.

[55] Marko KI, Ganju N, Brown J, Benham J, Gaba ND. Remote prenatal care monitoring with digital health tools can reduce visit frequency while improving satisfaction [3]. Obstet Gynecol 2016;127:1S. https://doi.org/10.1097/01.AOG.0000483620.40988.df.

[56] Krapf JM, Gaba ND, Ganju N, Marko KI, Martinez AG. Remote capture and monitoring of clinical data during pregnancy [54]. Obstet Gynecol 2015;125:26S. https://doi.org/10.1097/01.aog.0000462736.04207.70.

[57] Denicola N, Sheth S, Leggett K, Woodland MB, Ganju N, Marko K. Evaluating patient satisfaction and experience for technology-enabled prenatal care for low risk women [1L]. Obstet Gynecol 2018;131:192S. https://doi.org/10.1097/01.aog.0000533541.36412.24.

[58] Peahl AF, Novara A, Heisler M, Dalton VK, Moniz MH, Smith RD. Patient preferences for prenatal and postpartum care delivery: a survey of postpartum women. Obstet Gynecol 2020;135(5):1038−46. https://doi.org/10.1097/AOG.0000000000003731.

[59] Nores J, Malone F, Athanassiou A, Craigo S, Simpson L, Dalton M. Validation of first-trimester telemedicine as an obstetric imaging technology: a feasibility study. Obstet Gynecol 1997;90(3):353−6. https://doi.org/10.1016/s0029-7844(97)00265-2.

[60] Kings Fund. General service and improvement tools. 2012. Available at: kingsfund.org.uk.

[61] The Health Foundation. Quality improvement made simple. What everyone should know about health care quality improvement. 2021. https://doi.org/10.37829/HF-2021-105. Available at:.

[62] NMC (Nursing and Midwifery Council). Changes to midwifery regulation. 2017. Available at: https://www.nmc.org.uk/about-us/policy/projects-were-involved-in/changes-to-midwifery-regulation.

[63] American College of Obstetricians and Gynecologists. ACOG practice bulletin no. 106: intrapartum fetal heart rate monitoring: nomenclature, interpretation, and general management principles. Obstet Gynecol 2009;114(1):192−202. https://doi.org/10.1097/aog.0b013e3181aef106.

[63a] Zhao X, Ren Y, Cheah KSL. Leading virtual reality (VR) and augmented reality (AR) in education: bibliometric and content analysis from the web of science (2018−2022). 2023. https://doi.org/10.1177/21582440231190821. Available from: https://www.researchgate.net/publication/373374242_Leading_Virtual_Reality_VR_and_Augmented_Reality_AR_in_Education_Bibliometric_and_Content_Analysis_From_the_Web_of_Science_2018-2022. Accessed Mar 01 2024.

[64] Kinsella SM, Winton AL, Mushambi MC, et al. Failed tracheal intubation during obstetric general anesthesia: a literature review. Int J Obstet Anesth 2015;24:356−74. https://doi.org/10.1016/j.ijoa.2015.06.008.

[65] Barnardo D, Jenkins JG. Failed tracheal intubation in obstetrics: a 6-year review in a UK region. Anaesthesia 2000;55:690−4. https://doi.org/10.1046/j.1365-2044.2000. 01536.x.

[66] Rahman, Jenkins JG. Failed tracheal intubation in obstetrics: no more frequent but still managed badly. Anaesthesia 2005;60:168−71. https://doi.org/10.1111/j.1365-2044.2004.04069.x.

[67] Hawthorne, Wilson R, Lyons G, Dresner M. Failed intubation revisited: 17-yr experience in a teaching maternity unit. Br J Anaesth 1996;76:680−4. https://doi.org/10.1093/bja/76.5.680.

[68] Sharon CR, Melissa EB, Thomas TK, et al. Multicenter Perioperative Outcomes Group Collaborators; frequency and risk factors for difficult intubation in women undergoing general anesthesia for cesarean delivery: a multicenter retrospective cohort analysis. Anesthesiology 2022;136:697−708. https://doi.org/10.1097/ALN.0000000000004173.

[69] Quinn AC, Milne D, Columb M, Gorton H, Knight M. Failed tracheal intubation in obstetric anaesthesia: 2 yr national case-control study in the UK. Br J Anaesth 2013; 110:74−80. https://doi.org/10.1093/bja/aes320.

[70] Lipman, Carvalho B, Brock-Utne J. The demise of general anesthesia in obstetrics revisited: prescription for a cure. Int J Obstet Anesth 2005;14:2−4. https://doi.org/10.1016/j.ijoa.2004.10.003.

[71] Rucklidge M, Hinton C. Difficult and failed intubation in obstetrics Continuing. Educ Anaesthesia Crit Care Pain 2012;12:86−91. https://doi.org/10.1093/bjaceaccp/mkr060.

[72] Palanisamy A, Mitani AA, Tsen LC. General anesthesia for cesarean delivery at a tertiary care hospital from 2000 to 2005: a retrospective analysis and 10-year update. Int J Obstet Anesth 2011;20:10−6. https://doi.org/10.1016/j.ijoa.2010.07.002.

[73] Crowhurst A, Plaat F. Why mothers die − report on confidential enquiries into maternal deaths in the United Kingdom 1994−96. Anaesthesia 1999;54:207−9. https://doi.org/10.1046/j.1365-2044.1999.00854.x.

[74] Royal College of Anaesthetists. Raising the standards: RCoA quality improvement compendium. https://www.rcoa.ac.uk/sites/default/files/documents/2020-08/21075% 20RCoA%20Audit%20Recipe%20Book_16%20Section%20B.7_p241-268_AW.pdf. Accessed 1 August 2023.

[75] Johnson RV, Lyons GR, Wilson RC, Robinson AP. Training in obstetric general anaesthesia: a vanishing art? Anaesthesia 2000;55:179−83. https://doi.org/10.1046/j.1365-2044.2000.055002179.x.

[76] Searle RD, Lyons G. Vanishing experience in training for obstetric general anaesthesia: an observational study. Int J Obstet Anesth 2008;17:233−7. https://doi.org/10.1016/j.ijoa.2008.01.007.

[77] Teixeira, Alves C, Martins C, Carvalhas J, Pereira M. General anesthesia for emergency cesarean delivery: simulation-based evaluation of residents Braz. J Anesthesiol 2021;71:254−8. https://doi.org/10.1016/j.bjane.2021.02.059.

[78] Balki M, Cooke ME, Dunington S, Salman A, Goldszmidt E. Unanticipated difficult airway in obstetric patients: development of a new algorithm for formative assessment in high-fidelity simulation. Anesthesiology 2012;117:883−97. https://doi.org/10.1097/ALN.0b013e31826903bd.

[79] Grande B, Kolbe M, Biro P. Difficult airway management and training: simulation, communication, and feedback. Curr Opin Anaesthesiol 2017;30:743−7. https://doi.org/10.1097/aco.0000000000000523.

[80] Cook DA, Hatala R, Brydges R, et al. Technology-enhanced simulation for health professions education: a systematic review and meta-analysis. J Am Med Assoc 2011;306:978−88. https://doi.org/10.1001/jama.2011.1234.

[81] Chan TPSJM, Gerard JM. Overview of serious gaming and virtual reality. In: Nesel D, Hui J, Kunkler K, Scerbo MW, Calhoun AW, editors. Healthcare simulation research. Switzerland: Springer International Publishing; 2019. p. 29−38.

[82] Chang TP, Weiner D. Screen-based simulation and virtual reality for pediatric emergency medicine. Clin Ped Emerg Med 2016;17:224−30. https://doi.org/10.1016/j.cpem.2016.05.002.

[83] Salzman MC, Dede C, Loftin RB, Chen J. A Model for understanding how virtual reality aids complex conceptual learning Presence. Teleop Virt 1999;8:293−316. https://doi.org/10.1162/105474699566242.

[84] Bielsa VF. Virtual reality simulation in plastic surgery training. Literature review. J Plast Reconstr Aesthet Surg 2021;74:2372−8. https://doi.org/10.1016/j.bjps.2021.03.066.

[85] Khan R, Plahouras J, Johnston BC, et al. Virtual reality simulation training in endoscopy: a Cochrane review and meta-analysis. Endoscopy 2019;51:653−64. https://doi.org/10.1055/a-0894-4400.

[86] Kassutto SM, Baston C, Clancy C. Virtual, augmented, and alternate reality in medical education: socially distanced but fully immersed. ATS Scholar 2021;2:651−64. https://doi.org/10.34197/ats-scholar.2021-0002RE.

[87] Putnam EM, Rochlen LR, Alderink E, et al. Virtual reality simulation for critical pediatric airway management training. J Clin Transl Res 2021;7:93−9. https://doi.org/10.18053/jctres.07.202101.008.

[88] Kolb DA. Experiential learning: experience as the source of learning and development. Englewood Cliffs, NJ: Prentice-Hall; 1984.

[89] Mushambi MC, Kinsella SM, Popat M, et al. Obstetric Anaesthetists' Association and Difficult Airway Society guidelines for the management of difficult and failed tracheal intubation in obstetrics. Anaesthesia 2015;70:1286−306. https://doi.org/10.1111/anae.13260.

[90] Krom AJ, Cohen Y, Miller JP, Ezri T, Halpern SH, Ginosar Y. Choice of anaesthesia for category-1 caesarean section in women with anticipated difficult tracheal intubation: the use of decision analysis. Anaesthesia 2017;72:156−71. https://doi.org/10.1111/anae.13729.

[91] Dicicco-Bloom B, Crabtree BF. The qualitative research interview. Med Educ 2006;40:314−21. https://doi.org/10.1111/j.1365-2929.2006.02418.x.

[92] Christensen N, Black L, Furze J, Huhn K, Vendrely A, Wainwright S. Clinical reasoning: survey of teaching methods, integration, and assessment in entry-level physical therapist academic education. Phys Ther 2017;97:175−86. https://doi.org/10.2522/ptj.20150320.

[93] Norman G. Research in clinical reasoning: past history and current trends. Med Educ 2005;39:418−27. https://doi.org/10.1111/j.1365-2929.2005.02127.x.

[94] Norman GR, Eva KW. Diagnostic error and clinical reasoning. Med Educ 2010;44:94−100. https://doi.org/10.1111/j.1365-2923.2009.03507.x.

[95] Higgs J, Jensen GM, Loftus S, Christensen N. Clinical reasoning in the health professions. 4th ed. Edinburgh: Elsevier; 2019.

[96] Schmidt HG, Mamede S. How to improve the teaching of clinical reasoning: a narrative review and a proposal. Med Educ 2015;49:961−73. https://doi.org/10.1111/medu.12775.

[97] Smith A, Laflamme E, Komanecky C. Pain management in labor. Am Fam Physician March 15, 2021;103(6):355−64.

[98] Anim-Somuah M, Smyth RM, Cyna AM, Cuthbert A. Epidural versus non-epidural or no analgesia for pain management in labour. Cochrane Database Syst Rev May 21, 2018;5:CD000331. https://doi.org/10.1002/14651858.CD000331.pub4.

[99] Smith LA, Burns E, Cuthbert A. Parenteral opioids for maternal pain management in labour. Cochrane Database Syst Rev June 05, 2018;6:CD007396. https://doi.org/10.1002/14651858.CD007396.pub3.

[100] Baldo BA. Toxicities of opioid analgesics: respiratory depression, histamine release, hemodynamic changes, hypersensitivity, serotonin toxicity. Arch Toxicol August 2021;95(8):2627−42. https://doi.org/10.1007/s00204-021-03068-2.

[101] Howlin C, Rooney B. The cognitive mechanisms in music listening interventions for pain: a scoping review. J Music Ther May 02, 2020;57(2):127−67. https://doi.org/10.1093/jmt/thaa003.5816307.

[102] Chow H, Hon J, Chua W, Chuan A. Effect of virtual reality therapy in reducing pain and anxiety for cancer-related medical procedures: a systematic narrative review. J Pain Symptom Manage February 2021;61(2):384−94. https://doi.org/10.1016/j.jpainsymman.2020.08.016.S0885-3924(20)30695-3.

[103] Lambert V, Boylan P, Boran L, Hicks P, Kirubakaran R, Devane D, et al. Virtual reality distraction for acute pain in children. Cochrane Database Syst Rev October 22, 2020; 10:CD010686. https://doi.org/10.1002/14651858.CD010686.pub2.

[104] Son H, Ross A, Mendoza-Tirado E, Lee LJ. Virtual reality in clinical practice and research: viewpoint on novel applications for nursing. JMIR Nurs March 16, 2022; 5(1):e34036. https://doi.org/10.2196/34036.

[105] Navarro-Haro MV, López-Del-Hoyo Y, Campos D, Linehan MM, Hoffman HG, García-Palacios A, et al. Meditation experts try virtual reality mindfulness: a pilot study evaluation of the feasibility and acceptability of virtual reality to facilitate mindfulness practice in people attending a mindfulness conference. PLoS One November 22, 2017; 12(11):e0187777.

[106] Andrikopoulou M, Madden N, Wen T, Aubey JJ, Aziz A, Baptiste CD, Friedman AM. Symptoms and critical illness among obstetric patients with coronavirus disease 2019 (COVID-19) infection. Obstet Gynecol 2020;136(2):291−9.

[107] Linowes J. Unity 2020 Virtual Reality Projects: Learn VR development by building immersive applications and games with Unity 2019.4 and later versions. Packt Publishing Ltd; 2020.

[108] Kim S, Chen J, Cheng T, Gindulyte A, He J, He S, Bolton EE. PubChem 2019 update: improved access to chemical data. Nucleic Acids Res 2019;47(D1):D1102−9.

[109] Aaij R, Abdelmotteleb ASW, Beteta CA, Abudinén F, Ackernley T, Adeva B, Celani S. Tests of lepton universality using B 0 → K S 0 ℓ+ ℓ− and B+ → K*+ ℓ+ ℓ− decays. Phys Rev Lett 2022;128(19):191802.

[110] Kosiborod MN, Esterline R, Furtado RH, Oscarsson J, Gasparyan SB, Koch GG, Berwanger O. Dapagliflozin in patients with cardiometabolic risk factors hospitalised with COVID-19 (DARE-19): a randomised, double-blind, placebo-controlled, phase 3 trial. Lancet Diabetes Endocrinol 2021;9(9):586−94.

[111] Momenyan N, Safaei AA. Immersive virtual reality analgesia in un-medicated laboring women (during stage 1 and 2): a randomized controlled trial. 2021.

[112] Frey CB. The technology trap: capital, labor, and power in the age of automation. Princeton University Press; 2019.

[113] Osman AI, Mehta N, Elgarahy AM, Hefny M, Al-Hinai A, Al-Muhtaseb AAH, et al. Hydrogen production, storage, utilisation and environmental impacts: a review. Environ Chem Lett 2022:1—36.

[114] Akin B, Yilmaz Kocak M, Küçükaydın Z, Güzel K. The effect of showing images of the foetus with the virtual reality glass during labour process on labour pain, birth perception and anxiety. J Clin Nurs 2021;30(15—16):2301—8.

[115] Daviu N, Bruchas MR, Moghaddam B, Sandi C, Beyeler A. Neurobiological links between stress and anxiety. Neurobiol Stress 2019;11:100191.

[116] Takagi Y, Sakai Y, Abe Y, Nishida S, Harrison BJ, Martínez-Zalacaín I, Tanaka SC. A common brain network among state, trait, and pathological anxiety from whole-brain functional connectivity. Neuroimage 2018;172:506—16.

[117] Karaduman S, Akköz Çevik S. The effect of sacral massage on labor pain and anxiety: a randomized controlled trial. Jpn J Nurs Sci 2020;17(1):e12272.

[118] Gönenç IM, Terzioglu F. Effects of massage and acupressure on relieving labor pain, reducing labor time, and increasing delivery satisfaction. J Nurs Res 2020;28(1):e68.

[119] Sharkawi MM, Safwat MT, Abdelaleem EA, Abdelwahab NS. Chromatographic analysis of bromhexine and oxytetracycline residues in milk as a drug analysis medium with greenness profile appraisal. Anal Methods 2022;14(41):4064—76.

[120] Zulman DM, Wong EP, Slightam C, Gregory A, Jacobs JC, Kimerling R, Heyworth L. Making connections: nationwide implementation of video telehealth tablets to address access barriers in veterans. JAMIA Open 2019;2(3):323—9.

[121] Almedhesh SA, Elgzar WT, Ibrahim HA, Osman HA. The effect of virtual reality on anxiety, stress, and hemodynamic parameters during cesarean section. Saudi Med J 2022;43(4):360—9.

[122] Ebrahimian A, Bilandi RR, Biland MRR, Sabzeh Z. Comparison of the effectiveness of virtual reality and chewing mint gum on labor pain and anxiety: a randomized controlled trial. BMC Pregnancy Childbirth 2022;22(1):49.

[123] Xu N, Chen S, Liu Y, Jing Y, Gu P. The effects of virtual reality in maternal delivery: systematic review and meta-analysis. JMIR Serious Games November 23, 2022;10(4):e36695. https://doi.org/10.2196/36695.

Further reading

[1] Wired. Why the coronavirus hit Italy so hard. Available at: http://www.wired.com/story/why-the-coronavirus-hit-italy-so-hard/. Accessed 18 June 2020.

[2] Chen L, Li Q, Zheng D, Jiang H, Wei Y, Zou L, Qiao J. Clinical characteristics of pregnant women with Covid-19 in Wuhan, China. N Engl J Med 2020;382(25):e100.

[3] W.J. Guan, Z.Y. Ni, Y. Hu, et al. Clinical characteristics of Coronavirus disease 2019 in China N Engl J Med 382:1708

[4] DOH (Department of Health). Health Committee second report: maternity services (Winterton report). London: HMSO; 1992.

[5] Godber G. The origin and inception of the confidential enquiry into maternal deaths. Br J Obstet Gynaecol 1994;1994(101):946—7.

[6] MBRRACE (Mothers and Babies Reducing Risk through Audits and Confidential Enquiries across the UK). 2018. Available at: https://www.npeu.ox.ac.uk/assets/downloads/mbrrace-uk/reports/MBRRACE-UK%20Maternal%20Report%202018%20-%20Web%20Version.pdf.

[7] House of Commons Health and Social Committee. NHS patient safety strategy. The safety of maternity services in England. 2021.

[8] Swanson JO, Plotner D, Franklin HL, Swanson DL, Lokomba Bolamba V, Lokangaka A, et al. Web-based quality assurance process drives improvements in obstetric ultrasound in 5 low- and middle-income countries. Glob Health Sci Pract December 28, 2016;4(4): 675−83. https://doi.org/10.9745/GHSP-D-16-00156.

[9] Kurup VKM, Matei VA, Ray JM. Role of in-situ simulation for training in healthcare: opportunities and challenges. Curr Opin Anaesthesiol 2017;30:755−60. https://doi.org/10.1097/ACO.0000000000000514.

Neuropsychiatry and mental health

7

Abstract

Neuropsychiatry as a field remains relatively nascent, having solidified only in the 20th century; however, the origins of both psychology and neurosciences can be traced back to Egypt, Babylon, and specifically the Greek civilizations. Ancient civilizations such as Egypt and Babylon have remnants of documented proof surrounding neuropsychiatric disorders but did not allude to causality or brain—body relationships in observing them. The exploration of the mind changed between the period of 460 and 370 BCE after Hippocrates alluded to the following ideas: (1) our affect and emotional or cognitive states are dictated by the brain, (2) mental illness such as epilepsy is often comorbid with negative mood, and (3) disease acts on humans over a course of time requiring consistent observation and monitoring.

Keywords: Epilepsy; Hemiplegia; Mental health; Metabolic encephalopathy; Neurology; Neuropsychiatry; Neurosurgery; Neurosyphilis; Psychoanalysis; Traumatic brain injury.

Key messages

- Neuropsychiatry explores disorders mostly originating from functional issues in the brain. It is a branch of Neurology combining neurological and psychological illness
- Psychiatric neurosurgery largely involved precision interventions to resolve any malfunctioning neural circuits. Image-guided technologies are often used as part of these procedures. Complex quality control steps may be required to ensure the procedures conducted on patients remain a priority
- Quality control steps required to design, develop, and deliver neuropsychiatry and mental health interventions are vast.

7.1 Background

Neuropsychiatry as a field remains relatively nascent, having solidified only in the 20th century; however, the origins of both psychology and neurosciences can be traced back to Egypt, Babylon, and specifically the Greek civilizations [1]. Ancient civilizations such as Egypt and Babylon have remnants of documented proof surrounding neuropsychiatric disorders but did not allude to causality or brain—body relationships in observing them [1,2]. The exploration of the mind changed between the period of 460 and 370 BCE after Hippocrates alluded to the following ideas:

Quality Assurance Management. https://doi.org/10.1016/B978-0-12-822732-9.00007-2

- Our affect and emotional or cognitive states are dictated by the brain.
- Mental illness such as epilepsy is often comorbid with negative mood.
- Disease acts on humans over a course of time requiring consistent observation and monitoring.

In a comparable vein of studying the mind's role in the human experience from a neurophilosophical perspective, Renee Descartes identified the pineal gland in the 17th century, hypothesizing it to be the center that links the dualism between the soul and body and documented his understanding of neural connections as it relates to the visual system [2,3]. Similar to Descartes, the beliefs of the Copernican Revolution identifying the scientific method as a unique way of knowledge procurement were resonant even in Rome [4]. The concept of empirically investigating the brain via tactual exploration was employed by Galen, a key physician during the Roman empire, who examined cranial nerves to bifurcate between nerve types such as sensory and motor and explored ventricles to arrive at a similar conclusion of the brain being imperative to our functions including sense perception, cognition, and memory [3,4].

In the 1600s, Thomas Willis coined the term "neurology" and created an association between disease or pathology in patients by examining organs postmortem to find what is now known as the Circle of Willis. Upon extracting the brain from the cranium, Thomas identified structures of the limbic system and noticed the striated bodies suggesting their role in motion, which was further reinforced by his findings from postmortem patients who suffered from motor diseases [2–5]. The Enlightenment era then paved the way for an increased interest in the brain with introductions to the classification of nervous disorders and the concept of "tabula rasa"— postulating that the mind at birth is a blank slate after which our experiences imprint logic systems and knowledge [4]. Given its strong emphasis on environmental impact, this concept is one side of the coin in the ongoing nature versus nurture debate. In the subsequent Romanticism period, there was a transition toward the modern thinking of an embodied evolution of the mind and numerous poets became occupied with studying the mind. One of them was Samuel Taylor Coleridge who identified the gut–brain connection, a common example of which includes the sensation of gut feelings and coined concepts such as the "unconscious" and "psychosomatic." The main figures during the Romantic period that were crucial for neural Romanticism included Erasmus, Darwin, Gall, and Charles Bell. Thus, it is no surprise that the common theme arising from their theories mirrored current-day Lamarckian principles that focus on brain–behavior relations via an evolutionary lens. Of these scientists, Franz Gall, widely known as the creator of phrenology, highlighted neural development through anatomical examination and founded principles that indicated the importance of the brain and its localizations in impacting psychological behavior [3,4]. This emphasis led to a mindset change in clinical evaluation by physicians as the focus on the need for and potential merit of examining patients behaviorally and physically became more apparent. In terms of clinical research, the Romantic period was characterized by experimentation via external electrical stimulation, a methodology that has since advanced and is employed in current-day neuroscience via methodologies such as deep brain stimulation, transcranial magnetic stimulation, transcranial alternating current stimulation, and most recently, temporal interference [2–4].

Although the intersection and interdisciplinary field of neuropsychiatry exists today, the coalescence of neuroscience, psychiatry, and neurology underwent significant evolution and was previously, predominantly separate globally [5]. In Paris, physicians were mainly witnessing monomania and degeneration in patients at clinics leading them to form early attempts at disease classification and begin actual data collection [4,5]. A prominent name in clinical neurology at the time was Jean-Martin Charcot, who contributed heavily to hysteria research and John Hughlings Jackson, who constructed principles of nervous action and insanity [5,6]. His understanding of CNS disorder symptomatology arose from his observations of a hierarchy across neural structures wherein, the brain stem parts were the lowest and frontal/posterior cortices were the highest in impacting pathology. Both Charcot and Jackson impacted Freud significantly via their hysteria research and theories on the dissolution of the brain's psychological processes based on hierarchies between organs [3–6]. These influences are reflected in Freudian psychodynamic theories and his book, Studies on Hysteria which recorded case studies of hysteria such as the famous Anna O case. Freud, who moved to Vienna and then the United States, created an opposing school of thought from neurology called Psychoanalysis, a psychologically focused psychiatry [5]. This diversion rapidly resulted in a dichotomy between neurology and psychiatry in the United States wherein numerous psychiatrists tended toward psychoanalytical patient management approaches while there was a parallel emergence of Behavioralist, Jungian and Humanistic ideologies [5]. The overall thematic timeline of neuropsychiatry ideologies can be summarized into movement from neurophilosophical to anatomical, physiological, and psychiatric-focused theories.

7.2 Introduction

7.2.1 Parallel developments in neuropsychiatric care: Neurology and neurosurgery

Intriguingly, practices in neurology and neurosurgery were also developed in parallel timelines and are reflective of the ideologies being explored at each time period, from trepanning in the late Stone Age to neurosurgical advancements in the 1900s. Trepanning was a practice observed in the Incas since the late Stone Age, resembling contemporary techniques. Initially performed predominantly on combatants, skeletal remains indicate high mortality rates in the early methods [7]. However, by the 1400s, the Incas had evolved into adept surgeons, achieving a remarkable 90% survival rate. Evidence suggests strategic modifications to avoid critical head areas and employ a less traumatic scraping method [8]. Medicinal herbs like coca and alcohol alleviated pain, while balsam and saponin served as antibiotics. The ancient Egyptian Edwin Smith papyrus delves into trauma surgery, offering insights and treatments for various injuries, including neurological issues. Descriptions encompass meninges, the brain's external surface, cerebrospinal fluid, and intracranial pulsations [7−9]. Throughout history, observations of neurological phenomena abound. Sumerians portrayed paraplegia resulting from physical trauma, while the Vedic period's Ayurvedic text discussed epilepsy symptoms and treatments. Hippocrates attributed epilepsy to natural causes, while the Greeks dissected the nervous system [9]. Aristotle distinguished between cerebrum and cerebellum, and Galen's experiments revealed the recurrent laryngeal nerves' significance. In ancient China, Hua Tuo, a pioneering physician, reportedly conducted neurosurgical procedures [10]. In Al-Andalus (936−1013 AD), Al-Zahrawi performed surgical treatments for various head injuries and conditions. Concurrently in Persia, Avicenna provided detailed insights into skull fractures and their surgical remedies. Post-Greek era, the Renaissance marked significant progress in neurology and neurosurgery [11]. The invention of the printing press facilitated the dissemination of knowledge through anatomical textbooks, exemplified by Johann Peyligk's 1499 work, depicting the dura mater, pia mater, and ventricles in woodcuts. The landscape of both neurology and general anatomy underwent a profound transformation with the publication of Andreas Vesalius's *"De humani corporis fabrica"* in 1543 [12]. This groundbreaking work featured intricate illustrations encompassing the ventricles, cranial nerves, pituitary gland, meninges, eye structures, vascular supply to the brain and spinal cord, and peripheral nerves. Notably, Vesalius departed from the prevailing belief of his time that assigned the role of brain function to the ventricles [11,12]. He argued against this notion by pointing out that many animals shared similar ventricular systems with humans but lacked true intelligence. Remarkably, Vesalius seldom separated the brain from the skull before dissection, with the majority of his diagrams depicting the brain within a severed head [11].

Renowned philosopher René Descartes (1596−1650) conjectured that every action of an animal stemmed from a necessary reaction to an external stimulus, connected through a distinct nervous pathway. Luigi Galvani (1737−98) demonstrated the correlation between electrical nerve stimulation and muscle contraction. The concurrent efforts of Charles Bell (1774−1842) and Francois Magendie (1783−1855) contributed to the conceptualization of the spinal cord's ventral horns as motor and dorsal horns as sensory. Microscopic cell identification marked a pivotal shift from rudimentary anatomical concepts [11]. In 1837, J.E. Purkinje (1787−1869) provided the inaugural description of neurons, a notable early account of cellular structures. Golgi and Cajal later stained the intricate branches of nerve cells, highlighting their capacity for synaptic connections. The brain's form was established, yet localized functions remained elusive [9−11]. The observation of a hemiplegic patient unable to speak spurred Paul Broca (1824−80) to propose anatomically localized functions in the cerebral cortex. Ivan Pavlov (1849−1936), noting modifications in his dogs' simple reflexes, recognized the influence of higher brain functions [8]. The synthesis and integration of these neurological concepts were achieved by the neurophysiologist Charles Scott Sherrington (1857—1952) [13].

The pioneers in the exclusive pursuit of neurology were Moritz Heinrich Romberg, William A. Hammond, Duchenne de Boulogne, Jean-Martin Charcot, and John Hughlings Jackson. The practical application of neurological ideas in medical practice depended on the development of appropriate tools and procedures for clinical investigation. This evolution unfolded gradually in the 19th century with the introduction of essential instruments such as the tendon hammer, ophthalmoscope, pin, tuning fork, syringe, and lumbar puncture [9—12]. Subsequent advancements included X-rays, electro-encephalography, angiography, and CAT scans. Clinical neurologists systematically correlated their observations during patients' lives with postmortem findings analyzed by neuropathologists [8—12]. One prominent figure in this realm was W.R. Gowers (1845—1915), renowned for his comprehensive two-volume text on the cerebrospinal tract. By the close of the 19th century, significant connections were established, linking stroke with hemiplegia, trauma with paraplegia, and the spirochete with the paralysis observed in individuals populating mental hospitals [13]. A breakthrough in neurosyphilis treatment occurred with the introduction of the first chemotherapeutic cure, salvarsan, specifically for syphilis. Fever induction became a method for addressing neurosyphilis. The advent of antibiotics further enhanced the effectiveness of treating neurosyphilis, marking a transformative phase in neurological therapeutics [8—12].

Neurosurgery, involving deliberate incisions into the head for pain relief, has a long history spanning thousands of years, with notable advancements emerging primarily in the last century. The historical timeline of electrodes in the brain began in 1878 when Richard Caton discovered the transmission of electrical signals through an animal's brain. In 1950, Dr. Jose Delgado pioneered the first implanted brain electrode, using it to control the movement of an animal. A significant milestone occurred in 1972 with the introduction of the cochlear implant, a neurological prosthetic enabling hearing for deaf individuals [11]. The year 1998 marked another milestone when researcher Philip Kennedy implanted the first Brain Computer Interface (BCI) into a human subject. The history of tumor removal in neurosurgery dates back to 1879 when Scottish surgeon William Macewen successfully removed a brain tumor solely based on neurological signs. In 1884, English surgeon Rickman Godlee performed the first primary brain tumor removal, employing Alexander Hughes Bennett's technique for localization. Victor Horsley made history in 1887 by being the first to remove a spinal tumor [14]. In 1907, Austrian surgeon Hermann Schloffer achieved the first successful removal of a pituitary tumor. Harvey Cushing, an American surgeon, contributed significantly by successfully removing a pituitary adenoma in 1909, marking a pivotal moment in treating endocrine hyperfunction through neurosurgery. Egas Moniz in Portugal pioneered the development of leucotomy (lobotomy) as a treatment for severe psychiatric disorders. Although popular belief attributes the inspiration for lobotomy to the case of Phineas Gage, evidence suggests otherwise, challenging the association between Gage's injury in 1848 and the development of lobotomy [14,15].

Neuropsychiatry as we know it today was initiated surrounding the 1980s with key texts such as Neuropsychiatry (1981), Clinical Neuropsychiatry (1985), and the establishment of associations such as The British Neuropsychiatric Association (1987), American Neuropsychiatric Association (1998), Japanese Neuropsychiatric Association (1996), and International Neuropsychiatric Association (1998) [15−17]. Neuropsychiatry has been defined by the International Neuropsychiatric Association as "the field of scientific medicine that concerns itself with the complex relationship between human behaviour and brain function, and endeavours to understand to understand abnormal behaviour and behavioural disorders on the basis of an interaction of neurobiological and psychological-social factors. It is rooted in clinical neuroscience and provides a bridge between the disciplines of Psychiatry, Neurology and Neuropsychology." Given the ever-increasing prevalence of neuropsychiatric disorders globally characterized by aging populations, suboptimal patient management for those with neuropsychiatric disorders, and lifestyle choices that act as risk factors to neural health, neuropsychiatry has become a greater priority and resultantly, became formally recognized by the United Council for Neurologic Subspecialties less than 10 years ago.

7.3 Neuropsychiatric disorders

Neuropsychiatric disorders are a domain of disorders that incorporates patient care for those suffering from cognitive, affective, and behavioral symptomatology due to a neurological or organic cerebral disease. In 2022, a study conducted at Harvard found that approximately 418 million disability-adjusted life years (DALYs) can be ascribed to mental disorders in the year 2019 and the associated economic cost of such disease burden was calculated to be approximately 5 trillion US dollars. Granted that these costs are approximately 8% of North America's gross domestic product (GDP) equivalent to 4% in Eastern sub-Saharan Africa, ensuring high-quality and standardized clinical evaluation as well as treatments for patient populations with mental health and neuropsychiatric disorders is essential [10,13]. The common themes seen across neuropsychiatric symptom presentation included comorbidity of psychiatric symptoms, presence of cognitive impairment as a primary concern, probable prodromal cerebral symptoms, and similar medical presentation to psychiatric disorders. The International Neuropsychiatric Association considers the following to be neuropsychiatric disorders [17,18]:

- Cognitive disorders such as dementias, predementia syndromes, and non-dementing cognitive disorders
- Seizure disorders
- Movement disorders
- Traumatic brain injury
- Secondary psychiatric disorders such as psychosis, depression, mania, and anxiety disorders, which are secondary to "organic brain disease"

- Substance-induced psychiatric disorders
- Attentional disorders
- Sleep disorders

On the other hand, the American Neuropsychiatric Association refers to delirium, dementias, and major primary psychiatric disorders such as developmental and motor function—focused manifestations as neuropsychiatric disorders. It has been postulated that provided neuropsychiatric disorders is a term applicable to brain diseases causing psychiatric symptoms, that, organic cerebral disorders such as those of a neurodegenerative nature including Alzheimer's disease, Huntington's disease, frontotemporal lobar degeneration, progressive supranuclear palsy, corticobasal degeneration may also be included [18]. The same may be applied to Creutzfeldt-Jakob disease, cerebrovascular disorders, subdural hematoma, encephalitis, traumatic brain injury, brain tumors, metabolic encephalopathy, intoxication, and normal pressure hydrocephalus [19]. The complexity of neuropsychiatric disorders being within the intersection of neuropsychiatric, neuropsychological, and neurological symptoms renders applying a confined definition majorly challenging thus, leading to differing classification systems, or identified clusters based on interpretation and geography [18,19]. The two major classification systems that currently exist for neuropsychiatric disorders stem from the Diagnostic and Statistical Manual of Mental Disorders fifth edition (DSM-5) in the United States and the International Classification of Diseases 11th revisions (ICD-11) in ex-US countries [20].

Both, the DSM-5, and the ICD-10 used an authoritative approach employing top-down clinical thresholds to determine the severity and number of symptoms in patient populations as determined by subject matter experts [21,22]. The benefits of such systems include the standardization of research and the resulting improved data acquisition, clinical thresholding allowing for targeted treatment to be investigated in clinical trials and enablement of improved clinical assessment practices including differential diagnosis. From a patient perspective, having the ability to name and communicate one's symptomatology by a specific label or syndrome that is equally understood across medical systems and interpersonally is key to gaining disease awareness and thus seeking appropriate medical management. It is key to note, however, that the lack of a unified, holistic classification system, limited treatment options, heterogeneity in defining syndromes, and underutilization of clinical scales or tools remain gaps within the current landscape.

In terms of classification systems, the most currently internationally recognized system is the ICD-11, which has made transitions to include dimensionality of disease to improve reliability and clinical utility compared to the previous revision [22—24]. To ensure normative human behavior is not pathologized, the system also takes the support of the ICD-11 Clinical Descriptions and Diagnostic Guidelines (CDDG) to elaborate on key clinical features of each disorder and create appropriate boundaries between what is considered pathology and simple deviance in normative behavior [24]. Some features that are now included across clusters

(Personality disorders, depression, and schizophrenia being key cases) with clinical use and translation in consideration are the incorporation of degrees of severity, use of qualifiers for specific symptoms, course qualifiers for noting the longitudinal nature of symptoms and lastly, episodic nature, and acuity of disease in terms of remission [25,26]. When reviewed in field studies, these changes were noted to have great interrater reliability and received positive evaluations from clinicians in terms of practical utility and diagnostic accuracy [26]. Still, there lies an inherent trade-off in the classification system between how detailed and complex the classification system is and its clinical viability or use case, which must meet the needs of the user: researcher, clinician, or specialist. As each user has specific requirements, a stepwise approach has been proposed, which incrementally increases in detail from clinician to specialty treatment or research-focused users [15,18]. For the latter, it is recommended that there be a classification that incorporates both, categorical diagnoses with dimensional assessments by including symptom profiles with details of psychopathology. Such incorporations have been made for some clusters such as personality disorders, mood disorders, schizophrenia, and primary psychotic disorders; however, there are numerous clusters that remain [23–26].

A recent review utilizing deep neural networks found that depression, Alzheimer's, and schizophrenia are the most frequently studied neuropsychiatric disorders, respectively [27]. The immensity of research being conducted on these disorders aligns with the DALYs and mortality witnessed globally because of them. In 2019, depressive disorders (46.9 million), anxiety disorders (28.7 million), Alzheimer's disease and dementia (25.3 million), and schizophrenia (15.1 million) were drivers of the burden of disease seen due to neuropsychiatric disorders [28,29]. Given that these disorders are on the rise and contribute to significant economic costs to both, patient populations and healthcare systems, it is imperative that appropriate assessments and classification be employed across all users [30,31].

By creating relevant symptom profiles of both, psychological symptoms presented by the primary diagnosis and the multimorbidity seen in correlation with the primary disorder must be considered and may be evaluated by considering genetics, cellular and molecular patterns, and brain circuit activity [31]. Based on alignment with the Research Domain Criteria (RDoC) Framework and the ideal use case for current classification systems to be viable from a clinical and research perspective, analyzing disorders with measurements other than solely self-report instruments and behavior may render earlier stage diagnosis and points of intervention as well as a more holistic clinical image of the patient's health [32].

In Section 1.3, I will summarize the current holistic classification framework (ICD-11) that exists and propose symptom profiling that incorporates genetics, cellular and molecular patterns, and brain circuit activity that support future profiling, diagnosis, and clinical guidance for neuropsychiatric disorders with the highest burdens: schizophrenia or other primary psychotic disorders, mood disorders, anxiety or fear-related disorders, and neurocognitive disorders (Alzheimer's disease and dementia).

7.3.1 Classification of neuropsychiatric disorders and proposed clinical considerations

7.3.1.1 Schizophrenia or other primary psychotic disorders

Primary psychotic disorders include schizophrenia, schizoaffective disorder, schizotypal disorder, acute and transient psychotic disorder, delusional disorder, symptomatic manifestations of such disorders, and substance-induced psychotic disorders [32,33]. These are mainly characterized by their compromised perception of reality that is hindered by overt or positive symptoms such as disruptive delusions, hallucinations, and cognitions and covert or reduced symptoms such as blunted emotional expression [34]. Schizophrenia, derived from the Greek words for split mind, is a long-term psychiatric disorder that presents itself early on with significant shifts in cognition, affect, and social capabilities. It is usually diagnosed between the ages of 16 and 20 after a person's first episode of psychosis as symptoms of psychotic disorders impact the patient's human experience and start resulting in disconnection from the reality perceived by others [34]. In terms of risk factors, schizophrenia is highly genetic with higher risk seen due to environmental influences such as maternally induced malnutrition, early usage of cannabis, and migration.

7.3.2 Categorical diagnosis and state of remission

The current primary classification is based on course specifics that support in identification of the course of the disease, which also includes whether the symptoms of concern by the patient meet the criteria for schizophrenia or whether it is in partial or full remission [35]. The three main categories of course specifiers are as follows:

i. First episode

This is employed when the patient is experiencing the first episode or clinical manifestation of schizophrenia that meets the diagnosis in terms of symptoms being reported and the duration of time of symptoms [35,36].

ii. Multiple episodes

This is employed when the patient has already experienced two episodes before that resembled the clinical manifestation of schizophrenia or schizoaffective disorder and meets the diagnosis in terms of symptoms being reported and the duration of time of symptoms. In between episodes, there must be periods of partial or full remission that last a minimum of 3 months, and the most recently reported episode must be schizophrenia [37].

iii. Continuous

This is employed when the patient has continuously experienced symptoms that meet the clinical diagnosis requirements of schizophrenia after the initial onset, with brief periods of subthreshold symptoms that are short compared to the longitudinal course of the disease itself. If this specifier is being employed after the first episode, the duration of schizophrenia should be a minimum of 1 year [37,38].

There are residual categories such as "Other specified episode of schizophrenia" and "Episode unspecified" to ensure inclusion when there are miscellaneous or uncommon features and ensure flexibility in case a patient's clinical manifestation needs accommodation [39].

Across all categories, patient states can present as follows:

i. Currently symptomatic

The state, "currently symptomatic" refers to all diagnostic requirements for the disorder being met—in this case, schizophrenia [37,38].

ii. In partial remission

The state, "in partial remission" refers to partial diagnostic requirements for the disorder being met with some clinically relevant symptomatology being present which may or may not render the patient functionally impaired [39].

iii. In full remission

The state, "in full remission" refers to diagnostic requirements for the disorder not being met within the past month with no clinically relevant symptomatology being present [35,37].

iv. Unspecified

Currently, the ICD-11 does not offer insight into the patient state this specifier may include.

7.3.3 Dimensional assessments: Clinical manifestation of primary diagnosed disorders

From a dimensional perspective [40], the ICD 11 incorporates symptom specifiers with the criteria as follows:

i. Positive symptoms

Positive symptoms in the case of psychotic disorders refer to distorted natural actions that generally resonate with the overt clinical presentation of the patient. Some examples of positive symptoms are delusions, hallucinations, disconnection from reality, disorganized speech (also known as word salad), and catatonia or altered movement [41,42].

ii. Negative symptoms

Negative symptoms refer to symptoms that lead to a loss or decrease in higher cortical behaviors and naturalistic functions such as emotional responses, cognition, and socialization capabilities in a person suffering from schizophrenia. Some examples of negative symptoms are lack of motivation for goal-directed behaviors, blunted affect, anhedonia, and social withdrawal [37].

iii. Depressive symptoms

Depressive mood symptoms refer to the depressed mood which can either be reported as a concern by the patient due to low mood or feelings of dejection or present itself physically by the patient's appearance. In employing this specifier, it is key to note that it is not used if these are the only symptoms being presented by the patient but can be employed regardless of whether the severity of depressive symptoms meets the diagnostic criteria of depressive disorder [40,41].

iv. Manic symptoms

Manic mood symptoms are the opposite of depressive mood symptoms and refer to moods characterized by increased energy, which may lead to hyper increases in goal-based activity, high levels of euphoria, and volatility in moods, depending on the severity of the mania [42,43]. The rating of these symptoms is independent of any requirement to meet the diagnostic criteria for bipolar disorder and emphasizes the severity of symptoms experienced by the patient [43].

i. Psychomotor symptoms

Psychomotor symptoms refer to extreme psychomotor activity and activation or in contrast, slowing which can clinically present as behaviors of fidgeting, moving, being restless, or the opposite, wherein the patient is visibly slower when moving or talking. Additionally, catatonic behaviors with a bodily resistance to being moved, lack of response to surrounding stimuli (either physically, vocally, or both), and a patient state that resembles closely to unconsciousness [44]. The rating of psychomotor symptoms focuses on the severity of the symptoms within the past week of the presenting patient.

ii. Cognitive impairments

Lastly, cognitive symptoms refer to disruptions seen in the following cognitive functions: processing abilities and velocity, ability to focus, orientation, judgment, idea construction and projection, learning (verbal or visual stimuli), and working memory [45,46]. The rating is also dependent on the severity within the past week of the presenting patient but cannot be attributed to a neurodevelopment disorder such as dementia or being a side-effect/adverse event to substance use including medication use and withdrawal [47].

7.3.4 Symptom profile: Clinical manifestation of secondary comorbid disorders that reinforce primary disorder

7.3.4.1 Genetic influences in schizophrenia

Given that schizophrenia is a chronic, long-term condition, it is imperative to consider the burden of comorbidity patterns that may burden those with schizophrenia and significantly contribute to their burden of disease. Last year, a US-based study assessing real-world, phenotypic data identified specific patterns within the schizophrenic population when compared to age, sex, and location-matched controls [48]:

i. First, findings showed that anxiety, posttraumatic stress disorder (PTSD), and substance abuse were common predecessors of a positive schizophrenia diagnosis within the adolescent and young adults' population [49].

ii. 10 significantly enhanced phenotypes were observed for preschizophrenia diagnosis in this population with 297.1, 296.1, and 301.2 associated with suicidal ideation, bipolar, and antisocial/borderline personality disorder being the most significant, respectively [50]. Patients with 291.71, 296.1, and 301.2 phecodes expression were 51.2, 361, and 18.4 times likelier to be diagnosed with schizophrenia than those who do not show this enriched expression [50].

iii. Middle-aged adults (30–59 years of age) were likelier to develop phenotypic expression correlated with respiration and renal failure, sepsis, convulsion, and pneumonia [49].

iv. On the other end of the age spectrum, patients who were 60 years old or older and diagnosed with schizophrenia were at high risk for delirium, alcohol abuse, and bone-related concerns such as pelvic fracture or osteomyelitis when compared to their counterparts.

v. Differences were found in the way comorbidities were presented between sexes. The prevalence of Type 2 diabetes, sleep apnea, and eating disorders was more common in women with preschizophrenia diagnosis. On the other hand, men were seen to suffer more commonly from acute renal failure, rhabdomyolysis, and delayed development.

vi. Postdiagnosis, women with schizophrenia were found to be likelier to develop encephalopathy and epilepsy and suffer from the side effects of drugs and allergic reactions compared with their male counterparts.

vii. On the other hand, men with diagnosed schizophrenia were found to be likelier to develop impulse control disorder, esophageal bleeding, and acute osteomyelitis [49].

viii. Lastly, the type of burden was also found to differ based on the subtype of schizophrenia the patient suffered from with schizoaffective being most associated with anxiety and obesity compared to patients with different subtypes.

7.3.5 Cellular/molecular in schizophrenia

A study conducted at the University of Oslo found numerous linkages across one's lifetime that may offer biological insights into the underlying mechanisms that may impact schizophrenia and its expression [51]. For instance, challenges beginning even before birth may impact the child and affect the likelihood of developing schizophrenia. From a neurodevelopmental perspective, early-stage "injuries" such as the mother having hypothalamic–pituitary–adrenal (HPA) dysregulation, higher glucocorticoids, and bodily inflammation are all indicators of chronic stress that can harm a baby [52,53]. Other actions that may cause injury to the fetus include prenatal infectious disease, undernutrition within the diet or the mother starving herself, limited growth of the fetus, and limited oxygen to the fetus or baby can all negatively impact neural development and raise the likelihood of developing schizophrenia as seen across multiple studies [54,55]. Research on animal models indicates that potentially dangerous downstream effects of undernutrition may include disrupted prenatal renin—angiotensin system, placenta, and epigenetics that impact how genes are expressed and can render long-term, associated disorders related to cardiovascular and metabolic functions [53,54]. Additionally, numerous genes involved in increased vulnerability to schizophrenia can be indicated by modified vasculature, and having to battle infectious disease during pregnancy not only renders negative repercussions for the mother but also may contribute to different neural development thereby impacting the likelihood of psychosis.

Clinical research conducted by Correll and colleagues has found that young patients with schizophrenia who do not have a history of using medication also showed a significantly higher risk of cardiovascular disease as well as an indication of elevated cholesterol and heightened insulin resistance as opposed to their counterparts without schizophrenia [55]. Research findings from schizophrenic patients who have not undergone medication-based treatment for their symptoms show that elevated insulin and resistance to insulin affect neurological functioning or development and thereby may play a part in contributing to schizophrenic pathogenesis. In similar findings, biomarkers of inflammation such as C-reactive protein (CRP), interleukin-6 (IL-6), interleukin 1-receptor antagonist (IL-1Ra), and tumor necrosis factor (TNF) have been shown to be elevated in patients of schizophrenia suffering with their first episode of psychosis [56—58]. In terms of neurotransmission, insufficiencies in dopamine and glutamatergic pathways may be an area of concern when connecting obesity and schizophrenia, both diseases with high comorbidity and significant depletion in quality of life for the patient [57,58].

Another factor that significantly impacts disease manifestation is the process of aging itself and how it contributes to not just the prevalence and incidence of disorders on a population level but also how it impacts patient experience and ability to cope with disease onset on an individual basis. Studies have suggested that schizophrenia is positively correlated with faster aging which may be attributable to shortened telomeres and has been shown using brain imaging methodologies from the first episode of schizophrenia to throughout one's life. In fact, links have been seen with higher amounts of endothelial markers and volume of basal ganglia in patients who suffer from psychotic disorders and have been reinforced by research that shows wider retinal venules in the case of schizophrenia as opposed to healthy counterparts that have been positively associated with neurological conditions such as stroke, dementia, and cerebrovascular diseases [59,60].

On a global level, neural morphology alterations, such as thinning of cortices, increase in the size of ventricles, and decrease in the volume of hippocampi, are often seen in patient cases with schizophrenia [61]. On a cellular level, one can see that these global changes are seen with structural shifts such as the presence of smaller pyramidal neuronal cell bodies, fewer dendritic spines, and decreased interneuron density and presence [59,60]. A study by Uranova and colleagues found that in the neural cortex, a postmortem of those with schizophrenia, abnormally thick capillaries, distorted basal lamina, and formation of vacuoles of the cytoplasm of endothelial cells, the basal lamina, and astrocytes end-feet are present thereby hinting the role of the blood—brain barrier (BBB) in schizophrenia [62,63]. Additionally, a study analyzing brain tissue postdeath indicated that in the small blood vessels of the brain in individuals with schizophrenia, the activity of certain genes significantly varied from that seen in people without the condition, and these variations were mainly seen across genes that were associated with inflammatory responses, thereby indicating the presence of interplay between inflammation and schizophrenia. However, a meta-analysis done in similar postmortem brain tissue showed the presence of various upregulatory and downstream effects of genes involved in varying functions, thus reinforcing the strong linkage between genes and schizophrenia as a whole [62—64].

7.3.6 Brain circuit activity in schizophrenia

With the advancement in neural imaging techniques and stimulation therapies, neuroscientists are ever-increasingly studying the brain from a neural circuitry perspective by dissecting the pathways, neural oscillations, and signaling that impact human cognition, in both healthy and disease states [62,64]. Research studies conducted in animal models have found that there are differences in the way that gamma, theta, and sharp wave ripples were present, and these differences are postulated to be associated with behavioral and cognitive symptomatology as seen in schizophrenia [65,66]. Variations including disorganized gamma activity with differing amplitudes and frequency, disrupted theta oscillatory amplitudes for higher-level communication within the brain, and irregular sharp wave ripple patterns that are necessitated for memory functions are notable across models of schizophrenia [67].

In terms of human studies, researchers at Beth Israel Deaconess Medical Center at Harvard Medical School have been investigating the neural circuitry underlying the negative symptomatology seen in those with schizophrenia. Of 44 patients who were diagnosed with schizophrenia, functional magnetic resonance imaging (fMRI) scans showed that patients with severe negative symptoms showed a worse connection between the prefrontal cortex region and the cerebellum, whereas such links were not found in the case of positive symptomatology [68,69]. In addition to these findings, the researchers questioned whether employing noninvasive brain stimulation could support treating the malfunctioning of neural networks that causes the symptoms by modulating the brain's network, which they found to be the case. Upon recruiting a second cohort of participants with schizophrenia and classifying their degree of severity in terms of symptomatology, the participants in the study section of the research were given brain stimulation for two sessions daily with breaks of 4 hours between each after which, brain scans were assessed [67,68]. These scans indicated that participants who had received this stimulation therapy as opposed to those who did not show improved activity within the neural circuit and an associated improvement in the degree of negative symptomatology; however, effect sizes were not equally distributed among participants—a key consideration in terms of personalization of stimulation therapy and healthcare interventions [69].

Such findings align with previous literature that suggests the role of association cortices embedding information from sensory experiences by primary cortices as well as employing information from brain regions associated with memory functions to create a model of experiences [70,71]. There are often four aspects of the brain that are discussed in terms of implications of schizophrenia including the cortex, the hippocampus, the thalamus, and the basal ganglia, respectively [72].

Changes in GABA (Gamma-aminobutyric acid) and dopamine-based pathways in the cortex, atypical functioning of the dorsolateral prefrontal cortex (DLPFC), and associated changed functionality of D1 dopamine and serotonin 5-HT2A receptors are also seen within cases of schizophrenia [73]. These findings are furthered by the results of a study investigating the differences between resting-state patterns of connectivity of the right anterior and posterior DLPFC that indicated there are differences in frontal cortex patterns for the front and back portions of the right DLPFC that is associated with executive functioning, and the parietal, temporal, and cerebellar portions showed variance with lesser connectivity of those regions with the striatum and occipital cortex, respectively, In fact, the larger difference in the posterior and anterior functional cortex for the left inferior frontal gyrus or anterior insula was associated with higher degrees of psychopathology, thus denoting the differences that may exist in seemingly similarly placed neural regions [74]. A molecular understanding of this that can help understand these observations was found by Arnsten et al. who elaborated upon certain molecular characteristics such as employing NMDA (N-methyl-D-aspartate) as opposed to AMPA (a-amino-3-hydroxy-5-methyl-4-isoxazolepropionic acid) receptors, calcium signaling mechanisms, and network connectivity-related signaling that influences the neurotransmission and modulation of layer three in a primate DLPFC, which may impair the region's overall resistance to certain genetic predispositions and environmental adversities and thus render pathological presentations—in this case, schizophrenia [74]. The aspects that are crucial to note from such findings include the implications they may have for the improvement of early screening, diagnosis, and treatments, respectively. For instance, a clinical study conducted by a team at Zhejiang University investigating correlations between DLPFC metabolites and cognitive functionality in patients experiencing or diagnosed with first-episode schizophrenia found reduced *N*-acetyl aspartate and creatine ratios in the left DLPFC region, which was correlated with cognitive deficits in such patients, thus providing an opportunity for early biomarking of schizophrenia-related cognitive deficits [73,74].

In terms of the hippocampus, research has indicated that fewer nonpyramidal cells in the CA2 area are associated with changed synaptic organization and plasticity, which may render the observed symptomatology for schizophrenic patients. Additionally, malfunctioning of the thalamic relay and mediodorsal nucleus can influence the way sensory data is perceived and processed in associated areas such as

DLPFC [75,76]. Similar findings regarding a key role of the hippocampus in schizophrenia presentation were found in a study conducted by Sid Chopra and team at Monash University, wherein researchers found that the anterior hippocampus is implicated and may represent an epicenter of early-stage pathology from which malfunctioning can spread pathology progressively via axonal connections in a network-based manner [77]. In the case of schizophrenia, it is unsurprizing that there are connectivity differences, and findings by Uscătescu and researchers at the University of Salzburg have shown that people who suffer from schizophrenia have increased connectivity from their left and right hippocampi to the dorsal anterior cingulate cortex (DACC), right anterior insula (RAI), left frontal eye fields, and the bilateral inferior parietal sulcus (LIPS and RIPS) as well as the bilateral anterior insula (LAI), RAI, right frontal eye fields, and RIPS, respectively [78–80]. However, even more interestingly, in comparing connectivity differences across three resting-state networks between controls and patients with schizophrenia, the researchers found that positive symptomatology and negative symptomatology may differ in their neural connectivity implications. In those with schizophrenia, the presentation of negative symptomatology was found to forecast the strength of connectivity from LHC to the DACC, left inferior parietal sulcus (LIPAR), and the RHC, whereas the presentation of positive symptomatology was predictive of connectivity strengths between the LHC and the LIPAR and between the RHC and the LHC, thereby indicating the role that hippocampal circuitry may play as a biomarker for schizophrenia pathology [81].

In the future, schizophrenia research could significantly benefit from integrating clinical data with findings from genetic studies, environmental influences, and advanced biomarker implementation. For example, ongoing research on specific blood biomarkers is uncovering promising leads such as PBMC-derived biomarkers in supporting differential diagnoses as well as neuroimmune biomarkers, which incorporate the majority of the future biomarkers being studied for schizophrenia diagnosis. These biomarkers are linked to the central nervous and the peripheral nervous system comprising of cytokine biomarkers such as interleukin-6 and interleukin-8 as well as C-reaction protein, interferon-gamma, interleukin 1 beta, interleukin-1 receptor antagonist, interleukin-4, interleukin-10, interleukin-12, soluble interleukin-2 receptor, transforming growth factor beta and TNF. Additionally, potential metabolic biomarkers for diagnosis of schizophrenia include neurotransmitters-related metabolites such as homovanillic acid, -methoxy-4-hydroxyphenylglycol, kynurenic acid, glutamate, glutamine, and the glutamine to glutamate ratio. Some other types include metabolic biomarkers that are fatty acids specifically polyunsaturated fatty acids, neuroactive steroids such as cortisol, pregnenolone and pregnenolone sulfate, dehydroepiandrosterone sulfate, and neutrophins such as brain-derived neurotrophic factor. Furthermore, given the strong heritability and genetic component of schizophrenia, investigating common genetic variants via the genome-wide association study, rarer genes such as copy number, single nucleotide, and rare coding variants through genome-wide analysis and whole-exome sequencing can provide strong indications toward schizophrenia early on. Ever-increasingly, polygenic risk scores, methylation, and transcriptomics are playing a larger role in terms of mental illness evaluation given the global change in lifestyles and the interactions between genes and the environment leading to pathology [79,80].

Similarly, including genetic susceptibility genes, biochemical indicators, electrophysiological stimulation, and monitoring of epigenetic changes with associated phenotypic patient presentations of schizophrenia can drastically change the way clinicians classify and approach schizophrenia. By using neuroimaging, clinicians can observe brain network dysconnectivity via various types of magnetic resonance imaging (MRI) including structural, diffusion, task-based functional, and resting-state functional imaging. Similarly, cortical loss of gray matter and reduced thickness can be observed via structural MRI, whereas pattern recognition and responses to auditory stimuli can be studied via combinations of MRIs and the use of magnetoencephalography (MEG) and electroencephalography (EEG), respectively [80,81]. From a neurotransmission perspective, the varying glutamate transmission can be measured via magnetic resonance spectroscopy as well. This can be furthered to explore schizophrenia on a cellular level by characterizing the neuroinflammation malfunction, hyperactive dopamine, and decreased density of synaptic vesicles through positron emission tomography. This holistic approach could facilitate a more nuanced understanding of schizophrenia's pathogenesis, leading to more accurate diagnoses and personalized treatment plans. By incorporating a wide spectrum of data, from variances in patterns within neural circuitry to molecular changes such as differing types of receptors in implicated anatomical regions, this integrated methodology holds potential for breakthroughs in screening, diagnosing, and effectively treating schizophrenia.

7.4 Mood disorders: Depressive disorder

Mood disorders incorporate numerous disorders such as bipolar disorders, depressive disorders, and substance-induced mood disorders [82]. These are mainly characterized by their sustained, significant disruption in effect with either strong lows such as depression or excessively elevated moods such as mania or hypomania, or both [83–85]. Major depressive disorder (MDD), also known as depression or depressive disorder, is one of the leading causes in terms of the burden of disease and is projected to be the leading cause in the next 7 years. Based on the severity and individual, it manifests as loss of pleasure of interest in activities, depressed mood with psychological symptoms ranging from poor concentration and self-worth to suicidal ideation, and physiological changes like disrupted sleep or change in appetite. With causation that is multifactorial in nature, the interplay of stressful life events, intrapersonal personality traits, familial history, pregnancy and childbirth or menopause, loneliness, substance abuse, and comorbidity with other chronic conditions may significantly impact a person's likelihood of suffering from depression [82,85].

7.4.1 Categorical diagnosis: Disease severity, presence of psychotic symptoms, and degree of remission

The current primary classification is based on the severity of depressive episodes, presence or absence of psychotic symptoms and remission specifiers for both, single episode, and recurrent depressive disorder. For instance, single episode depressive disorder can present in patients as mild, moderate, or severe in terms of severity and may be with or without psychotic symptoms. Disease severity specifiers range from mild to moderate and severe, respectively [86]. These degrees are dependent on the intensity of symptomatology and impact on the patient's functionality; however, a rating scale has not yet been developed to reliably employ for delineating between degrees.

7.4.2 Dimensional assessments: Clinical manifestation of primary diagnosed disorders

Additional features of specification that allow for the elaboration of the presentation or characteristics of both, single and multiple depressive disorders are as follows:

  i. With prominent anxiety symptoms
 ii. With panic attacks
iii. Current depressive episode persistent
 iv. Current depressive episode with melancholia
  v. With seasonal pattern

Additionally, there are two additional contexts with diagnostic codes for depressive episodes that may be impacted by pregnancy or begin 6 weeks postdelivery that are bifurcated by the presence or absence of psychotic symptoms. The diagnostic codes are as follows [87−89]:

 i. Mental or behavioral disorders associated with pregnancy, childbirth, or the puerperium without psychotic symptoms
ii. Mental or behavioral disorders associated with pregnancy, childbirth, or the puerperium with psychotic symptoms

7.5 Symptom profile: Clinical manifestation of secondary comorbid disorders that reinforce primary disorder

7.5.1 Genetic influences in depressive disorder

Depression disorder is a significantly varied ailment and can occur due to numerous reasons rendering different symptomatology being manifested across patient pools as a result of specific pathogenetic mechanisms [90]. There are numerous ways in which depression can differ and the identified sources are as follows: combinations of symptoms, severity and episodic or longitudinal nature of disease, presence of comorbidities, age of onset, biological sex, and individual's previous history that may reflect current triggers for depressive episodes among others. It is no surprise that there is a role of both genetics and environmental factors that impact the presence of and experience an individual has with depressive disorder [91,92]. A review by Sridhar Prathikanti and Daniel R Weinberger of the Clinical Brain Disorders Branch, Genes, Cognition, and Psychosis Program at the National Institute of Mental Health (NIMH) forecasted the role that genetic research and pharmacogenomics would play in supporting improved classification of patients by analyzing the alleles that render them susceptible to neuropsychiatric disorders [93]. The review also mentions how the 5-HT transporter, known as 5-HTTPR, and brain-derived neurotrophic factor (BDNF) are implicated in neuropsychiatric disorders. This is unsurprizing given that the key function of 5-HTTPR is coding for serotonin transport and BDNF is responsible for the modulation of neurotransmitters.

Specifically, studies have shown short 5-HTTLPR alleles to be correlated with decreased expression of the serotonin transporter, decreased serotonin reception, elevated neuroticism, and higher risk of depression upon experiencing adverse events or challenges as opposed to others however, there are mixed results on the predisposition or response to such events [94]. Functions associated with this gene based on studies employing neural imaging are moderating emotional regulation, cognitive skills relating to sociability, and affective reactivity to triggering stimuli with connectivity mostly between the anterior cingulate cortex and amygdala regions. Similarly, the Val66Met variation in BDNF negatively impacts the BDNF release and is correlated to levels of resistance to stress as well as higher anxious responses that are treatment resistant to selective serotonin reuptake inhibitors (SSRIs) such as Prozac in animal models. In humans, meta-analysis studies have shown that both of these polymorphisms do not affect hippocampal volume in a significant manner but decreased hippocampal volumes were repeatedly seen in the case of bipolar disorder, indicating there may be subtypes where effect sizes are larger by virtue of the subtype being more heritable overall.

Interestingly, a study by Caspi and colleagues showed that a functional polymorphism or variation in the protomer portion of the 5-HT gene impacts the expression and transcription of the transporter protein. This appears to impact the response of adverse events and potentially, the risk of depression [95,96]. The study investigated over 900 participants who were monitored from birth till over the age of 25 and results focused on those who were carriers of the allele that predisposed individuals to depression [96]. The participants who underwent stressors or adverse events with the allele had a 3 times higher likelihood of suffering from an episode of clinical depression within a 5-year period as opposed to those who were noncarriers of the risk allele. The study highlighted the idea that the presence of genes themselves does not render the depression; however, it may predispose the reactions and impacts that adverse events have on those with the at-risk genotype, especially during more preliminary stages of life, whereas those without risk alleles may present with some resistance toward adverse environmental challenges [97].

Given the risk that genetic makeup may render in terms of depressive disorder, there is growing interest and effort being devoted to understanding and identifying the genetic variants that may be associated with the subtypes of clinical presentations or types of depressive disorders. One way these variants may appear is in the form of endophenotypes—inherited characteristics that are quantitative in nature and evaluated by lab-based methods as opposed to observation clinically which may offer answers regarding genetic factors and how they affect the pathogenesis of depressive disorders. It is worth noting that the different subtypes may be more impacted by genetic risk as opposed to others with bipolar depression being highly inheritable (approximately 60%−85%), whereas unipolar depression is not as interlinked (35%−40%). Findings of Wray et al., a large-scale meta-analysis, indicated that 44 independent loci associated with 153 genes are correlated to excitatory neurotransmission, synaptic function, and dendritic spines, and notably, six loci that were common to 108 risk variants in studies exploring schizophrenia, thus indicating the potential of using transdiagnostic models.

The use of neuroimaging technology and larger data sets have enabled researchers to explore depression by using large-scale genome-wide association studies, it remains difficult to explore how predominant single nucleotide polymorphisms impact depressive disorder, and increasingly, this is being approached through investigating multiple genes. A polygenic risk score indicates the approximate impact that numerous genetic variants may have on an individual and their risk of disease—in this case, depressive disorder. Preliminary studies employing this approach have explored depression and its associated symptomatology such as lapse in executive functions such as working memory. Yüksel and team explored if the polygenic risk for depression also impacted performance on working memory and brain activation was recorded with patterns within the right prefrontal cortex being impacted by depression. These findings indicate that there is a link between the presentation of depression and associated memory implicated that may be impacted by genetic variants that either play the role of endophenotypes or directly impact the underlying mechanism of depression, and finding the temporal sequence of onset of disease and genetic impacts on individual presentation of depression can further allude to the underlying mechanisms of depressive disorder.

Other identified risk gene variants for MDD include methylenetetrahydrofolate reductase (MTHFR), neuronal growth regulator 1 (NEGR1), solute carrier family 6 member 3 (SLC6A3), serotonin receptor (HTR1A), dopamine receptor D4 (DRD4), G protein subunit beta 3 (GNB3), Olfactomedin 4 (OLFM4), leucine-rich repeat and fibronectin type III domain-containing 5 (LRFN5), RNA Binding Fox-1 Homolog 1 (RBFOX1), and 5-HT transporter (5HTTLPR). Other than the previously discussed genes, these variants have been associated with the following functional roles in terms of depression, respectively:

i. When MTFHR is present, migraine with aura in individuals with depression if a C677T variant is present and a higher risk of depression by 1.2 times post-early trauma if an individual has a T-allele

ii. When NEGR-1 is knocked off, murine models have shown depressive behaviors and lower hippocampal neural growth

iii. Presence of DAT/SLC6A3 variants has been correlated with deficits in attention and time blindness with a higher overall prediction of mental states

iv. In the case of HTR1A, rs6295 (a single nucleotide polymorphism) has been correlated with adverse life events in MDD in adults aged 20–29

v. LRFN5 single nucleotide polymorphisms are correlated with MDD and risk of depression in older adults

Although the presence of genes associated with depression and findings regarding neurotransmission offer points of intervention, one population that remains a challenge within the landscape are those who are treatment resistant. Fabbri and colleagues explored the features of treatment-resistant depression (TRD) from a genetic and clinical perspective by using medical records from UK Biobank (UKB) and EXCEED. They found MDD to be significantly correlated with MDD polygenic risk score, whereas TRD was positively correlated with polygenic risk scores (PRSs) of factors such as attention deficit hyperactivity disorder (ADHD), lower socioeconomic status, obesity, more neuroticism, and other poor clinical features.

Building on the findings of various single nucleotide polymorphisms and genetic variants, the incorporation of genetic research into the study of depressive disorder marks a critical advancement in understanding its complex symptomatology and clinical presentation. By unraveling the intricate genetic underpinnings of depression, researchers are now better equipped to comprehend the variability in individual responses to treatment and the diverse manifestations of the disorder across patient pools. Genetic investigations, particularly through genome-wide association studies (GWASs) and the analysis of PRS, have illuminated the significant role of hereditary factors in predisposing individuals to depression. This genetic perspective offers insights into why certain individuals exhibit resilience or vulnerability to environmental stressors, a key element in the onset and progression of depressive episodes. Moreover, genetic research has paved the way for personalized medicine in mental healthcare, enabling clinicians to tailor treatments based on an individual's genetic makeup. This approach promises more effective and targeted interventions, potentially improving outcomes for patients with treatment-resistant forms of depression. Furthermore, understanding the genetic correlations between depression and other psychiatric or physical health conditions can lead to a more holistic approach to treatment. In essence, the integration of genetic research into the field of depression represents a transformative step forward, promising to enhance our understanding of this complex disorder and improve the efficacy of therapeutic interventions.

7.5.2 Cellular/molecular in depressive disorder

The interaction between the genetic features of an individual consisting of a genome constituted of epigenome, transcriptomes, and proteomes, the cellular and molecular features consisting of biochemical pathways, and synaptic structures on a cellular level are key constructs to an individual experience. When combined with adverse life events, these predisposed or unique combinations can lead to depressive disorder in people and associated symptomatology. With this hierarchy in mind, Fries and team investigated synaptic activity as an integral piece of pathways and how they contribute to our current understanding of MDD.

On a cellular level, MDD is characterized by changes in astrocytes, oligodendrocytes, and microglia. A review article by Czéh and Magy investigated these abnormalities across cell types employing clinical literature across three data types: in vivo imaging, postmortem molecular data, and postmortem cellular data. Regarding astrocytes, in vivo imaging data has indicated decreased glucose metabolism in the prefrontal cortex, amygdala, thalamus, and lateral temporal and parietal cortex in MDDs. Other studies have reported similar findings with lower blood flow and glucose metabolism in the brains of patients suffering from MDD and disrupted TCA cycle functioning, leading to lower energy being produced and hence, potentially worsening depressive symptomatology.

Additionally, studies employing postmortem molecular and cellular data in astrocyte-specific biomarkers from people with mood disorders have also indicated decreased Glial fibrillary acidic protein (GFAP) expression in the PFC, locus coeruleus, cerebellum, and lowered GFAP mRNA in the thalamus and caudate nucleus. Additionally, across studies, there was a reduction in gene expression seen for gap junction protein (GJA1), potassium and water channels (KCNJ10 and AQP4), as well as downregulation in connexin 30 and 43 expression across brain areas. In fact, larger astrocytes with bigger cell bodies and more offshoot process in the anesthesia critical care (ACC), decreased density in the amygdala, lower areal fraction, and density of astrocytes in the dorsolateral PFC were seen in young subjects versus their older counterparts with higher areal fraction and packing density of astrocytes.

In terms of oligodendrocyte abnormalities, diffusion tensor imaging (DTI) research has described lowered fractional anisotropy within the corpus callosum as well as numerous frontal and temporal regions and modified magnetization transfer ratios (MTRs) depicting disintegration of myelin in MDDs. Similarly, Wang et al. found lowered N-acetyl aspartate to creatine ratio (NAA/Cr) in the DLPFC white matter in first-episode patients who have never received depression treatment. Additionally, in MDD, mRNAs and proteins associated with myelin have shown modified expression in the ventral PFC's white matter. Similarly, studies utilizing postmortem cellular data have found decreases in the number and density of oligodendrocytes in the PHC, lower immunoreactivity of the myelin basic protein in the anterior frontal cortex, and higher axonal myelin thickness in the genu of the corpus callosum in association with major depressive disorder.

Changes in microglia associated with major depressive disorder have also been seen across studies with in vivo imaging studies showing higher translocator protein (TSPO) in the PFC based on PET scans and high availability of TSPO in the anterior cingulate cortex and insula when comparing patients with suicidal thoughts versus those with no ideation. Studies have also discovered that in the case of suicide victims, there is an upregulation of gene expression of Iba-1 and MCP-1 as well as increased cytokines such as interleukin-6 (IL-6), interleukin-1β (IL-1β), tumor necrosis factor-alpha (TNF-α), and toll-like receptors in the PFC.

Evidently, there is ever-increasing evidence of the contributions of microglia, oligodendrocytes, and astrocytes in being indicative of or impacting the experience of depressive symptomatology, thereby providing novel avenues to target depression. Examples include SSRIs such as Fluoxetine that enhances GFAP expression and other astrocyte-specific neurotrophic factors and Riluzole that increases glutamate uptake through GLTI1 similar to Ceftriaxone, which has similar effects. Studies also suggest the impacts of such medications have downstream effects on the neural environment, global brain health, and lower stress. That being said, the complexity of MDD and depressive disorders lies in its multifaceted molecular interplay, a subject that is pivotal to enhancing clinical approaches for its diagnosis and treatment. The pathophysiology of depressive disorder is not linear and involves various interconnected molecular pathways, each adding layers to its complexity. The understanding of such pathways and their functional implications is crucial for the evolution of personalized medicine in treating depression.

At the forefront of the onset of depressive disorder is often the impact of chronic stress, which deregulates the HPA axis. This dysregulation leads to persistent stress hormone secretion, affecting brain function and structure and potentially triggering other molecular events. The stress response is closely followed by an inflammatory response, where increased stress hormones contribute to immune system dysregulation, heightening proinflammatory cytokine production. This inflammatory state not only alters brain function but also shapes the structural changes associated with MDD.

A significant aspect of depressive disorder is the alteration in neurotransmitter systems as stress and inflammation often directly influence key neurotransmitters such as serotonin, noradrenaline, dopamine, glutamate, and GABA. These changes are critical in the manifestation of mood and cognitive symptoms in MDD. Accompanying these are alterations in neurotrophins, particularly BDNF, which is essential for neuronal growth and synaptic functioning. In fact, decreased BDNF levels as a consequence of stress and inflammation lead to synaptic dysfunction, which is a hallmark of depressive disorder. Additionally, stress and inflammation can induce mitochondrial dysfunction and oxidative stress, exacerbating neuronal damage and contributing to MDD symptoms. The disorder also encompasses metabolic factors and the gut–brain axis, wherein gut microbiota metabolites impact brain function and mood.

Notably, genetic and epigenetic factors play a role in potentially influencing an individual's susceptibility to these pathways. These pathways are not isolated but interact bidirectionally, creating complex feedback loops. For instance, neurotransmitter systems can both influence and be influenced by inflammation. This model is a higher-level understanding that underscores the need for an integrative approach to depression treatment. The variability in primary dysfunctions among patients, influenced by factors like genetics, environment, lifestyle, and previous stress or trauma, calls for personalized treatment strategies with the intricate order and prominence of these pathways contributing to the clinical heterogeneity seen across depression patients. Therefore, a deeper understanding of these complex molecular interactions is key to advancing clinical translation, and improving diagnosis, treatment, and overall management approaches for depression.

7.6 Brain circuit activity in depressive disorder

One of the key strategies under RDoC is the exploration of dimensional approaches to understanding psychiatric conditions, and modern-day neuroimaging technologies have enabled researchers and clinicians alike to focus on the identification of individual differences seen across the spectrum of clinical symptomatology due to depressive disorders and validate or quantify these presentations through measures of brain structure and function as opposed to simply comparing healthy controls to disease states. For instance, Xia et al.'s study utilized functional MRI measures of brain connectivity to identify dimensions of psychopathology that correlate with specific psychiatric symptoms and behaviors. Their analysis, involving a diverse cohort, revealed four distinct brain—behavior dimensions that correlated with various combinations of symptoms like mood, psychosis, fear, and externalizing behaviors. This study underscores the potential of data-driven approaches in delineating the complex symptomatology of psychiatric disorders. Similarly, Mihalik et al. investigated the relationship between psychopathology dimensions and changes in functional brain connectivity during adolescent development. Their findings revealed two distinct modes of brain—behavior covariation, associated with externalizing/internalizing behaviors and emotional well-being versus distress, respectively. These modes exhibited distinct age-related patterns and connectivity profiles, offering insights into the neural underpinnings of developing psychopathology in two key patient pools: adolescents and young adults. Transdiagnostic meta-analyses have further expanded our understanding of common underlying mechanisms across different psychiatric conditions. For example, Zhang et al. examined the neural correlates of anhedonia or "general disinterest" across MDD and schizophrenia. In doing so, they identified decreased activity in the basal ganglia and abnormalities in fronto-striatal networks, indicative of shared neural substrates across these disorders. Similar studies have identified commonalities in cognitive control, emotion regulation, and meta-cognition, providing a more integrated perspective on psychiatric symptomatology.

An alternative to dimensional analysis is the categorical clustering of subjects. Price et al.'s study exemplifies this approach. Using fMRI scans, they identified distinct subgroups of depressed patients based on brain activity during a positive mood induction task. Their findings revealed subgroups distinguished by functional properties of specific brain networks, offering the potential for more tailored diagnostic and treatment strategies.

A hybrid approach, combining both dimensional and categorical strategies, has also been explored. Drysdale et al. for instance, used resting-state fMRI data to identify dimensions predictive of specific depressive symptoms, subsequently clustering TRD patients along these dimensions. This approach revealed distinct subgroups with unique patterns of connectivity and symptom profiles, highlighting the utility of integrating both approaches for a more comprehensive understanding of MDD. In another notable study, Tokuda et al. utilized a Bayesian coclustering technique on a multimodal data set, incorporating functional connectivity, gene expression, and clinical symptoms. They identified distinct subtypes with unique functional connectivity patterns and treatment responses, illustrating the potential of integrating genetic and neuroimaging data for enhanced understanding and treatment of psychiatric disorders.

These studies collectively represent a significant paradigm shift in psychiatric research, moving away from broad, categorical diagnoses toward a more refined, individualized understanding of mental disorders. This shift is particularly pertinent for disorders like MDD, characterized by heterogeneity in symptomatology and etiology. The integration of diverse methodologies—from neuroimaging to genetics—offers a more holistic view of these conditions, paving the way for improved diagnostics, targeted treatments, and ultimately, better clinical outcomes.

In clinical practice, the identification of distinct brain–behavior dimensions and subgroups within disorders like depression can lead to more personalized treatment strategies. For instance, the identification of specific functional connectivity patterns associated with certain symptoms or treatment responses can guide clinicians in selecting the most effective interventions for each patient.

Furthermore, the integration of developmental perspectives into these models is crucial. Understanding how brain connectivity patterns evolve during adolescence and young adulthood can inform early intervention strategies and prevent the full onset of psychiatric disorders.

The RDoC initiative, therefore, stands as a testament to the evolving landscape of psychiatric research, one that embraces complexity and individual variability. By acknowledging and systematically exploring the multifaceted nature of disorders like MDD, this approach holds promise for more effective and personalized mental healthcare.

The integration of insights from brain circuit activity, genetics, and cellular molecular mechanisms heralds a transformative era in the clinical management and research of MDD. Advances in understanding brain circuitry, particularly the neural networks implicated in mood regulation and cognitive functions, offer a roadmap for targeted interventions. This knowledge, coupled with genetic profiling, can facilitate personalized medicine approaches, tailoring treatments to individual genetic makeups and specific circuit dysfunctions. The growing body of genetic data, including the identification of susceptibility genes and polymorphisms such as 5-HTTPR and BDNF, paves the way for predictive models of MDD, potentially allowing for early intervention strategies. On a cellular level, the exploration of molecular mechanisms, such as neurotransmitter imbalances, neuroinflammatory processes, and glial cell functions, has opened new therapeutic avenues. This includes the development of novel pharmacological agents that act on specific neurotransmitter systems or neuroinflammatory pathways and astrocytes, microglia, and oligodendrocytes, as well as nonpharmacological interventions like deep brain stimulation, which directly modulate brain circuits. Future research should focus on the synergistic integration of these domains, leveraging high-resolution neuroimaging, genomics, and advanced cellular studies. Such a multidisciplinary approach is poised to unravel the complex etiology of MDD, offering hope for more effective, individualized, and preventative treatments, ultimately improving patient outcomes in this challenging and prevalent mental health condition.

7.6.1 Psychiatric surgery

In 2014, the Mayo Clinic released an online video showcasing a unique scenario: a musician playing the violin while undergoing brain surgery performed by a neurosurgeon. The surgical objective was to target a specific area in the thalamus using electrodes, aiming to alleviate an essential tremor through electrical stimulation. The musical performance served as a real-time test to ensure the accurate placement of the electrodes, confirming success in achieving the desired outcome. The application of deep brain stimulation (DBS) for treating severe tremors in Parkinson's disease dates back to 1987, and it has proven effective in addressing severe dystonia as well. Since then, tens of thousands of individuals have undergone DBS procedures for various movement disorders, gradually replacing earlier lesion-based methods. The procedure has extended its reach to address "benign" essential tremors, emphasizing its relatively low side-effect profile and positive patient acceptance. In 1999, a Belgian team explored the use of DBS in three individuals with treatment-resistant obsessive-compulsive disorder (OCD), yielding favorable results. Subsequent trials have explored DBS applications across a spectrum of psychiatric conditions, accompanied by a more modest increase in ablative procedures. The renewed interest in psychiatric neurosurgery aligns with significant shifts in our understanding of the brain. At the onset of the 20th century, anatomist Santiago y Cajal asserted a perspective that once brain development concludes, the potential for growth and regeneration of axons and dendrites irreversibly diminishes. Throughout much of the past century, this notion of neurons being fixed and immutable dominated brain science, despite dissenting voices, particularly between the World Wars. DBS has revolutionized the treatment and understanding of various brain disorders by directly intervening in pathological neural circuits [98]. DBS involves surgically implanting electrodes into specific brain targets and delivering constant or intermittent electricity from an implanted battery source. With over 160,000 patients globally undergoing DBS for various neurological and nonneurological conditions, its clinical application continues to expand. DBS offers advantages such as its nonlesional nature, the ability to adjust stimulation parameters, and the direct interaction with circuit pathology, making it a versatile therapeutic and scientific tool [99]. As a clinical tool,

DBS is advantageous due to its nonlesional nature, adjustable parameters, and direct targeting of circuit pathology. It is particularly effective for movement disorders like Parkinson's disease (PD), where randomized controlled trials have shown its superiority in controlling motor symptoms. However, challenges persist, such as its limited efficacy in addressing nonmotor symptoms and the potential for serious risks, including infection and hemorrhage [98–100]. Although DBS is a standard treatment for movement disorders, its application in other conditions is limited to highly refractory cases and remains within the realm of expert multidisciplinary care and clinical research. Although DBS has shown remarkable success in PD, it also highlights challenges, such as the need for more comprehensive interventions to address dysfunction across multiple circuits. Technical innovations are sought to improve practicality, extend battery life, design smaller devices, and develop more tailored and adaptive stimulation methods. Clinically, challenges include meeting the needs of an aging global population and expanding DBS indications to conditions beyond PD, such as depression and Alzheimer's disease (AD) [100].

Several hypotheses have been proposed to elucidate the mechanisms underlying the efficacy of DBS. The prevailing theories center around the idea that DBS disrupts pathological brain circuit activity, with effects occurring at the ionic, protein, cellular, and network levels to produce symptomatic improvements. Although it remains unclear which specific effects of DBS are necessary and sufficient for therapeutic outcomes, it is evident that high-frequency ($\sim$ 100 Hz) trains of short pulses ($\sim$ 0.1 ms) generate network responses distinct from those produced by low-frequency ($\sim$ 10 Hz) stimulation. At the ionic level, an electrode polarized to a negative potential (cathode) is implanted into the brain to redistribute charged particles (e.g., Na+ and Cl− ions) in the extracellular space, creating an electric field that can manipulate sodium channel proteins' voltage sensors in neurons' membranes [101]. At the cellular level, the opening of sodium channels can induce an action potential, typically initiated in the axon. Stimulated action potentials propagate in both the orthodromic and antidromic directions to the axon terminals of the neuron [102]. Although many axons can be stimulated during DBS, high-frequency signals may lead to synaptic exhaustion and depression in axon terminals. Additionally, stimulated synapses may become low-pass filters, suppressing the transmission of low-frequency signals. This phenomenon, known as "synaptic filtering," might play a crucial role in DBS, hindering the propagation of oscillatory activity patterns within associated brain networks [98]. The basic biophysical effects of DBS provide a framework for interpreting observed network activity patterns in patients. As stimulation frequency remains constant during DBS, the information content of the stimulation signal is effectively zero, creating an "information lesion" in stimulated neurons. According to this hypothesis, DBS-induced action potentials override intrinsic activity in stimulated neurons, limiting the propagation of oscillatory activity through the network. The concepts of information lesion and synaptic filtering may work together to robustly suppress low-frequency signals in stimulated brain circuits [97].

However, advancements in technology, such as MRI, fMRI, and other techniques at the century's end, demonstrated the brain's capacity for structural adaptation and regeneration. Simultaneously, simplistic ideas of functional localization are evolving into a more nuanced understanding involving task-related systems and 'default' networks. Over the past 25 years, there has been a profound transformation in our comprehension of glial cells. Previously perceived as mere brain scaffolding and housekeepers, they are now recognized as contributors to brain development, shapers of responses to injury, modulators of synaptic transmission, and operators of an independent chemically based communication system.

The majority of current procedures in psychiatric neurosurgery employ the insertion of electrodes into the brain, with only two exceptions: vagus nerve stimulation (VNS) and gamma knife capsulotomy. In most cases, a stereotactic cage is affixed to the head to guide electrodes to specific brain locations identified through MRI mapping. For VNS, the surgical process entails isolating the left vagus nerve within the carotid sheath in the neck and encircling it with two electrodes. Subsequently, these electrodes are connected to a programmable stimulator positioned subcutaneously in the upper chest wall. This arrangement allows for the precise modulation of neural activity through electrical stimulation, demonstrating a distinct approach compared to the more common intracranial electrode insertion procedures.

Each electrode in psychiatric neurosurgery consists of both an anode and a cathode. The application of electrical current in this setup causes the brain tissue between these electrodes to become part of the circuit. In DBS, voltages typically range from 3 to 5 volts, with pulse frequencies exceeding 100/s. At such frequencies, the brain tissue immediately surrounding the electrodes experiences deactivation or depolarization. However, just beyond this region, volume conduction occurs, leading to electrical stimulation of axons. This stimulation propagates both upstream to cell bodies and downstream to synapses, resulting in the interruption of local brain function and the generation of effects at more distant sites. When using frequencies below 100, such as 15 pulses/s in VNS, stimulation also occurs in the tissue immediately surrounding the electrodes. The experimental use of electrodes to stimulate brain tissue in humans dates back to the late 1940s. Additionally, electrodes have been employed to create lesions through thermocoagulation, as seen in procedures like anterior cingulotomy. In this context, a 10 mm exposed portion of the electrode is heated to 85°C for 60 s. In gamma knife surgery, a different approach is taken. Multiple narrow beams of gamma radiation converge at a premapped point within the brain, eliminating the need to open the skull. This method provides a noninvasive alternative for precise interventions in targeted brain regions.

Brain imaging and EEG play pivotal roles in pinpointing the precise position of DBS electrodes during surgical interventions. In the initial stages, a rudimentary electrical system was employed for brain stimulation. Since 1950, a single-wire probe has been widely utilized for both stimulation and extracellular recording. In this setup, multiple electrodes were derived from an array situated on a ceramic plate. Advancements in integrated circuit and thin film technologies led to a breakthrough when Wise and colleagues applied these methods for developing microelectrodes. This marked the commencement of a new era in research on implantable neural interfaces. Despite the considerable progress in interface technology, the clinical success of brain stimulation hinges on factors beyond interface development. Critical elements include the quality of stimulation and the precise localization of the electrode within the targeted brain area. The integration of brain imaging and EEG not only facilitates the identification of the electrode's exact position but also contributes to enhancing the overall effectiveness and accuracy of DBS interventions.

Although systems utilizing brain stimulation technologies have proven useful and practical in various cases, they are not without drawbacks. The inherent variability in the brain structures among individuals poses a challenge, as employing a common stimulation program for different people may yield divergent responses and, in some instances, lead to severe complications. In recent decades, efforts to address these limitations have given rise to the development of closed-loop and flexible systems. As a result, the quality control steps required are complex. In these innovative systems, the stimulation current can be automatically adjusted in proportion to recorded brain physiological signals. This adaptive approach is believed to be more effective than previous fixed procedures. However, these advanced systems face substantial challenges, including the requirement for large batteries to sustain the system, necessitating surgery for replacement several years after implantation. Another issue is the constraint on the use of electrodes, often mandating the placement of a single electrode for both signal stimulation and recording. Additionally, determining the precise coordinates of the target area within the brain poses a challenge, especially when aiming to stimulate small regions such as the subthalamic nucleus. Beyond the subthalamic nucleus (STN), other targets for DBS in PD include the globus pallidus interna and the ventral intermediate nucleus of the thalamus (VIM). Controversies persist regarding the optimal region with minimal side effects and maximal effectiveness for DBS in neurological disorders.

Randomized trials evaluating DBS in PD reveal a spectrum of outcomes, with variations reported in different studies. A recent review compiled results from several studies investigating both STN and globus pallidus internus (GPi) DBS. For STN DBS, encompassing 943 patients across nine studies, the mean improvement in UPDRS III scores ranged from 29% to 49%, and PDQ-39 index scores showed improvement ranging from 8.3% to 26.4%. In the case of GPi DBS, involving 377 patients, mean improvements in the same outcome measures ranged from 29% to 39% for UPDRS III scores and from 6.3% to 17.5% for PDQ-39 index scores. The variability in response, even within renowned hospitals where efforts are made to optimize procedures, can be attributed to factors such as patient differences in anatomy and physiology at a millimeter scale. Operational differences, including the trajectory planning process and heuristics used to determine an acceptable lead location, can also contribute to the observed variability. These challenges highlight the complexity of DBS and the need for a personalized approach to optimize outcomes for individual patients [103].

7.6.1.1 Neural interphase

A neural probe is a microstructure designed to establish a connection between neural tissue and external electrical, optical, or chemical systems. Key considerations in designing these structures include size, thickness, dimensions, and impedance, all aimed at minimizing brain damage during and after implantation. Thickness, dimension, and stability against breakage or bending during implantation are critical factors to address [104]. The reduction in the cross-section of conductive metals in the probe can increase electrode impedance, leading to elevated Johnson noise within the structure. The integration of stimulation and recording sites in a small volume adjacent to each other is achieved through micromachining techniques and thin film nanotechnology. Microelectromechanical system-based (MEMS-based) technology probes typically have body lengths ranging from 200 µm (200 µm) to a few millimeters (mm) and thicknesses between 10 and 200 µm [105]. Since the 1970s, when Wise and Angle first utilized MEMS techniques for neural electrode production, ongoing studies have been conducted each year to enhance electrode functionality, focusing on aspects such as biocompatibility, stability, and low noise. In the past decades, a thin film of iridium oxide coating the probe's body has been employed to prevent direct contact of incompatible metals with brain tissues. However, prolonged use of high-level voltage can lead to delamination and the loss of this protective layer. Zhang et al. [105a] addressed this issue by utilizing carbon nanotubes, known for their excellent mechanical stability and more effective connection with neural cells [106]. Furthermore, the combination of gold nanotubes with carbon nanotubes has been shown to significantly reduce electrode impedance. The probe production process involves micromachining, where the probe is immersed in a gold nanoparticle bath, and a layer of carbon nanotubes with a 2-µm thickness forms on the electrode body [107]. Finally, ultrasonic waves are used to homogenize nanoparticles and complete the probe structure. This innovative approach represents a continuous effort to enhance the functionality and performance of neural probes in neuroscientific research and medical applications. These emerging fields require rigorous and expansive testing with well-designed clinical research [108].

One of the significant challenges in using implantable electrodes for brain stimulation is the potential reduction in stimulation and recording quality due to blood aggregation and coagulation around the implanted region. To address this issue, an anticoagulant liquid is often employed as a solution. In the design of these probes, multiple parallel channels are incorporated, typically created through glass deposition. The process begins with the etching of approximately 5—20 µm of a silicon surface. Subsequently, a glass layer is deposited on the probe using thin film techniques, serving as a protective and separating layer for the channels from the external environment. This design allows for the controlled flow of the anticoagulant liquid through the channels, mitigating the impact of blood aggregation and coagulation around the implanted region. By incorporating such features, these implantable electrodes aim to maintain optimal functionality and recording quality in the dynamic environment of the brain.

Presently, open-loop systems are widely integrated into DBS procedures, allowing trained physicians to adjust relevant parameters such as frequency, amplitude, and duty cycle. In this approach, stimulation parameters are initially set for the first few months of the treatment period and can be readjusted based on the patient's condition and treatment outcomes. The goal of this readjustment is to identify and provide optimal parameters for more effective treatment results with minimal side effects. However, a closed-loop system represents a more advanced approach, continuously receiving feedback from the patient's brain through a programmed algorithm for effective stimulation parameter adjustments. Experimentally adjusted parameters may not be universally applicable across various genders and races due to differences in brain structures. Closed-loop systems aim to address this variability by automatically delivering therapeutic parameters based on real-time detection of brain signals. Challenges associated with these systems include the need for compact size, low energy consumption, and minimizing surgical injury during implantation procedures. Various system designs have been developed to overcome these challenges. Rhew et al. [108a] introduced a microchip designed to convert input signals into logarithmic form and perform mathematical calculations on a logarithmic scale within a closed-loop feedback system. This conversion reduces volume calculation requirements, resulting in benefits such as lower power consumption and extended battery life. The system comprises a logarithmic analog-to-digital converter (Log-ADC), digital signal processors (DSPs) for calculations, a clock pulse generator, stimulator, and power components, all integrated into a compact 2×2 mm electronic chip. In this system, electrical current serves as the stimulation factor, delivering a uniform and constant charge to tissues without changes in electrode impedance. Stimulation parameters can be adjusted automatically in a closed-loop fashion or manually via radio frequency (RF) and serial peripheral interface (SPI), using an external computer under specialist supervision in an open-loop condition. Power management poses a significant challenge in implantable devices for DBS, as implanted batteries typically require replacement every few years through surgical procedures. The connection of implanted electrodes to the device and battery pack, located under the patient's skin in the chest, involves a wire passing through the patient's neck, leading to some movement difficulties in the neck region. Researchers are actively exploring innovative technologies that address challenges such as power consumption, device size, and stimulation effectiveness. Wireless energy transfer technology is a noteworthy advancement in this regard. Lee et al. introduced a system designed to power a head-implanted device using mutual electromagnetic induction, with the energy source mounted on the back of the patient's ear. Stimulation in this system is achieved through capacitive switch technology, involving the injection of balanced electrostatic charge into the tissue. The waveform has been adjusted from a common square to an exponential form, contributing to lower power consumption and more effective results. Charge injection is executed by capacitors discharging through electrodes in contact with the targeted tissue. Additionally, the system includes an array of light-emitting diodes (LEDs) capable of optical stimulation. The associated chip is manufactured using 35 μm complementary metal-oxide semiconductor (CMOS) technology, with a total size of 12 mm^2, including its connection pads, This system delivers signals with amplitudes in the range of 1, 3, 5, 130–180 μs and frequencies of 7–244 Hz. With an efficiency of about 80%, this system demonstrates excellent performance compared to similar stimulation systems. These advancements in wireless energy transfer technology signify a promising trajectory, and it is anticipated that, in the near future, implanted devices may no longer necessitate batteries for power. The rapid growth of these systems holds the potential to revolutionize the field of implantable devices for DBS.

7.7 Anxiety or fear-related disorders: Generalized anxiety disorder

Anxiety or fear-related disorders include generalized anxiety disorder, panic disorder, agoraphobia, specific phobia, social anxiety disorder, and substance-induced anxiety disorders. These disorders are mainly characterized by the fear of the stimulus or event that triggers a specific fear or anxiety and can range from a niche fear or phobia such as agoraphobia—a fear of spiders, to more general classes of fears such as generalized anxiety disorder. For this case study, I will be discussing generalized anxiety disorder—a common disorder in which the person has generalized worry and anxiety that is not caused by a recent stressor. This presents clinically as feelings of being under threat, restlessness, agitation, sleep-related changes, and symptoms of stress such as heart beating, mouth dryness, and perspiration. From an etiological perspective, stress, physical disorders or comorbidities, genetic predisposition, substance abuse, and environmental factors such as child abuse may significantly affect a person's likelihood of suffering from generalized anxiety disorder [109].

7.8 Categorical diagnosis and disease severity

The key specifier or feature within these disorders is related to the disorder-specific focus of apprehension, which is essentially the triggering stimulus or situation that initiates fear or anxiety [110]. The diagnostic features heavily focused on in this cluster of disorders are the essential symptoms, clinical features, course features about onset and severity, and developmental presentations with notes on cultural or gender-based specificities as this may impact patient concerns, thus resulting in diagnosis.

7.8.1 **Dimensional assessments: Clinical manifestation of primary diagnosed disorders**

Additional features of specification that allow for the elaboration of the presentation or characteristics of generalized anxiety disorders are as follows:

i. Marked anxiety symptoms with general worry that is not due to a specific circumstance and extreme worry about negative events across domains of daily life (for instance, familial, occupational, health, financial, etc.)

ii. Anxiety accompanied by additional symptoms like motor tension/restlessness and sympathetic autonomic overactivity as seen via gastrointestinal signs (nausea, abdominal tension, cardiovascular symptoms like palpitations, shaking, and dry mouth)

iii. Experiencing being tense, edgy, restless

iv. Struggling with focus and attention

v. Agitation

vi. Sleep disruptions (insomnia, lacking restful sleep)

7.9 **Symptom profile: Clinical manifestation of secondary comorbid disorders that reinforce primary disorders**

7.9.1 **Genetic influences in generalized anxiety disorder**

Anxiety disorders are a significant global health burden across age groups and the importance of genetics in understanding and treating GAD is increasingly recognized in psychiatric research. GAD, characterized by excessive and uncontrollable worry, poses significant challenges due to late diagnosis, high comorbidity with other disorders, and treatment resistance. Clinical genetics studies have found a notable genetic heritability for GAD, indicating a substantial genetic component in its etiology. For instance, children of parents with GAD have a significantly higher risk of developing the disorder. Additionally, twin studies have shown a high genetic correlation between GAD and traits like neuroticism. Molecular genetics research, including GWAS and candidate gene studies, further elucidates the complex genetic underpinnings of GAD. These studies have identified specific genetic variants and loci associated with GAD and related traits, highlighting the polygenic nature of the disorder. For example, variants in genes related to the serotonergic and monoaminergic systems like SLCGA4 (serotonin transporter) and HTR1A (serotonin 1A receptor) have been linked to GAD and anxiety-related phenotypes, thereby alluding to the potential for further research on such targets for specified interventions in this patient population.

A report by Meier and Deckert reviewing the genetics of anxiety disorders found that these disorders are not attributable to a single gene mutation, but rather multiple genes that contribute in different ways. Although current research on candidate genes related to neurotransmitter and stress responses has been mixed and not replicable,

GWASs that have explored an unbiased assessment of genetic variants have found numerous risk loci such as the transmembrane protein 132D (TMEM132D) gene for panic disorder. Genes such as thrombospondin-2 gene (THBS2), membrane-associated guanylate kinase, WW and PDZ domain-containing protein 1 (MAGI1), calmodulin-lysine N-methyltransferase (CAMKMT), chromosomal band 3q12.3, and genetic loci on chromosomes 19q13, 21q22, and 22q11 among other findings have been associated with GAD.

Studies have shown that in people from Hispanic and Latin American lineage, the rs78602344 polymorphism in the THBS2 gene impacts GAD but may need to be reexamined across other ethnicities. Studies examining neuroticism via linkage analysis and meta-analysis of GWAS have found potential loci on 19q13, 21q22, and 22q11 associated with severely neurotic traits and the rs35855737 polymorphism in MAGI1 associated with higher neuroticism scores. Similarly, the rs1709393 polymorphism in a noncoding RNA locus on chromosomal band 3q12.3 has been correlated with a lifelong diagnosis of GAD, and the rs1067327 polymorphism in CAMKMT on chromosome 2p21 was seen in a GWAS study to be correlated with anxiety disorders. Similarly, five genome-wide correlations were identified among people with European lineages from UKB who appear to have an anxiety disorder diagnosis or GAD. DSM-4 loci was linked to SNPs rs10809485 at 9p23, rs1187280 in neurotrophic receptor tyrosine kinase 2 (NTRK2), rs3807866 upstream of transmembrane protein 106B (TMEM106B), rs2861139 on chromosome 5, and rs4855559 in the myosin heavy chain 15 (MYH15) gene. It is key to note that genetic studies providing risk assessments for patients based on their genetic expression would be key to more upstream intervention and assessment of generalized anxiety disorder. A review by Julia Tomasi et al. also suggests, similarly to findings in depressive disorder, employing endophenotypes to improve our diagnosis of the genetic variants that may align with specific treatment responses, investigating genes found via animal epigenetic research in human participants, and using PRS to find patients that would respond to treatments to find indicators of health and treatment outcomes for GAD patients.

7.9.2 Cellular/molecular in generalized anxiety disorder

Cellular and molecular research is deepening our understanding of GAD by illuminating the intricate biological processes underpinning it, identifying key molecular pathways as well as cellular mechanisms and molecular signaling that could be targeted for therapeutic intervention, and differentiating the contributions of heritable factors from environmental influences in the etiology of GAD. Notably, studies focusing on serotonin-related markers have revealed decreased platelet 5-HT-reuptake-site binding in GAD patients, suggesting alterations in serotonin metabolism although serotonin binding in lymphocytes remains unchanged. This dichotomy underscores the complexity of serotonin's role in GAD and its potential as a therapeutic target. Additionally, GAD's interaction with the HPA axis, a central stress response system, appears to be distinct from other anxiety disorders. Unlike in PTSD or MDD, GAD does not consistently demonstrate marked HPA-axis dysregulation. This finding is exemplified by variable cortisol responses in GAD patients, which sometimes correlate with comorbid MDD. This variation indicates a nuanced relationship between GAD and stress physiology, which could influence treatment strategies, particularly those targeting the HPA axis. An example is Agomelatine, a drug primarily used in treating major depression that has shown promising results in treating GAD with minimal side effects, as indicated in both murine models and clinical trials. Its unique mechanism as a melatonin receptor agonist and a 5-HT2C receptor antagonist differentiates it from traditional GAD treatments like benzodiazepines and serotonin reuptake inhibitors. This distinct action involves modulating stress-sensitive glutamatergic circuits and altering neuropeptide release in key brain regions, contributing to its anxiolytic effects. Agomelatine's effectiveness in GAD, especially in cases of severe illness and in relapse prevention over short and extended periods, along with its low adverse effect profile, underscores its potential as an effective alternative therapy for GAD management.

Further, immunological factors like elevated CRP levels in some GAD studies point to a possible inflammatory component in the disorder. However, the inconsistent findings across different studies emphasize the need for further research to elucidate the role of immune system dysregulation in GAD. From a clinical translation perspective, these neurochemical biomarkers offer promising avenues for personalized medicine in GAD. Understanding individual differences in serotonin system functioning and HPA-axis regulation could lead to more tailored pharmacological interventions. For instance, patients exhibiting specific serotonin transport or HPA-axis anomalies might respond better to certain types of antidepressants or psychotherapies. Moreover, the potential involvement of immune responses in GAD opens up new therapeutic possibilities, such as antiinflammatory treatments.

7.9.2.1 Brain circuit activity in generalized anxiety disorder

Neuroimaging research on GAD has revealed significant insights into the structural and functional neuroanatomy of the disorder, shedding light on the brain circuit activities associated with it. Structural brain morphology studies indicate GAD is marked by notable anatomical changes in regions key to anxiety neurocircuitry. For instance, increased gray matter volume in the amygdala has been observed, particularly in females, which is linked to attentional impairments. Other findings include a larger gray matter volume in the right putamen and distinct differences in the left precuneus/posterior cingulate cortex between males and females. Adolescents with GAD exhibit changes such as increased volumes in the right precuneus and precentral gyrus and decreased volumes in the left orbital gyrus and posterior cingulate. Additionally, a reduction in white matter volumes in the DLPFC and decreased hippocampal volumes suggest issues in structural connectivity.

Functional MRI studies further explore these changes by examining neuronal responses to emotional stimuli and resting-state connectivity. Key observations from these studies include greater amygdala activation in pediatric GAD patients, which correlates with the severity of anxiety. Abnormal activities have also been identified in regions like the amygdala, anterior cingulate cortex, and medial prefrontal cortex. Interestingly, functional abnormalities in the ventral cingulate and amygdala are common in both major depression and GAD. Moreover, there are alterations in functional connectivity patterns, such as lower prefrontal-limbic connectivity and higher prefrontal-hippocampus connectivity, which underscore the complex neural underpinnings of GAD.

From a clinical translation perspective and discussing the use of potential biomarkers for treatment response to tailor therapy, Julia Tomasi and colleagues discuss neuroimaging studies that have identified specific brain region activation abnormalities in GAD patients, such as a hyperactive amygdala in response to environmental threats and deficits in prefrontal attenuation of fear responses. Similarly, a study conducted by Goldstein-Piekarski and colleagues provided significant insights into the neural circuit dysfunctions associated with GAD. Their research highlighted a key role of the salience circuit, where hypoconnectivity, particularly between the left anterior insula and the left amygdala, was strongly predictive of anxious avoidance symptoms. This pattern is also related to a broader spectrum of symptoms, including anhedonia, negative bias, threat dysregulation, and cognitive dysregulation, underscoring the multifaceted impact of salience circuit dysfunction in GAD. Additionally, contrary to initial expectations, hyperconnectivity in the default mode circuit did not correlate with rumination. Instead, global hypoconnectivity within this circuit was significantly associated with severe negative bias and anhedonia, indicating varied influences of connectivity patterns on mood and anxiety disorders. The study also shed light on the predictive value of certain neural circuit markers for treatment responses. It found that pretreatment connectivity patterns in the default mode and negative affect circuits could differentiate responses to antidepressants, while patterns in the attention circuit predicted the effectiveness of behavioral interventions. These findings emphasize the potential of neural circuitry analysis in refining treatment approaches for GAD, marking a step toward personalized psychiatric care. These findings have significant implications for understanding the neurobiological basis of GAD and may inform future therapeutic strategies targeting specific brain regions and circuits.

This comprehensive body of neuroimaging research on GAD, encompassing both structural and functional aspects of brain circuitry, provides a deeper understanding of the disorder's neurobiological underpinnings. The observed alterations in gray and white matter volumes, along with changes in functional connectivity and neuronal response patterns, highlight the complexity of GAD at a neural level. These insights not only enhance our comprehension of GAD's pathophysiology but also open new avenues for clinical application with there being potential of using specific neural circuit markers as biomarkers for diagnosing GAD and predicting treatment rendering improved personalized therapeutic strategies, optimizing treatment efficacies and patient outcomes for those with GAD.

7.10 Neurocognitive disorders: Alzheimer's disease and dementia

Neurocognitive disorders include delirium, mild neurocognitive disorder, amnestic disorder, dementia due to AD, cerebrovascular disease, Lewy body disease, fronto-temporal dementia, or dementia due to psychoactive substances and medications among other disorders. Neurocognitive disorders are mainly characterized by a developmental, general decline in memory and cognitive functioning, which may progress to severity levels that impair a patient's daily functioning. For this case study, I will be discussing AD—a neurodegenerative disease in which the patient suffers from a progressive decline in cognitive function and presents clinically as significant memory loss, loss of executive function including higher functions like speech and motor movements, and behavioral alteration. From an etiological perspective, the disease remains idiopathic however, both genetic and environmental factors contribute to the likelihood of a patient developing Alzheimer's [111]. Mutations in amyloid precursor protein (APP), PSEN1, and PSEN2 as well as occupational hazards (exposure to pesticide, electromagnetic fields, volatile anesthetic), chronic conditions (cerebrovascular disease, high blood pressure, diabetes, traumatic brain injury, depression, cancer), and lifestyle risk factors (smoking, substance abuse, physical and cognitive inactivity) can all affect and impact the probability of developing AD.

7.10.1 Categorical diagnosis and disease severity

The primary distinction between neurocognitive disorders and other disorders that render similar cognitive deficits is that the main features of these disorders are cognitive in nature, which is the first-level classification. The second level of classification that occurs within neurocognitive disorders stems from identifying the etiology which can then support further specific diagnosis. For example, dementia due to Lewy body disease is mainly characterized by the presence of Lewy bodies in four brain parts: brain stem, limbic area, forebrain, and neocortex. Each dementia category is characterized by degree of severity into mild, moderate, and severe and is characterized as part of the clinical descriptions and diagnostic requirements (CDDRs) for dementia. The severity is based on clinical exams and data collected regarding the patient via a caretaker or guardian who has experience with the patient and is segregated as follows:

i. Mild dementia: Patients who are categorized as having mild dementia generally may reside alone with limited support required and can partake in social settings without much assistance or distinguishment compared to someone without dementia. On the other hand, complex or higher-order functions such as organizational and financial planning as well as judgment or problem solving may be diminished.

ii. Moderate dementia: Patients who are categorized as having moderate dementia generally require assistance to be outside the home and may struggle with daily functioning activities such as bathing and dressing and will have noteworthy memory function impairment. Similarly, complex or higher-order functions such as organizational and social judgment are significantly reduced with socialization becoming increasingly challenged with potential behavioral changes.

iii. Severe dementia: Patients who are categorized as having severe dementia are generally dependent completely on others for basic functions including bathing, feeding, and defecation due to potential incontinence. The severe memory loss (depending on the cause) leads to a lack of spatial awareness and an inability to make decisions across contexts.

7.10.2 Dimensional assessments: Clinical manifestation of secondary comorbid disorders that reinforce primary disorders

The key specifiers within dementias refer to behavioral and psychological disturbances that may be employed when of severity in a manner that they represent a focus of clinical intervention and are as follows:

i. Psychotic symptoms in dementia

This specifier is employed when clinically relevant delusional or hallucinatory concerns are presented by the patient in addition to cognitive impairments of dementia.

ii. Mood symptoms in dementia

This specifier is employed when clinically relevant mood symptomatology such as depression or elevated moods are presented by the patient in addition to cognitive impairments of dementia.

iii. Anxiety symptoms in dementia

This specifier is employed when clinically relevant concerns of anxiety and worry are presented by the patient in addition to cognitive impairments of dementia.

iv. Apathy in dementia

This specifier is employed when clinically relevant concerns surrounding lack of interest or apathy are presented by the patient in addition to cognitive impairments of dementia.

i. Agitation or aggression in dementia

This specifier is employed when clinically relevant psychomotor control issues that are extreme in correlation to higher tension and violent behavior are presented by the patient in addition to cognitive impairments of dementia.

ii. Disinhibition in dementia

This specifier is employed when a clinically relevant lack of inhibition in terms of social norms, impulse control, and risk management is presented by the patient in addition to cognitive impairments of dementia.

iii. Wandering in dementia

This specifier is employed when clinically relevant wandering is presented as risky in addition to cognitive impairments of dementia.

iiii. Other specified behavioral or psychological disturbances in dementia

This specifier is employed when clinically relevant, severe behavioral or psychological concerns are presented by the patient in addition to dementia and cannot be captured appropriately above. There is also a specifier when the case of such disturbance is nonspecific known as behavioral or psychological disturbances in dementia, unspecified. Additionally, when describing specific dementias, for instance, with AD, specifiers include timing of onset (early or late or unknown/unspecified) and whether it is a mixed type of dementia containing two of the common types or not (with cerebrovascular disease or other nonvascular etiologies).

7.11 Symptom profile with details of psychopathology: Clinical manifestation of secondary comorbid disorders that reinforce primary disorder

7.11.1 Genetic influences in dementia

Various dementias including AD have been discussed within the context of genetic contributions focused heavily on the apolipoprotein E (APOE) gene, specifically APOE4. APOE4 was associated with contributing to the risk of developing AD as well as early onset of the disease. AD can either start impacting individuals early or late, also known as, early-onset AD (EOAD) and late-onset AD (LOAD) of which the earlier onset type makes up a small portion of all AD patients. EOAD is familial and occurs when symptoms or clinical manifestation is before 65 years old for the patient, wherein most of EOAD cases are due to genetic mutations of APP, presenilin 1 (PSEN1), and presenilin 2 (PSEN2). On the other hand, in late-onset AD that is seen majority of the time, genetic interactions such as phosphatidylinositol binding clathrin assembly protein (PICALM), clusterin (CLU), translocase of outer mitochondrial membrane 40 (TOMM40), complement receptor 1 (CR1) bridging integrator 1 (BIN1), and sortilin-related receptor L (SORL1) have also been identified to impact likelihood of AD. These have additionally been studied from a polygenic approach in mind by amalgamating various genetic loci to create polygenic risk scores (PGS), which increase the number of cases of AD, transition rates of mild cognitive impairment (MCI) to AD, and the likelihood of cognitive decline.

Similarly, a study conducted in South China by Jiao and team investigated dementias across 1795 patients and found 39 pathogenic or likely pathogenic (P/LP) variants in 14 different genes, and these were seen in 2.2% of AC and 10.9% of frontotemporal dementia, which is a diagnostic rate of 2.6%. Across the patients, the gene that was mutated in almost half of the cohort was PSEN1, and then PSEN2 and APP, respectively. However, there is still research that must be conducted as one-third of the variants identified were novel and patients who had the presence of such variants presented with dementia almost a decade earlier than patients who did not possess the variants. Another study also found that genome-wide significant associations for an amyloid-beta 42 to 40 ratio in COPG2 and WWOX genes have been seen. Additionally, a study investigating plasma biomarkers and genetics in the diagnosis or prediction of AD found that combining biomarkers, sex, APOE, and PGS has a very high accuracy with an area under the curve of 0.81 in the prediction of AD status. Similarly, Koriath et al. explored the use of next-generation genetic sequencing (NGS) in diagnosing and improving our knowledge of dementias by targeting 17 genes. The researchers found 354 deleterious variants (DVs) in 12.6% of patient samples collected, with 39 of those being novel. However, 71 DVs showed signs of lower penetrance, and DVs were often discovered in genes that were not connected to the patient's diagnosis; however, this also indicates the potential for them to be used across diverse cases. This being said, it is still equally crucial to keep exploring what genes are characteristic of specific dementias that do present differently, for instance, frontotemporal dementia that has been correlated with mainly chromosome 9 open reading frame 72 (c9orf72), microtubule-associated protein tau (MAPT), granulin precursor (GRN), and TANK-binding kinase 1 (TBK1) and clinically manifests with familial frontotemporal lobar degeneration. Evidently, these studies advocate for gene-panel diagnostics in dementia, frequent genetic testing, and investigation of variants as well as clinical predictors and symptoms. These large-scale studies in dementia genetics significantly impact clinical practice by emphasizing the role of genetic factors in dementia. The research emphasizes the necessity for continued investigation into the pathogenicity and penetrance of dementia-related genetic variants, highlighting the importance of sharing clinical and genetic data for accurate genetic classifications. Clinically, it guides the use of gene-panel diagnostics in all early-onset dementia cases and in late-onset dementia with a family history, aiding in better counseling and decision making regarding genetic testing in dementia. This shift toward a genetics-informed approach necessitates enhanced training for healthcare professionals in genetic counseling and interpretation. Overall, these insights advocate for a more personalized care approach in dementia, focusing on individual genetic profiles.

7.11.2 Cellular/molecular in dementia

Advancements in cellular and molecular research have significantly transformed the landscape of diagnostics and therapeutics in dementia, paving the way for more precise and effective approaches to tackling this complex and multifaceted disorder.

Regarding the underlying cellular and molecular mechanisms underlying dementia, literature primarily discusses the amyloid β (Aβ) hypothesis, tau pathology, the role of mitochondrial disruption and oxidative stress, proteasomal malfunctioning, neuroinflammatory responses, and presence of risk factors. The former most being rather central to our understanding of AD in that amyloid-beta build-up renders formations of neurofibrillary tangles and associated long-term cognitive deficits and these amyloid-beta peptides as a result of the disintegration of APP, discussed previously, tend to clump into oligomers that are toxic and plaques that are insoluble in nature. A review by Hampel and team discussing the evolution of AD healthcare emphasizes the need for the use of blood-based biomarkers (BBBMs) in this disease across diagnosis and treatment for patients. With Aβ42 and 40 being fundamental to AD aggregation, utilizing the plasma ratio of both of these peptides allows for visibility into their presence and aggregation within the brain. To measure the Aβ42/40 ratio, concentrations of both peptides are compared in blood samples, and the lower the ratio, the higher the Aβ42 amount, denoting a higher likelihood for plaque formation as this peptide is likelier to accumulate compared to Aβ40. Having capabilities to employ noninvasive, accessible biomarkers for earlier detection of AD is crucial due to its lengthy, "silent" prodromal stage before clinical symptomatology and may be even more important for use in MCI patients whose risk of AD transition and progression is higher. Clinically, such a biomarker would offer improved risk evaluation of incoming patients, better detection, and guide improved clinical decision making by healthcare professionals (HCPs).

Similarly, tau which is a neuronal microtubule-associated protein tends to degrade in its capacity to stabilize microtubules and becomes hyperphosphorylated leading to the creation of neurofibrillary tangles (NFTs), characteristic of AD. In fact, there have also been observations regarding the interplay of both tau and neuroinflammation with emphasis on the idea of continuous inflammation in glia or neurons worsening tau pathology, thereby adding to the progression of AD. Tau increasingly became an important target for AD treatment over time with the development of active vaccines such as AADvac1 and ACI-35/ACI-35.030 and the use of passive immunotherapies or tau-targeting antibodies such as gosuranemab, tilavonemab, zagotenemab, and semorinemab that were trialed among others. In the context of diagnosis and detection, the use of phosphorylated tau (pTau) isoforms such as pTau181, pTau217, and pTau 231 have been explored for indicating increased levels of pTau within the bloodstream as these have been associated with neural tau pathology. The use of such isoforms may be especially useful in differential diagnosis of AD compared to other types of dementias or tau-related disorders which present differently and may also support research through monitoring of treatment effects as indicated via decreased pTau levels in AD pathology.

Additionally, there are two other key mechanisms that are potentially implicated in AD and lead to neuronal death: mitochondrial and proteasomal dysfunction. Aβ clumping disrupts mitochondrial activity, which impacts energy production negatively and leads to higher oxidative stress as well as neuronal death. Comparably, the presence of damaged or suboptimal functioning of ubiquitin-proteosome pathways in AD renders accrual of improperly folded or clumped proteins, thereby leading to death of neuronal cells. A study investigating the metabolic alterations in the brain correlated to AD has found that 298 metabolites across numerous pathways such as bioenergetics, metabolism of cholesterol, neuroinflammation, and neurotransmission are impacted by AD-correlated metabolic dysregulation and that these associations are heavily attributable to tau pathology. Lastly, a key focus is on neuroinflammation as can be witnessed by the activation of glia including astrocytes and microglia, a common feature of AD, and the reactivity of such cells as well as inflammatory responses aggravate $A\beta$ as well as tau pathology. Within neuroinflammation, GFAP, a protein seen primarily in astrocytes has been shown to be elevated in AD as astrocytes respond to damage of neuronal cells and $A\beta$ accumulation and thus is increasingly becoming of interest as a BBBM. Similarly, to tau and amyloid, levels of GFAP have been positively correlated with the degree of neuroinflammatory alteration in the brain and thus can support disease progression or treatment effectiveness monitoring.

The current treatment landscape for AD, which includes cholinesterase inhibitors like Donepezil and Galantamine, NMDA antagonists such as Memantine, and their combination formulations, has recently been augmented with the advent of disease-modifying immunotherapies like aducanumab and lecanemab. These newer therapies target the clearance of abnormal $A\beta$, marking a significant shift toward addressing the underlying pathology of the disease.

Expanding on this, the integration of blood-based biomarkers (BBBMs) into clinical practice offers a transformative potential not only in the realm of early detection but also in the continuous monitoring of disease progression in existing patients. With biomarkers such as plasma $A\beta42/40$ ratio and various pTau isoforms, clinicians now have the ability to track the biological changes occurring in the brain more closely. This enables a more dynamic approach to patient care, where treatment regimens can be tailored and adjusted based on real-time insights into the disease's progression. Additionally, the use of BBBMs facilitates a more nuanced understanding of individual patient responses to specific treatments. For example, the monitoring of specific biomarkers can reveal the efficacy of immunotherapies in reducing amyloid plaque burden, thereby guiding clinical decisions regarding treatment continuation or modification. This approach aligns with the principles of precision medicine, ensuring that patients receive therapies most suited to their unique disease profile and biological response.

7.11.3 Brain circuit activity in dementia

With the advent of improved technologies, AD research is increasingly able to focus and emphasize understanding of AD symptomatology that may occur due to dysregulations or disruptions in neural circuitry. A study by Grieco and researchers that emphasized the use of novel technologies such as single-cell, spatial, and circuit omics to probe neural circuit mechanisms in AD found that dysregulation early on within the entorhinal-hippocampal system is significantly associated with the progression of AD and thus provides insight to a circuit that may be a potential target for early-stage AD interventions. Additionally, research has found that changes in hippocampal circuitry are notable in AD with modulation in dendritic spine density of oriens lacunosum-moleculare (OLM) interneurons as well as a global increase in hyperactive and silent neurons in the cortex and hippocampal CA1 regions in AD models being found. Furthermore, in terms of tau pathology, results from Alzheimer's Disease Neuroimaging Initiative (ADNI) studies have shown a specific pattern of spread across neural circuitry that generally starts with clumping within the entorhinal cortex and continues spreading to other regions eventually, entering the hippocampus and cortical regions as well. This pattern, deduced as per PET imaging is also associated with the functional decline witnessed clinically [97]. Lee et al. further explored these patterns via cross-sectional analyses and the use of neuroimaging data that remote communication between amyloid- and tau-positive areas of the brain that are neuroanatomically linked support early spreading of tau, whereas closer interaction of amyloid and tau increase the progression of tau spreading outside of the entorhinal cortex [112].

Furthermore, studies using functional MRI have indicated changes in the functional memory network specifically, in the medial temporal lobe, responsible for declarative memory, in patients at risk of and with AD. In alignment with these findings, ADNI studies have also indicated changes such as decreased connectivity in the default mode network (DMN) in the context of AD, thereby reflective of the associated cognitive deficit progression and memory impairments. Neuroimaging modalities not only remain instrumental in the visualization of neuroanatomical regions impacted across stages of progression but have also been useful in the identification of biomarkers for clinical utility. As put forward by Lee et al., numerous modalities and associated findings must be further researched and utilized clinically to support the use of noninvasive, less costly biomarkers as opposed to the standard of care, PET. For instance, structural MRI has shown atrophy in the entorhinal cortex and hippocampus; however, it is key to note that, in MCI, one can expect a loss of gray matter in these regions, whereas, in AD, this atrophy would reach frontal, parietal, and temporal lobes. Similarly, DTI findings have shown damage of microstructures in white matter tracts with lower corpus callosum integrity and similarly reduced cohesion in the temporal brain area as well as the superior longitudinal fasciculus in AD that can be further analyzed by measuring quantitative metrics such as fractional anisotropy (FA) and mean diffusivity (MD). Moreover, the use of fMRI has also revealed changes in the activation and connectivity of the brain with hyper- and hypoactivation patterns seen in the medial temporal lobe as well as posterior cingulate gyrus when engaging in memory tasks. In addition to these circuit-based indicators, biomarkers based on alterations in metabolites such as lower levels of N-acetyl aspartate (NAA) as seen via magnetic resonance spectroscopy (MRS) and hypoperfusion in certain brain areas such as temporoparietal regions and posterior cingulate cortex as seen via arterial spin labeling (ASL) and single photon emission computed tomography (SPECT) may support research-based or clinically focused decision making regarding AD or other dementias.

Evaluating such findings is crucial as often disorders do not exist in a vacuum, and thus the impact of comorbidity can be seen even in the case of dementia on a circuitry level. For instance, Song et al. found that the amygdala-hippocampus connectivity that is necessary for affective memory and cognitive functioning is impacted by metabolic diseases due to an imbalance in fatty acids that render cognitive repercussions as well as anxious behaviors. Regarding dementia, they found atrophy in the amygdala to be correlated with impairment in memories tied to emotion; however, knowledge of contributors from multiple perspectives offers new avenues for multitargeted or layered detection, diagnosis, treatment, and ongoing management of this clinical population.

In summarizing the pivotal role of neural circuitry in AD, it is evident that a detailed understanding of changes in specific brain regions like the hippocampus, amygdala, and the DMN is crucial. These areas are intimately linked with the cognitive decline and neuropsychiatric symptoms characteristic of AD. Advanced neuroimaging techniques have shed light on these disruptions, revealing alterations in functional connectivity and neural network integrity even in early disease stages. Integrating these insights with biomarker-based classifications, including amyloid-beta, tau proteins, and genetic profiles, offers a comprehensive approach to diagnosis and management. This strategy enables the identification of distinct AD subgroups, facilitating personalized treatment plans tailored to individual disease progression. However, it is essential to recognize the influence of social determinants of health on dementia presentation and progression. This multifaceted approach, combining neural circuitry understanding with biomarker-based classifications and socio-health considerations, heralds a new era in AD management, aiming at more targeted therapies and improved patient outcomes.

7.12 Quality assurance and quality control in neuropsychiatry

7.12.1 Importance of quality in neuropsychiatry and mental health

The American Psychological Association (APA) defines quality assurance (QA) as a "*systematic process that is used to monitor and provide continuous improvement in the quality of health care services by evaluating the services in terms of effectiveness, appropriateness, and acceptability as well as offering feedback and implementing solutions to correct any identified deficiencies and assessing results.*" Although assumed to be interchangeable terms, the term, quality control (QC) refers to the "*process associated with research, production, or services that are designed to reduce the number of defective measurements and products.*" In a nutshell, quality assurance is an evaluation mechanism or framework to ensure goals of healthcare services are met and operational gaps are minimized to improve healthcare outcomes—in this case, related to mental health and neuropsychiatric diagnosis and care; whereas, quality control is the "gates" or checkpoints within this process that allows for improvements to occur and defective measurements or products to be reduced. Inherently both must be employed in conjunction with one another for optimal healthcare outcomes and sole focus on one or the other renders ineffective results. Without continual feedback, gap analysis and patient-centric framework in mind, healthcare systems cannot develop and evolve in the long term; whereas, without daily or annual quality control measures, stakeholders operating in the confines of the framework may not have visibility on how to ensure they are maximizing quality of care provided to patients. It may not be obvious as to how the quality of care can be measured or what this refers to. In this chapter, I will the quality of care based on the Donabedian framework, which would incorporate structure and organization of care, the impact of structure on clinical processes of care delivered via providers, and lastly, patient-based healthcare outcomes. This triad of mental health quality measures including structure, process, and outcome is reflected within national guidelines even today. The terms structure, process, and outcomes allow for the following questions to be answered, respectively:

i. Are sufficient healthcare personnel, theoretical and practical trainings, appropriate facilities, quality-enhancing infrastructure, information and technological systems, and systemic policies present to provide proper care?

ii. Are the processes based on evidence and are they being delivered?

iii. Is the care being provided improving clinical outcomes?

Quality assurance and quality control in mental health and neuropsychiatry both serve the purpose of tracking progress in differing temporal scales and continually evaluating mental health or neuropsychiatric services such as diagnosis, treatment, and ongoing clinical management of patients within these domains. The aim of QA and QC is to ensure that the performance of medical systems and healthcare practices are as close to *ideal standards of care* as possible and to provide the healthcare professional or other relevant parties indications toward areas for improvement. In 2001, the US-based report, "Cross the Quality Chasm" emphasized the six goals of improving healthcare quality which was for care to be "safe, effective, patient-centric, timely, efficient and equitable."

Given the high burden of disease of mental health disorders and severe disorders such as schizophrenia or bipolar disorders have led to premature mortality by 8—25 years compared to controls, it is no surprise that addressing health disparities and improving outcomes is a serious global priority. In fact, historically, literature concerning the quality of care and the patient's general check-ups regarding mental health and neuropsychiatric disorders has indicated significant variance between differing geographical regions and healthcare providers, which may not align with proposed standards by the healthcare profession. It is key to note that this difference in what is implemented during clinical practices and what is proposed by national guidelines or frameworks is an important opportunity to improve and optimize both, quality of care for patients and reduce the overall cost burden presented due to medical negligence or overtreatment. This being said, a study conducted in 2018 found that levels of quality for mental healthcare still remain relatively low, and the speed with which improvements have been made within the field is slower than for other medical domains, which have been mainly attributed to the lack of systematic methods for quality assessment. Kilbourne and team also acknowledged the following as challenges in establishing a systematic, standardized quality assessment:

I. Lack of consistent technology-based data sources
II. Limited scientific proof for measuring the quality of mental healthcare
III. Healthcare providers not getting enough training and support
IV. Cultural barriers that make it hard to combine mental healthcare with general healthcare.

Based on these challenges, authors have also suggested recommendations for improved mental healthcare such as providing healthcare insurers and payers patient-centric outcomes to measure improvements across disorders, integrating homogenous data types and features in existing information technology systems for medical records, and regularizing mental health check-ups to reduce any stigma or separation of mental health from the overarching medical infrastructure. Having a reliable and valid methodology to assess quality would enable one to effectively address gaps and support groups being burdened the most as a result of systemic gaps. However, these recommendations must consider the reality of mental health burden and pertinent quality assurance, or control also lies in the social context it is in and implementation, adherence, and uptake of quality measures. Although training and support for healthcare providers may be provided, the global shortage of mental health personnel and the lack of past capacity building remain a blockade in the context of low and middle-income countries (LMICs) wherein 85% of patient populations have no accessibility to care. Endale et al. found that challenges for quality assurance in LMICs include convolution in measuring an intervention's effect or results, variances in the language used, assessing, or providing treatment in informal delivery settings, and the presence of emergencies like natural disasters regionally, which can all impact the outcomes of interventions employed. From a resource perspective, QA and QC can be intensive and require spending on infrastructure-based changes or the addition of better technology or adaptation to account for aforementioned contextual realities, which can also reduce QA capacity by constraining how regular or what type of assessments are used. Second, a participant in the study emphasized the requirement to have benchmarks to understand quality assurance results and monitoring or evaluations to make investment, implementation, and thresholding decisions for assessments and interventions. A trade-off between the flexibility to maximize appropriateness and sustainability of clinical practice versus the need to strictly follow evidence base to ensure reliability and higher supervision was noted during implementation.

To create unified processes for quality that may eventually be globally employable, there must be increased research activity within this niche to assess the health benefits that may be conferred by injecting funding and improving resource allocation for quality assurance and control. However, a recent study did show that there exists a positive correlation between indicators of higher research activity with better quality of care outcomes in psychiatry and this was also indicated clinically by lowered rates of readmissions for individuals with psychoses, accounting for 8.2% of variation when considering impact of other factors. Similarly, the study by Endale and team also found that using impactful frameworks to document pathways and processes to implement is considered to as a key success factor for quality assurance implementation. Additionally, longitudinal tracking and monitoring of progress after the initial implementation and integrating the service to appropriately transition to a governmental healthcare system were also seen as success factors for enhanced clinical translation of interventions for wider patient populations. Regardless of challenges, examples of research-centric projects being clinically translated with quality assurance and patient-centricity exist in both high-income countries (HICs) and LMICs. Two patient-centric, lasting research projects conducted in German outpatient psychotherapy systems assessing a QA and feedback system for feasibility into routine care systems and a new methodology for QA utilizing electronic documentation of patient features and outcome parameters. Across both studies, a triadic collaborative effort between mental healthcare personnel, researchers, and health providers such as insurers and service institutions lead to successful outcomes. In addition to these findings, patients were also interested in and receptive toward incorporating psychometric data collected into clinical translation and felt more engaged given their assigned mental healthcare professional was encouraging of it. Comparably, a quality assurance model called QualiND, a multilevel, video-assisted iterative model utilizing remote evaluation, feedback system, and supervision, was rolled out to evaluate the possibility of systematizing neurodevelopment evaluation in sub-Saharan Africa. By providing workshop training with the support of QA center staff who were sufficiently experienced in the domain, delivering refresher training annually regarding best practices and processes and reviewing standard operating procedures (SOPs) on a quarterly basis, high levels of compliance, and test completion were achieved with valid, reliable, and consistent test results.

Benchmarking the efficiency and performance of the medical system around prediction, diagnosis, treatment, and clinical management into measurable outcomes can allow for enhanced understanding for healthcare professionals and policymakers alike while also informing them where improvements can be made from an interpersonal and systemic level, respectively. In the 1990s, approximately 6% of the National Health Service costs in England were driven by patients with schizophrenia, and thus actions to minimize both, costs to medical systems and governances, as well as a burden on patient populations and their caretakers, have since remained a fundamental priority. Similarly, a year later, a study examining patterns of care in schizophrenia against the patient outcomes research treatment recommendations at the time surveyed how patient treatment aligned with the recommendations that were in place and found that they were not conformed to more than 50% of the time with adherence being higher for pharmacological interventions as opposed to psychosocial and even lower overall for patients who were ethnic minorities. Several other studies have also demonstrated that among people suffering from mental disorders, the inequalities in terms of quality of care received and related mental health outcomes are more severe among racial as well as ethnic minorities and those who are from a lower socioeconomic status. Clearly, there are high costs to patients, payers, and providers when quality assurance and control measures are not in place for mental health and neuropsychiatric disorders from a clinical perspective. The dearth of implementable systems is only further exacerbated on the research side, which is siloed and responsible for the generation of the knowledge necessary to implement optimal systems. The gap in terms of information on how severe mental disorders are addressed across various countries, the quality of care being provided across different medical systems, and investment in measurement or calibration of quality and reporting feedback systems is immense. Additionally, Mainz and Bartles have previously found that investing in the measurement and systems would significantly increase opportunities for quality enhancement. Evidently, the information and implementation gaps must be addressed by quality assurance research in neuropsychiatric disorders and mental health disorders as well as translated effectively to clinics for patients who need it the most. This chapter aims to not just call for action in this niche but also provide further insights into the conceptual frameworks and practice-based applications that may be employed for quality assurance and control to enhance quality in clinical care and research within neuropsychiatry.

7.13 Importance of quality for neurology/neurosurgery in clinical research

Evidence-based neurosurgery represents a practice paradigm where the best available evidence guides the principles of diagnosis and treatment. This approach, rooted in evidence-based medicine (EBM), relies on high-quality evidence, categorized as level I and level II evidence, to inform clinical decisions. Despite EBM being the gold standard in medicine, studies estimate that only 10%−25% of clinical decisions in various medical fields, including neurosurgery, are based on such high-quality evidence. In 2011, the Grading of Recommendations Assessment, Development, and Evaluation (GRADE) system was introduced, offering an outcome-centric approach to rate the quality of evidence derived from diverse study types. Although GRADE guidelines enable the assessment of evidence quality and the strength of recommendations in systematic reviews and clinical guidelines, neurosurgery still predominantly employs the traditional levels of evidence rather than GRADE guidelines.

Noteworthy investigations by Rothoerl et al. [113] and Yarascavitch et al. [114] into the levels of evidence in neurosurgical literature for the years 1999 and 2009−10, respectively, revealed that only a modest percentage (22.8% and 10.3%) of evidence was categorized as higher-level evidence (level I or level II). Particularly, level I evidence from randomized controlled trials with consistent results was scarce, found in only 3.8% and 2.1% of the evaluated papers in the respective studies. These findings suggest a potential shift in surgeon engagement with research, as indicated by decreasing grant applications, reduced publication activity, and a perceived diminished role of research in their professional responsibilities compared to a decade or two ago. It is emphasized that participation in research not only enhances the rigor of surgeons' daily work but also contributes to the assessment, maintenance, and enhancement of the overall quality of work within the surgical community.

Martens et al. conducted a ground-breaking study, representing the first comprehensive evaluation of neurosurgeons' opinions on evidence usage in multiple countries. Despite the global acknowledgment of level I and level II evidence as high quality, only 48.5% of respondents (84/173) considered either level I or levels I and II to be of high quality. Interestingly, the majority of neurosurgeons seem to utilize all levels of evidence, with some expressing concerns about the scarcity of evidence in neurosurgery. Historically, neurosurgical advancements were often driven by technical innovations advocated by pioneers without rigorous clinical trial assessments. This led to technology-driven changes in clinical practice rather than strictly evidence-based approaches. The study highlights a potential misalignment between everyday clinical management in neurosurgery and the best available evidence.

Comparing neurosurgery with other medical specialties, the study reveals that while neurosurgery employs a higher percentage of high-level evidence than certain specialties, it still lags behind others. The transition from rating guidelines using levels of evidence to the GRADE system is noted, with the GRADE system offering advantages in rating evidence quality and strength of recommendations. Noteworthy findings include the observation that some neurosurgeons feel that neurosurgery relies more on eminence than evidence, emphasizing the importance of critical appraisal of scientific evidence. The study also underscores the need for formal training in EBM within the neurosurgical curriculum to enhance the interpretation of statistical outcomes. Additionally, the study advocates for the integration of shared decision making (SDM) alongside EBM, recognizing the importance of patient and caregiver knowledge in treatment decisions. Despite some limitations in response rates and potential biases, the study provides valuable insights into the state of evidence-based practice in neurosurgery and highlights the necessity for ongoing efforts to bridge gaps between evidence-based principles and clinical decision making in the field.

The healthcare landscape in the United States is undergoing significant changes, necessitating a demand for quality data across various aspects of neurological surgery. With a shift toward incorporating quality into payment calculations, both public and private insurers are emphasizing value over quantity. The healthcare industry is witnessing rapid consolidation as hospitals and healthcare systems strive to position themselves effectively in the evolving landscape of accountable care organizations and patient-centered medical homes. Consumers are increasingly seeking information about the quality of care they receive. The US Department of Health and Human Services (HHS) is taking steps to measure quality through programs like CAHPS, Physician Compare, and Hospital Compare. However, there is recognition that these initiatives may fall short in providing comprehensive information about neurosurgical quality. The uncertainty of the future has led many physicians to opt for the safety of employment within hospitals or physician groups. Medical practices are grappling with the challenge of navigating both fee-for-service reimbursement and the transition to value-based contracting and bundled payments in the post-ACA era.

Amid these challenges, neurosurgery is actively addressing the need for quality data. The NeuroPoint Alliance has developed the National Neurosurgery Quality and Outcomes Database (N2QOD), the first national risk-adjusted quality and outcomes database for organized neurosurgery. In its early years, N2QOD has shown promise in validating procedures, predicting outcomes, and educating patients about potential surgical results. The database is continuously evolving to encompass a broader range of conditions, starting with modules focused on the lumbar and cervical spine, with plans for vascular and spinal deformity modules. For socioeconomic data, several sources collect information on salary, call pay, and productivity voluntarily from participants. Entities like Sullivan Cotter and the Medical Group Management Association (MGMA) conduct surveys on hospitals, health systems, and medical practices. The Neurosurgery Executives' Resource Value and Resource Society (NERVES) produces the largest neurosurgery socioeconomic survey, focusing exclusively on neurosurgery practice. Although discrepancies may exist among the survey results, these data points play a crucial role in negotiations, especially concerning compensation and call pay. As healthcare costs rise, and resources become constrained, the importance of quality data becomes increasingly vital. The future necessitates active participation from providers in obtaining accurate and meaningful data to inform decision making. Relying on third parties for data collection may result in inaccuracies and unfavorable outcomes.

A study conducted in Germany by Schumann et al. in the field of neurosurgery showed a significant aspect of the daily routine involves addressing emergency room admissions and acute cases from various departments or external hospitals. Despite the crucial nature of this acute care, it is often not accounted for in performance metrics or budget management, and its quantitative and qualitative aspects are not systematically analyzed for neurosurgeons. To address this gap, a comprehensive 1-year study was conducted in a large northern German city, where all acute care cases handled by two on-call neurosurgical teams were meticulously recorded and analyzed. This initiative resulted in a substantial database of 1819 entries, allowing for in-depth examination using descriptive statistics. The treatment of additional patients requiring acute care, sourced from the emergency room or other healthcare facilities, is an integral part of the daily responsibilities of neurosurgical units. Unfortunately, this critical work is frequently overlooked in performance evaluations that typically focus on easily accessible measures such as hospital occupancy, admission rates, duration of stay, and annual operation numbers. The efforts of on-call teams, often comprised of surgeons fulfilling additional duties alongside their elective responsibilities, are not adequately reflected in these conventional metrics.

The study aimed to shed light on the often-ignored daily activities of neurosurgical on-call teams, emphasizing the need for a more nuanced approach in assessing the quality and impact of their performance.

The research focused on the daily activities of two neurosurgical on-call teams in Hannover, Germany, with the objective of documenting and analyzing the quantity and quality of neurosurgical on-call activities. The resulting databank comprised over 1800 patient contacts and 114,500 data entries, representing a substantial portion of neurosurgical acute care and emergency cases within the city over 1 year. The findings highlight the importance of addressing deficits in the treatment chain and gathering epidemiological data on acute neurosurgical diseases. Additionally, the study advocates for a more comprehensive understanding of the challenges faced by neurosurgical departments, especially in the context of budget constraints and resource limitations outlined in current public health policies. The study revealed that while traumatic brain injury and intracranial hemorrhage were prevalent, they constituted only 50% of all cases. The incidence of traumatic brain injury in the studied population was notably lower than in the United States, attributed in part to the exclusion of minor head injuries treated in peripheral hospitals. Subarachnoid hemorrhage, with a presumed incidence similar to other western countries, was less common than intracerebral hemorrhage. The data also highlighted demographic differences between patients from peripheral hospitals and those admitted through the emergency room, emphasizing the need for targeted approaches in neurosurgical care.

In conclusion, the study underscores the critical role of neurosurgical on-call teams in addressing acute cases and emergencies. It emphasizes the necessity of recognizing and analyzing the often-overlooked aspects of their work to improve overall patient outcomes, resource utilization, and the reputation of neurosurgical departments. The findings suggest a need for increased resources, staff, and a dedicated team structure to meet the demands of neurosurgical acute care effectively.

Neurocritical care (NCC) stands as a multidisciplinary subspecialty intersecting neurology, neurosurgery, and critical care, dedicated to the intricate treatment of critically ill patients grappling with life-threatening neurologic and neurosurgical conditions. The evolution of NCC into a distinct subspecialty has become apparent over the last 2 decades. This is marked by the establishment of dedicated neuro-ICUs (NCCUs) designed to cater to the specific needs of its patient demographic. The emergence of neurointensivists and specialized nurses trained in NCC, the formation of the Neurocritical Care Society (NCS) in 2002, and the creation of unique board certifications and fellowships through organizations such as the United Council of Neurologic Subspecialties (UCNS) and the Accreditation Council for Graduate Medical Education (ACGME) further solidify NCC's status. Additionally, the field has seen the development of clinical and translational research networks, along with the publication of clinical guidelines and performance measures for various NCC pathologies.

Concurrently, advancements in implementation science and quality improvement (QI) have been instrumental in shaping the landscape of NCC. Influential works such as the Institute of Medicine's "Crossing the Quality Chasm" and the Agency for Healthcare Research and Quality's "Making Healthcare Safer" have provided a framework for understanding healthcare quality. The six domains of healthcare quality—safe, effective, patient-centered, timely, efficient, and equitable—established by the IOM have become a cornerstone in QI programs and performance measure development. The Centers for Medicare and Medicaid Services (CMS) have also played a role through initiatives like the Hospital Inpatient Quality Reporting Program, defining QI as a systematic approach to standardize processes and structures, aiming to reduce variation and enhance outcomes. Comparatively, subspecialties like stroke and critical care have made significant strides in QI research. Stroke, for instance, has witnessed the formulation of disease-specific guidelines, certifications, and performance improvement programs, fostering evidence-based practices and improving patient outcomes. Critical care has similarly seen advancements with intensivist-led staffing models and structured processes, as evident in guidelines and toolkits.

In the realm of NCC, the focus has shifted from demonstrating the impact of subspecialty providers on patient outcomes to a broader scope of QI initiatives. Noteworthy publications now include detailed recommendations for NCCU structures, evidence-based guidelines, performance measure sets, and investigations into optimal NCCU structure, staffing, education, and process improvement. The establishment of the NCS Quality Committee in 2016 signifies a commitment to furthering NCC QI initiatives and research, underscoring the ongoing maturation and commitment to excellence in neurocritical care.

The PRINCE study marked a pivotal moment in understanding the global landscape of NCC delivery. This point prevalence study, encompassing 257 centers across 47 countries, unveiled the spectrum of neurocritical conditions admitted to neurocritical care units (NCCUs). The most prevalent diagnoses included acute ischemic stroke, intracerebral hemorrhage (ICH), subarachnoid hemorrhage (SAH), traumatic brain and spinal cord injuries, neuromuscular weakness, status epilepticus, and hypoxic-ischemic injury. Strikingly, the study revealed a wide variance in the specialties of providers caring for NCC patients globally. In the United States, for instance, the study found that 21% of providers identified their specialty as NCC, while 38% were from pulmonary critical care medicine (PCCM), 16% from ACC, 5% from surgical critical care (SCC), 2.5% from neurosurgery, and 17% from other specialties. The study highlighted that, depending on the geographical region, a single nonintensivist often served as the primary provider for 3 to 10 patients. Moreover, NCCUs reported utilizing disease-specific treatment protocols between 40% and 90% of the time, depending on the specific pathology. Given the substantial morbidity and costs associated with these neurocritical conditions, the existence of numerous evidence-based guidelines, and the diverse array of providers involved, there is a compelling case for leveraging QI techniques to enhance NCC patient care. However, the state of QI efforts in NCCUs remained largely unknown until a survey by Lele et al. in 2020. This survey, drawing responses from 225 Neurocritical Care Society (NCS) participants, revealed that 45% reported having a dedicated

NCC QI program, and 44% had dedicated NCC QI personnel. Intriguingly, 88% reported the presence of a dedicated hospital-wide QI program, indicating a potential discrepancy in the attention given to NCC within broader institutional QI initiatives. The survey also identified insufficient resources from hospitals or academic departments as the primary self-reported barrier to QI efforts. Additionally, awareness of NCC-specific performance measures (PMs) was varied, with 88% for Comprehensive Stroke (CSTK), 57% for Trauma Quality Improvement Program (TQIP), and 54% for the American Academy of Neurology (AAN) Inpatient and Emergent Neurology Measure Set. The findings underscored the need to enhance awareness of existing NCC PMs and expand QI resources, emphasizing the importance of aligning these efforts with the unique challenges and complexities of neurocritical care.

The existing variability in organizational structures and patient care models, coupled with geographical differences in access to care, has the potential to magnify health disparities. Numerous studies have underscored the impact of organizational factors on the quality of NCC and subsequent patient outcomes. For instance, research by Suarez et al. revealed that the implementation of an NCC team led by a neurointensivist was associated with a significant reduction in mortality and length of stay. Similarly, a systematic review by Kramer et al. demonstrated lower mortality and improved neurologic outcomes in specialty NCCUs, led by neurointensivist-led teams. These specialized teams also showed additional benefits such as cost savings and a decreased need for ventriculoperitoneal shunts in patients with SAH. The correlation between patient volume and clinical outcomes has been established in various NCC conditions. Low-volume centers, treating fewer than 10 cases per year for SAH, were associated with worse outcomes compared to high-volume centers treating more than 35 cases per year. Similarly, centers with higher volumes of ICH cases demonstrated increased survival rates. High-volume centers for ischemic stroke thrombectomy were linked to better survival and functional outcomes. Recognizing these volume-outcome associations, The Joint Commission (TJC) includes the presence of an NCCU as a prerequisite for achieving designation as a comprehensive stroke center. To address the challenges faced by low-volume hospitals, the American Stroke Association recommends implementing processes to facilitate the transfer of stroke patients to experienced high-volume centers with neurosurgical and NCC capabilities when necessary. In the realm of traumatic brain injury (TBI), research by Grieve et al. indicated that early transfer of TBI patients to a specialist neuroscience center was associated with reduced mortality and higher quality of life compared to late or no transfer. Moreover, the management of TBI patients in a dedicated NCCU, as opposed to a general ICU, was deemed likely more cost-effective. These findings underscore the importance of organizational structures, team expertize, and patient volume in shaping the quality of NCC and highlight the need for standardized approaches to optimize patient care and outcomes in diverse healthcare settings.

Several NCC disease conditions stand to benefit significantly from care in a dedicated NCCU due to the severity of illnesses and the requirement for highly specialized resources. Some of these conditions include large hemispheric and cerebellar strokes necessitating hemicraniectomy or suboccipital craniectomy, severe aneurysmal SAH, and ICH requiring interventions like external ventricular drain (EVD), decompression, clot evacuation, aneurysm coil embolization, or clip ligation, refractory status epilepticus demanding continuous electroencephalogram monitoring, and severe TBI necessitating intracranial pressure monitoring, intracranial hypertension management, and/or decompression. Given the importance of directing NCC patients to the appropriate level of care, it is crucial to design systems that recognize institutional capabilities, leveraging local resources and clinical networks to ensure optimal patient care. For acute stroke, stroke program certification standards, such as The Joint Commission's Comprehensive, Thrombectomy-Capable, and Primary Stroke Center designations, provide a framework for delivering care in the best environment and establishing benchmarks for data-driven performance improvement. The American Stroke Association's "Recommendations for the Establishment of Stroke Systems of Care" details how Emergency Medical Services (EMSs) and hospitals can use these designations for triaging stroke patients from the field and for hospital-to-hospital transfers. Recognizing the need for a similar framework for other NCC disease conditions, the NCS published "Standards for Neurologic Critical Care Units" in 2018. These standards outline best practices for structural measures, categorizing NCCUs into levels I, II, or III based on their care capabilities. Level I NCCUs provide comprehensive services for the care of the most complex patients, including advanced monitoring, surgical and medical therapies, fellowship-trained neurointensivists, and training capabilities for physicians and advanced practice providers. Level II NCCUs deliver comprehensive neurocritical care but may not have the same advanced monitoring or dedicated neurocritical care fellowship-trained personnel as Level I NCCUs. Level III NCCUs are equipped to evaluate and stabilize neurological emergencies and facilitate transfer to Level I and II centers. The NCS NCCU standards offer detailed recommendations on interprofessional care and teamwork, quality and safety infrastructure, clinical operations and administration, equipment, and education and training. Leadership structures, interprofessional teams, and equipment are tailored to the level of care provided. The development of a culture of safety, supported by leadership, adverse event reporting, and closed-loop communication strategies, is emphasized to achieve high reliability of care within the NCCU. To advance QI programs, formal education and training are widely available. The Institute for Healthcare Improvement (IHI) Open School and online training in Lean Six Sigma methodology offer resources, and health organizations increasingly provide programs embedding core QI concepts within local systems. When developing an NCC QI program, a structured approach is recommended, considering elements such as defining priorities, establishing structure and leadership, implementing information technology, allocating resources, collecting and analyzing data, and disseminating information.

Standardizing processes of care is crucial in improving outcomes in the Neurocritical Care Unit (NCCU). Several approaches and interventions have been explored to enhance care quality and patient safety in the NCCU context:

1. Adaptation of critical care bundles: Similar to general critical care, the NCCU benefits from the implementation of evidence-based strategies. For instance, the Society of Critical Care Medicine's (SCCM) "ICU Liberation Campaign" emphasizes spontaneous awakening and breathing trials, and early mobility to reduce harm from common ICU conditions. However, these interventions need to be adapted to the unique characteristics of NCC patients, considering factors such as elevated intracranial pressure

2. Prevention of hospital-acquired infections (HAIs): NCC patients, with nervous system dysfunction, are particularly vulnerable to infections. Strategies to reduce HAIs, including catheter-associated urinary tract infections (CAUTIs), catheter-associated line infections (CLABSIs), and ventilator-associated events (VAEs), have shown success. Interventions may involve reviewing urinary catheter use, reeducating personnel, and minimizing patient transports for procedures

3. Prevention of ventriculostomy-related infections (VRIs): Patients with EVDs in the NCCU are at risk of ventriculostomy-related infections. Implementation of comprehensive EVD bundles, emphasizing aseptic techniques, has been shown to significantly reduce VRI rates

4. Use of standardized pathology-specific order sets: The use of standardized order sets tailored to specific pathologies, such as stroke and TBI, is recommended. These sets improve adherence to best practices and can lead to better patient outcomes

5. Implementation of bedside rounding tools and standardized handoffs: Standardized communication tools and handoffs have been shown to improve information transfer and positively influence patient, provider, and organizational outcomes. Electronic multidisciplinary rounding tools and structured handoffs using established formats contribute to improved communication

6. Prevention of rapid returns to the ICU ("Bouncebacks"): NCCU patients are susceptible to rapid returns to the ICU after transfer to a floor service. Interventions to prevent bouncebacks include risk stratification, enhanced handoff processes, and transfer checklists

7. Improvement of interhospital transfers (IHTs): Given the complexity and financial impact of IHT, interventions such as guideline dissemination, process redesign, and electronic enhancements have been effective in reducing emergency department boarding times and improving overall efficiency

8. Optimization of other NCCU processes: Various QI strategies have been applied to other NCCU processes, including the transition to comfort care, clinical documentation strategies, palliative care consultation, and deep vein thrombosis (DVT) chemoprophylaxis

These QI strategies underscore the importance of tailoring interventions to the unique characteristics and challenges of neurocritical care, ensuring that they align with the specific needs of NCC patients. Standardization, adaptation, and continuous evaluation are key elements in enhancing the quality of care provided in the NCCU.

7.13.1 Performance measures as quality control steps

Monitoring and tracking PMs in critical care settings, including NCC, is crucial for ensuring the delivery of high-quality care and improving patient outcomes. Institutions may focus on various critical care-specific PMs. These include fundamental measures such as hand hygiene to reduce healthcare-associated infections (HAIs). Patient outcomes measures encompass parameters like ICU mortality, length of stay (LOS) exceeding 7 days, average ICU LOS, average days on mechanical ventilation, and evaluations of pain management and patient/family satisfaction. Process measures involve assessing the effectiveness of pain management, appropriate blood transfusion use, prevention of ventilator-associated pneumonia, sedation practices, and prophylaxis for conditions like peptic ulcers and deep venous thrombosis. Access measures include evaluating rates of delayed admissions, delayed discharges, canceled surgical cases, and emergency department bypass hours. Complication measures involve tracking rates of unplanned ICU readmission, central line-associated bloodstream infections (CLABSI), and resistant infections. Additionally, rates of various HAIs, including CLABSI, CAUTIs, surgical site infections (SSIs), and VAEs, are monitored. Other general critical care PMs encompass 30-day mortality, mortality index, in-hospital falls, adherence to daily rounding checklists, percentages of elevated glucose values, ICU LOS, head-of-bed elevation, lung-protective ventilation, early and adequate antibiotic therapy, and early enteral nutrition. Regularly monitoring these measures enables healthcare institutions to identify areas for improvement, implement targeted interventions, and enhance overall patient care and safety in critical care and NCC units.

The distinct subspecialty focus of NCC, coupled with the increasing prevalence of evidence-based practices, has led to the development of specific PMs tailored to NCC patients. These PMs address various neurological conditions and are formulated by authoritative bodies such as TJC, the American Heart Association/American Stroke Association (AHA/ASA), the AAN, the NCS, and the TQIP. Notably, these PMs encompass measures related to stroke, inpatient and emergency neurology, NCC, and TBI. The existence of these specialized PM sets reflects the evolving understanding of NCC and the need for targeted metrics to assess and enhance the quality of care provided to patients in this subspecialty.

Effectively utilizing PMs can lead to improvements in patient outcomes, as demonstrated by initiatives such as the preprocedure checklist for reducing CLABSIs. This checklist, initially tested at Johns Hopkins Medical Institutions and subsequently implemented widely across US hospitals, has become a reportable PM to the Centers for Medicare and Medicaid Services (CMS). The Agency for Healthcare Research and Quality's (AHRQ) national scorecard on Hospital-Acquired Conditions highlighted improved patient care associated with PM tracking, with reductions in *Clostridium difficile* infections, venous thromboembolism cases, ventilator-associated pneumonias, CLABSIs, CAUTIs, and falls in hospitals between 2014 and 2017. Among NCC measures, the adoption of Get with The Guidelines (GWTG) measures was linked to significant reductions in mortality at 6 months and 1 year, as well as increased discharges home at 1 year. Additionally, a study comparing stroke patients receiving thrombectomy directly admitted versus secondarily transferred found better outcomes for directly admitted patients. Although NCC measures are not currently reportable to CMS, the positive impact on patient care suggests that adopting robust NCC PMs in the future could further enhance outcomes. Managing a large number of PMs can be challenging and implementing a PM dashboard can provide a visual tool for organizing and monitoring QI initiatives. Creating a PM dashboard involves several crucial steps, including determining its type and purpose, assembling a dedicated team, setting objectives, defining included PMs, establishing benchmarks, specifying PM details, devising a data collection plan, deciding on display methods, establishing a dissemination plan, developing a review and action plan, gathering baseline data, determining a pilot period, and continually exploring new PMs for inclusion. Quality tools commonly used in dashboards include run charts, control charts, bar graphs, and pie charts.

7.14 Conceptual frameworks and practice-based applications used to optimize quality assurance in neuropsychiatric clinical care and optimizing mental healthcare

In 2015, the European Psychiatric Association (EPA) issued a guidance regarding quality assurance in mental healthcare consisting of 17 graded recommendations bifurcated into three groups: structures, processes, and outcomes, also in resonance with the Donabedian framework referred to previously. The recommendations were also further categorized by vantage point and layer of analysis into macro-, meso- and microlevels. In this case, the macro level refers to national or regional policy as it pertains to mental health and the way it is organized including fairness, continuity, and exhaustiveness. Second, analysis was conducted on a meso-level, which refers to the setting in which the healthcare service is provided including but not limited to primary care facilities and outpatient or inpatient psychiatric hospitals Lastly, the most detailed or core level analyzed for the recommendations is in regard to the individual direct healthcare benefits conferred by people that suffer from mental disorders such as psychotherapy, pharmacological interventions, psychotherapy or specialized formats of support such as cognitive behavioral therapy (CBT), dialectical behavior therapy (DBT), and eye movement desensitization and reprocessing (EMDR) therapy.

In 2017, the need for benchmarking practices was a major call to action vocalized by the Organization for Economic Cooperation and Development (OECD), which then developed a report called A New Benchmark for Mental Health Systems to support countries in their imminent goal of providing high-quality care via highly efficacious mental health systems. This report was a global effort with collaboration between numerous stakeholders and key opinion leaders (KOLs) across countries in the OECD. The following consensus was achieved as to the functional role of a highly efficacious mental health system:

- Being individual-centric, focused on the patient or person who is undergoing the experience of distressed mental health
- Providing accessible and high-quality mental health services
- Approaching mental health from a unified and multisectoral perspective
- Preventing mental illness and disorders as well as promoting individual's mental well-being
- Holding robust leadership and proper governance
- Having foresight and remaining focused on future innovations

Although measures were recognized per dimension to track the progress and performance of mental health systems, it is crucial to note that in terms of practical feasibility, only two measures out of 23 were found to be available for every OECD country. These two measures were life satisfaction and death by suicide; whereas, challenges were seen in areas of importance including measuring stigma, coverage of services by insurers, and improvement due to the intervention and as seen in outcomes and experiences by patients as well as healthcare personnel or carers.

Thus, in 2018, the OECD Mental Health System Performance Framework created the values or aims and the criteria for how to achieve such goals to benchmark the performance of a mental health system.

To achieve the first goal of being individual-centered, the framework focuses on making sure the person feels like they have autonomy of the decision making process linked to their care. This ensure the person feels respected and where appropriate, their caretakers, family members' feelings are included as part of their patient journey. Additionally, the emphasis in mental health must lie in personalized healthcare and be personalized to the individual's requirements from the treatment, healthcare personnel, and well-being goals in a manner that is culturally, age- and gender-wise appropriate. Lastly, the patient as a result must feel empowered and supported to actualize their own capabilities and feel that they can function and contribute to society. To ensure neuropsychiatric treatment is enhancing a person's quality of life and not just confined to symptomatic remission, it is crucial to incorporate these treatments into a holistic intervention that finds itself stemming from the biopsycho-social model. According to findings by Rief and team in 2016, medications need to be employed in conjunction with socially supportive environments to be completely impactful. A study by Whitley and Drake recognized five lenses through which recovery may be observed, that is, clinical, existential, social, functional, and physical, which may support in viewing individual health holistically. Thus, the goal of individual-centered has validity in ensuring personal growth and development values in contrast to institution-focused or population-focused care systems, which may forgo personal needs to offer one-size-fits-all interventions.

The second measure of a high-performing mental health system lies in its ability to be accessible and provide mental health services of high quality. This is in alignment with the metrics employed to measure our progress on the provision of Universal Health Care as defined by the World Health Organization (WHO), in measuring how countries ensure that everyone has access to the healthcare they require appropriately in terms of timeliness, geographical accessibility and with undue financial duress to achieve healthcare services. According to the OECD framework, high-quality services must be based on evidence and created closely to the community of impact and provided in a timely fashion. Additionally, these services must remain inclusive of and respectful toward the patient population being addressed and provide enhancement of the patient's conditions in a safe manner and ideally be integrated within the overarching medical system's infrastructure to allow continuity of care.

However, a major practical consideration that must be accounted for is the financial limiters that often exist granted that prescribers have a certain number of interactions with a patient and have to rely on information transmission via social workers or other mental healthcare personnel in regard to the patient's progress to help understand what treatments to prescribe, what the patient response and profile looks like at any given time point and for the duration for which the patient must remain on the treatment. Additionally, given that the mental health personnel who partake in quality assurance and improvement (QA/I) are key to health outcomes, it is imperative to understand how they perceive their role within the system to ensure high-quality services, what their roles incorporate, what milestones or targets for QA/I resemble in terms of a system with high-quality services, and what their contributions to ensuring these systems are. A study conducted at Washington University in St. Louis found that there were major discrepancies in how personnel conducting QA/I activities portrayed their role with some focusing on chart and data review while others emphasized survey data and monitoring. Not just daily tasks but even overall objectives were focused on varying aspects of the QA/I role with some personnel focused on creating a strategy to meet objectives, whereas others emphasized gap analysis in processes and optimization; however, a common theme was ensuring external frameworks or guidance correlated with national accreditation standards are met. Targets were mainly in place to track and enhance the provision of services, safety, patient perspectives and health outcomes, internal staff outlook and challenges, community perspective, and maximizing overall yield while optimizing finances, but the degree to which one or another target was emphasized differed across agencies. By and large, a common consensus among QA/I personnel was that most targets did not focus on metrics that denote high-quality service provision such as the sensitivity of interpersonal interactions between healthcare personnel and client or technical skill of the providers. Instead, measures of success emphasized the presence of a treatment plan for the patient, the presence of progress monitoring notes regarding the patient, and the assessment of the appropriateness of the selected treatment for the associated medical concern or diagnosis as opposed to evaluating the reliability of evidence-based interventions. Generally, there remains a lack of consensus on the function of QA/I across agencies conducting this work within the mental health field and has steered from its intended purpose of enhancing quality to ensuring compliance, thus, would greatly benefit from a mindset shift to reframe objectives to refocus on improving quality of care and patient health outcomes or experiences.

From a macrolevel, an effective mental health system approaches an individual's mental health from an integrated, multisectoral manner which essentially means that mental health is accounted for across policies being implemented. The system ensures that all individuals' physiological or physical requirements are being catered to as well and allows for the affected individuals to be linked to the appropriate healthcare resources, services, and medical personnel who can adequately support their conditions. Lastly, mental healthcare systems must not be limited to returning a patient state to full remission only but also have methodologies or systems of social support and protection for individuals that support their venture into or return to work, education, or otherwise. Having such a focus can allow for the patient to not just heal from the disorder but also integrate into society effectively and feel supported in this transition. In fact, in the past 51 years, the mental healthcare landscape has been evolving toward accessible community-based mental healthcare and these reforms have notably been documented across five countries: Serbia, Turkey, Ukraine, Georgia, and Kyrgyzstan. A common theme emerging across the case studies of these countries is the gaps in mental healthcare for young children and adolescents, that is, within the fields of child psychiatry who require special mental healthcare and inefficient financial prioritization. Similarly, to initiatives being undertaken by respective governments, there is a focus required on capacity building from mental health personnel and availability of care facilities perspective.

For instance, a National Strategy for Development of Mental Health Care that was permitted in 2007 recognized deinstitutionalization and creation of community service as key features that could support transforming neuropsychiatric healthcare in Serbia. In alignment with approaching mental healthcare in an inclusive manner, the Ministry of Health (MOH) of the Republic of Serbia identified community mental healthcare to be provided at centers specialized for mental health and thus, opened five such centers however, this only provided coverage for 2.3% of the entire geographical region. The goals set out by the National Program for Protection of Mental Health in the country aimed for 2026 incorporate strategies such as restructuring the network of psychiatry centers, enhancing current mental health services across hospitals, and a steady decrease in number of institutionalized patients associated with a corresponding decrease in hospital beds for the same purpose. In doing so, their focus is also on the progression of the preventive measures for psychiatric disorders, shifting focus upstream in terms of tackling neurodevelopmental and mental health illness in younger populations, providing support for reassimilation into the workforce, assisting geriatric populations, and capacity building for improved mental healthcare services to increase coverage by 13.7%.

Similarly, Turkey introduced a consolidated program in 2006 to provide accessible community healthcare services, and due to this, 177 community mental health centers have been established in collaboration with state hospitals, wherein personnel can get formal education and training as well as academic centers and mental health hospitals. Akin to Serbia, these efforts occurred simultaneously with the restructuring and reduction of mental health beds within inpatient facilities. Like Serbia, in alignment with the priorities placed on targeting interventions and care for younger patient populations, the Ministry of Family and Social Policies addressed autism spectrum disorder (ASD) by focusing on dedicated healthcare for the disorder and associated progressive delay in younger children.

These challenges in terms of lack of development for child and adolescent mental healthcare, psychosocial support for patients suffering from mental illness, and lack of specialized or trained mental healthcare personnel can also be witnessed in the case of Georgia. In fact, in 2018, it was revealed that of 102,977 people with officially registered mental illness, which is significantly lower than the representative prevalence still, only 49,789 people utilized mental healthcare services. The burden significantly manifested as mostly psychotic or intellectual disability with patients suffering from mood disorders and anxiety only presenting at 7% and 9% in terms of diagnoses, however, these stark differences are attributable to levels of social stigma, low-quality services, and inadequate accessibility in terms of location and affordability. A concurrent challenge with tackling these factors, as mentioned previously, surrounds the challenges of measuring how much each factor contributes to health outcomes and diagnosis in a society in the first place. Regardless of these challenges, the Government of Georgia published two key policies regarding mental healthcare as follows: the *Concept on Mental Health Care* and *Universal Health Care and Quality Control for the Protection of Patients' Rights.* In terms of financial injections, there was an increase of €3 million to fund community-based healthcare services specifically outpatient and mobile healthcare. In fact, it is crucial to note that the introduction of new services for outpatient facilities did lead to an enhanced uptake by 51% in community care with more people opting for community care as opposed to institutional.

The fourth tenet of the OECD Mental Health System Performance Framework highlights the prevention of mental disorders and promotion of mental well-being by placing policies that aim to decrease the incidence and prevalence of suicides and create awareness and literacy surrounding mental health. On an environmental level, the policies must create environments that encourage resilience and enhance good mental health in academic and work settings for children and adults, alike while ensuring people who feel the need to seek mental health support can do so easily. Lastly, key stakeholders to identify and address mental distress within the population effectively. In 2001, the Malaysian MOH introduced the Mental Health Act followed by Mental Health Regulations in 2010 reorganized how psychiatric healthcare services are delivered across private and public institutions. The Mental Health Act and Regulations also supported community-based mental health services and assisted development of their growth as well as protecting patients by allowing for discharge at any point and placing safety mechanisms for those being placed under mandatory psychiatric treatments within national and international human rights benchmarks. In 2020, a 5-year national strategic plan for mental health and similar disorders was introduced with Strategy 5 and Strategy 6 being focused on the prevention of mental disorders and promoting mental health and well-being across settings and numerous target populations. Some quality assurances or monitoring within strategies is assured by bifurcating them into actions, activities, indicators, and associated time frames and responsible parties as well as associated funding donors or partners.

For instance, Strategy 5 focuses on establishing and cultivating sectoral collaboration within and across sectors and encompasses the following:

i. Promotion of mental health to decrease stigma and provide education or increase awareness within the population by providing ongoing education to relevant agencies. The indicator for success or progress would be if there is a presence of a minimum of one article or publication related to mental health within the media including social media once a month. The time frame provided was once every 4 months for a minimum of 1 hour being sufficient for target achievement of 100% and agencies responsible for this include the Ministry of Communication and Multimedia, MOH, a nongovernmental organization called the Malaysian Mental Health Association and other related ministries.

ii. Promotion of mental health educational resources through large social media platforms and collaborating with currently utilized platforms to provide visibility on the mental health programs conducted via these platforms. The indicator for success in this case would be to post once a month from 2020 to 2025 and the same ministries or stakeholders would be responsible alongside NGOs such as Laman Minda, Medtweet.my, and Medical MythBusters.

iii. Prevention of mental illness focused on reducing risk and incorporating awareness pertinent to depression, suicide, and disaster management within the academic curriculum. Different age groups were targeted with varying actions, for example, couples were provided stress and conflict management courses and predivorce therapy based on marital status with one 30-minute session of management in every premarital course as provided by the Department of Islamic Development Malaysia (JAKIM), MOH and religious departments statewise. Similarly, preretirement populations receive coping mechanisms to transition effectively into their retirement period. On the opposite end of the spectrum, children receive mental health education as part of the school curriculum; however, both older and younger populations are targeted to receive 20% of the overall training by 2023. Community heads and religious leaders were also trained in mental health with at least one being trained per district. Lastly, non-MOH agencies were given training on psychological first aid (PFA) with a minimum of two non-MOH agencies state-wise trained by 2023.

On the other hand, Strategy 6 focuses on encouraging good mental health and well-being across populations in various settings such as communities, schools, students, NGOs, workforces, and political or nonpolitical leaders in the following ways:

i. To encourage communities a campaign called Let's TALK Minda Sihat was implemented as well as a Malaysia Mental Health Film Festival with indicators focused on maximizing the number of campaigns, booths, and participants across the campaign and festival, respectively. In 2021 this was limited to one booth on a state level but by 2023 this was projected to half of all districts and is predicted for all districts to have a minimum of one booth in the next 2 years.

ii. To promote mental health knowledge and equip students across various levels (preschool and primary school, secondary and tertiary school) regarding mental well-being by employing infotainment approaches and e-mental health approaches for pre- and primary as well as secondary and tertiary school, respectively. The key indicator for this revolves around engagement levels on social media between 2020 and 2025.

iii. Students are empowered for positive mental health and encouraged to seek help by provision of training regarding affect regulation, communication, and interpersonal skills via Program Siswa Sihat (PROSIS) and Pendidikan Rakan Sebaya. Indicators of success focus on the number of trainings held and students hosted with feedback sessions before and after trainings and success is seen as half of the training hosted in facilities.

iv. To encourage NGOs and groups that advocate for mental health to improve awareness and earlier screening, or intervention is instructing and providing Echo training for NGO's and community groups as well as general promotion via campaign, providing language to discuss mental health and via religious groups.

v. Provide the workforce with adequate awareness, outlook and skill sets regarding mental well-being and enable them to detect mental illness within group settings and find work-life balance via training on both, mental health, and work-life balance through training, KOSPEN Plus (a program to develop stress management capabilities), promotion activities (Campaign, Convention, Lectures), and advocacy work.

vi. Lastly, inspire political and nonpolitical heads via existing platforms for instance Majillis Belia Negara by conducting promotional activities including campaigns and dialogue as indicated by a certain number of mental health promotive campaigns.

By providing national-level strategies with specific actions to enhance awareness of mental health and encourage mental well-being within the various populations using targeted strategies, the National Strategic Plan by the MOH of Malaysia is a key example of how an environment supportive of such aims can be created. Additionally, the placement of key indicators per goal and action allows for measurable tracking of progress and offers a quantitative quality control measure as well as assigning responsibility to specific stakeholders and parties responsible for funding of each action. From a quality assurance perspective, a government may hold an audit for QI while upholding a culture that places quality care at the center of its activities. An example of this is the MOH of Malaysia, which has both, national indicator approaches (NIAs), key performance indicators (KPIs), clinical audit containing workload data, and other QI activities incorporating client satisfaction surveys among other constituents. These can then be aligned to supplement specific clinical goals in mind such as improving awareness and identification of and early treatment of disorders like depression, schizophrenia, attention deficit hyperactive disorder, and dementia across public and private healthcare settings.

However, a key factor in the execution of an effective and high-performing mental health system lies in having strong leaders and suitable governance, which is the fifth principle of the OECD Mental Health System Performance Framework. The leadership must ensure that mental health is heavily prioritized on a systemic level by advancing expenditure to provide a high-performing mental healthcare system with lower levels of stigma regarding mental disorders and mental health. To do so, an optimal allocation of resources is needed in a manner that is geographically equitable across targeted populations and varying disorders. In 2020, experts from Oxford University stated the importance of QI being at the forefront of priorities by leadership in healthcare. In the National Health Service (NHS), the nurse that was interviewed voiced how being part of QI projects allowed for flexibility to enhance her work, and when studied across NHS staff, it became evident that healthcare personnel feel less valued and that there is limited prospect of systematic change within the structure. As QI is dependent upon mental healthcare personnel and their judgment to preempt or understand patient needs to facilitate positive outcomes, leaders must provide encouragement within the workforce to carry out the same. A study by Burgess and team outlines a governance that is learning focused and exemplified by collaborations that push the same attitude such as NHS Improvement and five other US-based trusts as well as building relations with regulators that lead to a paradigm shift in how QI and governance are discussed in the long run. Some key factors to consider in the practical implementation of quality being at the center of leadership and governance are as follows:

i. Acceptance in a paradigm shift as it relates to how leaders view QI and their roles within the ecosystem. This would involve putting trust within the workforce to not just follow certain guidelines or comply with standards, but rather shift their focus to furthering and enhancing the standards of care for better healthcare outcomes.

ii. A holistic focus on people management for overall improvement that incorporates building of trust within teams, the presence of interdisciplinary teams, and integrating processes that retain, attract, and develop valuable members, among other strategies.

iii. Educating senior leadership to transition management styles and best behaviors or models of thinking to adapt to influence the workforce and build a culture focused on QI characterized by high-quality processes, services, and resulting outcomes.

iv. Investing in quality management systems and giving the patients a voice in terms of catering higher quality to what is aligned with patient needs.

In fact, when 10 senior multidisciplinary leaders when questioned about the necessary skill set required by a leader in any respective field, the overarching consensus was found to be that to achieve large-scale or systemic changes can be created via "soft power" usage. The strategies that such leaders highlighted to cause systematic change were engaging with healthcare personnel to create an understanding of the need for QI and drive workflows to support the change, collaborating with patients and their caregivers to identify where changes need to occur, maintaining a balance between consistency in terms of purpose of activities and adaptability of services alongside how these changes may be implemented and providing a stable and reliable leadership for the medical system. The mental healthcare system must remain focused on the long term and remain innovative in nature with the emphasis being on the provision of evidence-based, optimized mental healthcare services and provision of care effectively and efficiently. To do so, investment in clinical research to support mental healthcare services, encouragement of creative solutions for challenges plaguing those with mental health concerns, building capacity in terms of the workforce for upcoming years, and creating resilient systems for information for mental health are mandatory.

In the United Kingdom, the NHS provides a framework guidance specifically focused on quality and outcomes on an annual basis. The Quality and Outcomes Framework (QOF) of 2023–24 edition outlines the QOF indicators, details regarding clinical and public health indicators such as why it was incorporated and what standards need to be met to achieve success, specificities regarding QI and process to flag questions correlated to QOF indicators and understanding them among other pertinent sections. Each framework outlines clinical domains or major disorders with dementia, depression, and mental health being relevant to the scope of this chapter.

The guidance under the umbrella of neuropsychiatric disorders and mental health is as follows:

i. Dementia:

To provide a high-quality diagnosis and treatment, healthcare personnel should maintain a register of all diagnosed dementia patients ensuring all diagnoses—across secondary care or the medical personnel's professional judgment—are recorded. Additionally, care plans should be reviewed for every dementia patient annually to update the patient's condition accurately and track progression. The review should consist of a comprehensive physical, mental, and social evaluation as well as a review of patient response to pharmacological treatments with note of adverse events or side effects and complying with the NICE guidance regarding antipsychotic use. Lastly, the patient's caregiver must also be recognized and support such as information sharing and resulting health check-ins may be conducted. To ensure quality is assured and validate the integrity of these processes, practices are focused on the presence of documentation regarding the review of planned care plans and whether key concerns are addressed. Quality indicators for dementia care include maintaining accurate and up-to-date records, achieving a set percentage of care plan reviews within 12 months, and meeting established thresholds for these reviews (35%–70%). Quality control may be conducted by occasional audits by commissioners who sample patient records to verify that care plans reviews are in alignment with and as comprehensive as demanded by regulation.

ii. Depression

To provide high-quality care for depression, healthcare professionals must diligently document every new diagnosis of depression in a dedicated register with a timely review to ensure that patients who are newly diagnosed with depression are reviewed between 10- and 56-days postdiagnosis to evaluate treatment efficacy, disease progression, and patient response and tailor care plans accordingly. The comprehensive assessment must also be carried out that includes not just symptom counting but also the quality of life considering functional impairment and duration of the depressive episode with an emphasis on continual reassessment for high-risk patients that have severe symptomatology or signs of suicidality. Collaboration is a key function when it comes to better patient outcomes and effective information transfer between primary care and mental health specialists is crucial for follow-up care to be seamless for the patient after specialist diagnosis. Quality assurance and control practices are focused on meticulous record-keeping and appropriate timing and content regarding patient reviews being conducted. Quality indicators for depression emphasize the initial management of patients 18 and over who have a new depression diagnosis who have been reviewed between 10 and 56 days after the date of diagnosis with a benchmark range of 45%–80% and further reviews if a patient's symptoms remain unresolved in a timely manner. Adjustments to care for personalization per patient may be applied by specialist mental health personnel, and if the patient is discharged, follow-ups by primary care teams must follow up and invite for a review as needed. To safeguard the quality of care, occasional audits may be performed by commissioners, who check the percentage of telephone reviews conducted and who provided them.

iii. Mental health (schizophrenia, bipolar affective disorder, and other psychoses)

High-quality care for mental health patients suffering from schizophrenia, bipolar affective disorder, and disorders characterized by psychoses require numerous key actions by healthcare systems such as established and maintaining medical records of patients with severe mental illness (SMI), including patients undergoing lithium treatment. Additionally, healthcare professionals must be diligent with creating comprehensive care plans and documentation of the same annually for patients with SMI in collaboration with the patients and their caregivers, as appropriate. With SMI, conducting regular health check-ups of physiological parameters such as blood pressure, body mass index (BMI), alcohol consumption, lipid profiles, and blood glucose or HbA1c level as well as doing a holistic physical check-up with the previously mentioned parameters, lifestyle, and medication assessment in line with the NHS long-term plan and NICE guidelines is crucial. To ensure quality assurance and control, practices are focused on the accuracy of documentation with indicators to benchmark the percent of patients reviewed within specified timeframes, and annual reviews are conducted for patients in remission to reevaluate the accuracy of diagnosis and whether they should remain within a certain diagnosis of other indicators. Indicators of quality are regarding if the contractor has created and maintained the presence of medical records for patients diagnosed with schizophrenia, bipolar disorder, or other psychoses-characterized disorders and patients being treated with lithium as well as regarding ongoing management of complex mental health disorders depending on the percent of patients with complete care plan documentation, percent of patients with records for physiological parameter reviews and holistic check-ups. Quality control measures for SMIs include auditing of patient records to essential health checks and comprehensive care plans that have been prescribed, monitored, and followed up appropriately, and these reviews must show annual recurrence. Similarly, patient's remission codes are reviewed to make sure they are coded correctly and that patients in remission do meet the criteria to be included within the classification. Lastly, protocol adherence may be rechecked to ensure that coding and clinician's judgment regarding patient plans have been conducted correctly.

7.15 Conceptual frameworks and practice-based applications used to optimizes quality assurance in neuropsychiatric and mental health research

The provision of evidence-based guidelines and resulting improved patient outcomes hinges upon advancing basic and applied research in neuropsychiatry and mental disorders. Research and development are crucial to understanding both, causality and risk factors that impact the manifestation of disease, which can further the ability of systems to support mental well-being on a population level as well as enable resilience by propagating healthy coping mechanisms. Additionally, analysis of existing standards of care and translation of research to create mental, pharmacological, and biological treatments, therapies and assistance for patients suffering from such diseases can directly support the alleviation of the burden of disease. In addition to developing innovative interventions, research also focuses on how these innovations can support those who need it most, how they must be managed, and how they can most effectively be integrated within the healthcare architecture in question (inclusive but not limited to healthcare settings, communities, occupational health, and intrapersonal contexts).

Thus, it is imperative that the research being conducted to advance neuropsychiatric and mental health prevention, diagnosis, treatment, and ongoing care be done with strict controls and a heavy focus on high-quality studies and clinical projects/trials. The National Institute of Neurological Disorders and Stroke (NINDS) and National Institutes of Health (NIH) provide general guidelines that serve the purpose of embedding QA processes in clinical research and support guidance of high-quality study implementation as well as troubleshooting of data quality or integrity concerns. The guidelines also provide a checklist that researchers can employ to plan and evaluate QA practices as well as a bibliography for references regarding QA.

General activities that support high-quality clinical research are documenting SOPs and providing Training and Certification Programs. SOPs allow researchers to note the major activities and operations within the research study that can be appropriately replicated to ensure studies are conducted in the same way to ensure results seen are valid and reliable. They generally incorporate protocol validation, IRB-approval steps, and best practices for safety monitoring, record storage and maintenance, equipment-related specificities, and data management. These are also useful for onboarding new members and liazing with collaborator centers. Similarly, upskilling and teaching researchers' courses on "Good Clinical Practice," "Clinical Research Coordinator (CRC)," and "Human Subjects Protection" allow them to carry out high-quality research in an informed manner.

To ensure reliable results and high-quality research practices, study protocols must be established, and key processes involved in maintaining the quality of a clinical research study involve:

i. Implementing study administration and manual of procedures (MOP)
ii. Governing conflict of interest (COI)
iii. Documenting drug and/or device-related procedures
iv. Documenting information related to participant materials or samples
v. Planning recruitment and retention of participants
vi. Prescreening and screening of participants
vii. Ensuring informed consent, randomization, and blinding of participants (as per study design)
viii. Collecting and managing data
ix. Monitoring safety and protection of human subjects

Regarding QA during these studies, there are four key aspects to consider:

i. Creating a quality control plan

The researcher's role during these studies involves evaluating the collected and reported data to routinely create reports that monitor the progress of the study and associated challenges to flag any potential concerns earlier in the study. Monitoring sites and reports and procedures identified for data review alongside documenting and evaluating the systems being used for the study are key aspects of quality control.

ii. Identifying QA concerns during a study

After the study has commenced, investigators conduct a critical analysis of numerous generated reports is conducted including those on screening, recruitment, enrollment, and retention to understand any challenges with recruitment or sites of study, protocol compliance to ensure there are no protocol violations, data quality to track any deviation in terms of data and protocol compliance, serious adverse events

(AEs) to make sure any AEs are raised correctly and as early as possible, and site monitoring and data to give feedback regarding site-related concerns and validate data across measures. Each site will undergo systematic visits involving checks for protocol compliance, which will be reported to NINDS and researchers describing the audit and any feedback.

iii. Setting quality standards and ongoing maintenance

By establishing quality standards, researchers can identify issues within the research pipeline. Some generally employed standards revolve around the percentage of participants that meet all screening criteria, the percentage of study enrollment goals achieved in a timely manner, attrition rate, error rate within data sets, and appropriateness of software employed for data analysis.

iv. Ensuring quality correction processes are introduced

Post identification of data quality and integrity concerns, there must be processes for correction of these errors. Some instances of these include an audited trail of tracked changes in data and changes of the system or documentation to ensure it is appropriate for the mental illness of concern, that is, any systematic changes that may render results reflective of reality. Similarly, changes in reports or procedures may be required to enhance the quality of a study such as using digital platforms to enhance recruitment reach, and if certain protocol-related concerns are found cross-site, retraining staff may be required.

Overall, the QA of a study ensures that there is a plan in place to control the quality of data and study noticed across numerous time points within a project wherein concerns are identified as the study progresses or are predicted based on indicators and consistent feedback is provided for improvement of the study. The general way maintenance of the study occurs is linked with the quality standards that must be followed, and during the timeline of the clinical research, quality correction when mistakes are made or protocol is not followed occurs.

An example of QA used in clinical research is exemplified by a quantitative cross-sectional study about behavioral and psychological symptoms of dementia conducted in South-Western Uganda. This study employed QA at various levels by appointing trained research assistants with prior experience in using research tools, who conducted comprehensive data collection, cleaning, analysis, and troubleshooting of identified challenges within the study. In fact, research is not limited to the use of research tools to drive understanding but also exists on the flip side of introducing new tools in our repertoire to handle neuropsychiatric disorders and mental illness. An example of the same is the use of dementia care mapping (DCM) as an audit tool that was utilized by the NHS as a QA strategy to audit outcomes of dementia care in formal healthcare settings. Now, it has been in implementation for more than 20 years but a consensus from review across studies was that DCM is likelier to be successfully utilized if the correct people are chosen to get training as mappers with proper education, continual support, and good leadership within the healthcare setting. On the other hand, the main optimization was in regard to the time taken to conduct a DCM cycle, which can be further reduced, and understanding the factors that make DCM utilization effective.

From the perspective of QA in academic settings where clinical research is often conducted as well, a case study evaluating the values of recommendations across QA literature extensively explored the practical considerations of quality management research to improve process quality wherein context is often not provided in detail. In terms of QA in academia, this is defined by Suvin and team as the methodical assessment and supervision of the standard of instruction provided by academic institutions.

The authors, Everard van Kemenade and Cuong Huu Nguyen outlined five major themes or learnings and two main practical considerations regarding quality management within academic settings of research findings which are as follows:

i. Stakeholder engagement is crucial, so all those involved in the QA process such as student researchers, professors, and management staff know the importance of their roles

ii. QA training remains key so that stakeholders can understand and be trained on what QA consists of and how they can comply with standards and maintain a quality-focused mindset across tasks and priorities

iii. Shift in the metric system from a "numbers game" to solely ensure compliance and transitioning to qualitative assessments based on the experiences of stakeholders with the processes and workflows

iv. QA centers allow for the identification of key factors of success for internal QA organizations, which may be commitment toward quality, presence of good governance, level of involvement by stakeholders across levels, accuracy of process itself, hybridization, and utilization of external QA processes

v. Encouragement of dialogue and creating a space that supports feedback across levels to support better outcomes or quality enhancement as well as reducing rigid management and stringent control

The authors recommend and identify the creation of learning communities within universities or cross-regionally so that collective inquiry can emerge and enhanced translatable research outcomes can be achieved. A key caveat to bear in mind, as discussed in previous sections, is to bear in mind the cultural contexts in which quality-related recommendations are being implemented, and the development of internal QA processes must be tailored by local experts who are well versed with regional best practices or the university's specific requirements.

7.16 Translation of improved quality in real-world contexts

Healthcare delivery systems such as NHS are shifting focus to quality with ever-increasing monetary and performance-based pressures to deliver quality care, which can benefit from a global improvement in quality via quality-enhancing techniques as opposed to local shifts. The common principles that are stagnant across contexts include skill building of mental health or healthcare personnel in using internal systems, employing available data sets to benchmark performance, providing staff members the space to voice and implement ideas to enhance quality, testing on smaller scales or prototypes to learn, and keeping patients or users centered behind all the efforts being conducted. In fact, a program called Getting It Right First Time (GIRFT) that focuses on eliminating service or practice-based differences across services and tracks executed changes to improve quality, practices, and productivity was implemented within the NHS. This program identified a total of between 20 and 30 million pounds of financial savings upon one visit with an additional 15−20 million predicted for the year 2017. Another example of the same is the program's identification of over prescription of antibiotic medications, which when changed could render £3.7 million annual savings through optimized prescription activities. Similarly, by focusing on quality, there is an optimization across features of the medical healthcare system such as under-, over-, and misplaced utilization of resources and their allocation. Provision of a national strategy (similar to the one published by Malaysia's MOH), appointing appropriate leadership, addressing gaps within the organization's structure, consistent and reliable measurement and responsibility measures, and skill building based on identified gaps must occur to see any true reform.

7.17 Managing quality optimization methods for neuropsychiatric populations

As neuropsychiatry is a growing field that aligns with the boom in medical technological advancements in the fields of neural imaging, genomics, neuroscience, data analytics, and artificial intelligence, it is no surprise that innovation is occurring at a rapid rate. However, a major gap remains between the innovative side of neuropsychiatry and the clinical or medical management of disease. This gap between research and clinic is only furthered due to limited quality management and pathways that could facilitate high-quality services being translated to the user or patient therefore, it is imperative that quality optimization methods be placed into mental health service systems and managed appropriately to support those suffering with mental illness and neuropsychiatric disorders.

A review of optimization in mental healthcare systems conducted by Noorain and team discussed the several crucial aspects and methodologies vital for enhancing quality in mental healthcare systems. The study delved into the various operational techniques, emphasizing adaptation to meet the specific challenges present in mental healthcare. An optimization model consists of an objective function, decision variables, and constraints to find the values per decision variable that can maximize or minimize an objective function while satisfying the provided constraints. For instance, one may want to minimize patient waiting times and maximize the utilization of mental healthcare providers. In such a case, the objective function or aim of the model would be the minimization of patient waiting times and maximization of the utilization of mental healthcare providers, whereas decision variables would be appointment times for patients and assignment of patients to the healthcare providers. This optimization may be constrained by the context of the mental healthcare setting thus, involving the availability of healthcare providers, the maximum number of patients a provider is feasibly able to see in a day and the specific care needs of patients to match the expertize presented by the providers. Another example of an optimization model could be one that has the objective function to maximize the utilization of beds while minimizing the refusal rate of admissions due to lack of space. In this case, the decision variables would include assignment of patients to beds in the psychiatric ward and discharge scheduling to free up the beds however, the setting may have constraints such as a limited number of available beds, a mandatory LOS as per the patient's evaluation condition and admission prioritization based on the urgency of each patient's mental health condition. On a regional level, concerns often surround the distribution of high-quality mental healthcare services wherein governances would prioritize maximization of mental health service coverage across a geographic region while minimizing operational costs. Therefore, they are required to research locations where new mental health clinics or service points must be introductions and how resources such as staff or equipment are to be allocation per site. However, they are often constrained by the budget for the introduction of such services, the geographic distribution of the most vulnerable populations that would benefit from the introduction, and the associated transport or accessibility to and from sites of care.

Such optimization models are created by using various research techniques and certain techniques can be employed to address major themes identified across the mental healthcare architectures. These key challenges may be addressed by employing the following methodologies:

(1) Confronting uncertainty and variability: This theme focuses on managing the unpredictable aspects of mental healthcare, such as fluctuating patient demand, variations in patient attendance (like no-shows), and the availability of healthcare staff. It recognizes the need for mental health services to be flexible and responsive to changing conditions and patient needs.

    a. Stochastic programming: Utilized for modeling the uncertainties in service demands, patient absenteeism, and the availability of staff.

    b. Robust optimization: Aids in creating systems capable of withstanding the unpredictability and variations inherent in mental healthcare.

(2) Ensuring prompt accessibility to care: This aspect emphasizes the importance of reducing wait times for mental health services and ensuring that patients can access care when needed. Efficient patient flow and reduced waiting times are crucial for effective mental healthcare, as delays can worsen health outcomes.

    a. Queueing Theory and Simulation Models: Applied to analyze and enhance patient flow, thereby diminishing waiting times and facilitating easier access to healthcare services.

(3) Maintaining continuity in care: Continuity of care is about ensuring consistent and ongoing treatment for patients, especially as they move between different levels or types of care (like transitioning from inpatient to outpatient care). It involves careful planning of patient pathways to maintain treatment consistency and avoid gaps in care.
  a. Network models and multistage programming: Effective for orchestrating patient transitions through different care stages, such as inpatient, outpatient, and community care.
  b. Markov decision processes: Suitable for sequential decision making to maintain continuous patient engagement and ongoing treatment.

(4) Handling integrated and complex systems: This theme acknowledges that mental healthcare often involves multiple interconnected components, including various healthcare providers, services, and care settings. Optimization in this context requires a holistic approach that considers the complex interactions and dependencies within the healthcare system.
  a. System dynamics and simulation: Employed to examine the interplay among various elements of the mental healthcare framework.
  b. Multicriteria decision analysis (MCDA): Supports decision making by weighing various objectives and criteria against each other.

(5) Optimizing resource allocation and usage: This is about using the available resources (such as staff, beds, and equipment) in the most effective and efficient way. It involves making strategic decisions on how to best allocate and utilize these resources to meet patient needs while also considering cost-efficiency.
  a. Linear, integer, and mixed-integer programming: Targeted at the efficient allocation of resources, including staffing, beds, and equipment.
  b. Goal programming: Strives to achieve a balance and fulfillment of multiple goals, such as cost-effectiveness, care quality, and patient satisfaction.

(6) Incorporating preferences of patients and staff: This theme recognizes the importance of considering the individual needs and preferences of both patients and healthcare staff in the planning and delivery of mental health services. It is about personalizing care to patient needs and ensuring staff workloads are manageable and aligned with their capabilities and preferences.
  a. Discrete event simulation: Capable of simulating individual patient pathways and preferences along with staff scheduling and workload.

(7) Adjusting to policy and environmental shifts: This aspect involves the ability of mental health services to adapt to changes in healthcare policies or external environmental factors. It is about being proactive and responsive to changes that could impact service delivery, such as new health regulations or societal shifts.
  a. Scenario planning and analysis: Utilized to evaluate the implications of potential changes in healthcare policies or environmental factors on mental health services.

(8) Leveraging predictive analytics: This theme is about leveraging data and predictive models to anticipate future trends in patient outcomes, service demands, and other key factors. Predictive analytics can inform better decision making and planning in mental healthcare, leading to improved patient care and resource management.

   a. Data mining and machine learning algorithms: Used for forecasting patient outcomes, service demands, and other critical variables that inform resource allocation and service planning.

These themes have been supported by results found in a study conducted by Samartzis and Talias in 2020 [115], which include indicators across seven dimensions of quality assessment: suitability of services, accessibility of patients to services, acceptance of services by patients, competence of HCPs in delivering services, efficiency of healthcare personnel, continuity of service longitudinally, and safety for patients and HCPs. The backbone of such complex algorithms and data analysis lies in the system, that is, the integration of electronic data collection and IT systems in the medical system for systematic data collection regarding patient outcomes and interventions, allowing for subsequent quantification or estimation of mental health data and its associated indicators. This not only opens the doors for real-time monitoring and analysis but also data standardization to have consistency in the way data is gathered so it is truly reflective of real-world scenarios and changes. This would ideally support reducing time or service-related redundancies as well as indicate areas of improvement for both, neuropsychiatric patients as well as medical care delivery or intervention. Similarly, the presence of such data enhances visibility regarding the patient for the respective HCP and can encourage cross-functional communication to ensure that care is continuous within the medical system for the patient in distress. Lastly, the availability of representative and consistent data can be employed in research or to effectively inform healthcare policy that supports better mental healthcare quality from evidence-backed strategies to address quality concerns. A quality control measure for the use of such IT systems may evaluate how much electronic health records and being implemented and how the technology is integrated with service delivery in a way that supports the mental healthcare delivery as opposed to introducing layers of complication to an existing complex system.

A key consideration in establishing such systems is ensuring the safety and personal data security measures by ensuring data and stakeholder behavior follow regulations. In the case of Europe, this is the General Data Protection Rule (GDPR) that provides regulation for how one's sensitive health data is collected, employed, shared, maintained, linked, or incorporated in data sets and deleted. It also ensures that consent is taken and that data collection only begins after permissions from authorized bodies are granted, which indicates the strength of the process in the medical system. The presence of it and the general target across medical systems expect full implementation of GDPR across areas as well as provision of areas where it may not be implemented to ensure it is.

Second, strategic plans or action plans are fundamental building blocks of health policy as they ensure the quality of services are planned and provided. These indicate progress in terms of the process with timescales, roles, and responsibilities outlined and the global or fixed budget (often seen as a percent of the whole state budget for healthcare). A common case against quality-centric interventions is stated due to the change management and perceived significant investment within new systems or interventions and initiatives that may render an opportunity cost for a different spend. However, the initial assessment of mental health services includes predominantly economic priorities to ensure sustainable development of the mental healthcare system with recruitment, funding, and source efficiencies being the key features emphasized during strategic planning. In fact, a measure known as Cost per Diagnosis Related Group (DRG) created at Yale University is built from the idea that every diagnosis based on the ICD-10 classification system is associated to a specific DRG, which is associated with standard specific costs for the hospital being examined and predecided. Hospitals are then reimbursed per patient hospitalization based on the patient DRGs predetermined by diagnosis on the patient discharge notes which are from either ICD-10 or ICD-11, classification systems discussed previously in Section 7.1. The hospital software then links the ICD and DRG codes that are a match, and the accounting office then gains the reimbursement from the responsible funding source such as the MOH, a fund, and an insurer. Such standardized and appropriately employed organizations can then indicate progress within the medical healthcare system. For example, quantifying how much of funding is incoming as a result of DRG organization is a clear indicator of economic organization. The utilization of tools such as the WHO Assessment Instrument for Mental Health Systems (WHO-AIMS) and WHO-Quality Rights can also support initial idea formation regarding the quality of mental healthcare systems.

Over time, there has also been a transition of viewing quality mental healthcare as just evaluating the presence of structures and services toward the diagnosis, treatment outcomes, and quantification of outcomes with consideration of the individual's social determinants of health. These can be assessed on how appropriate the service is and how accessible it is for the individual. Structural indicators point toward the adequacy or lack in terms of a mental health service. Some examples include investigating the number of chronic patients hospitalized in psychiatric wards as opposed to being in rehabilitation within outpatient units, preventable cases of hospital admission if provided adequate external interventions, and the number of patients who get treated in the correct health setting with personalized treatment. For such indicators, performance targets focus on reducing hospitalization burden and preventable hospitalizations by providing community services and support more upstream in the patient journey thereby, preventing severe outcomes for neuropsychiatric patients. Similarly, another performance objective is ensuring that all patients receive the correct treatment at the correct facility. In terms of accessibility, indicators depict the waiting times/days for various healthcare settings (Accident and Emergency Department, Outpatient and Clinic Settings) as well as the overall coverage of the health system on a population level. Performance targets focus on minimizing waiting times to ensure timely treatment and check-up of patients, eliminating waiting lists and maximizing coverage across the population having access to health services. Lastly, evaluations in terms of the effectiveness of treatments also serve as direct quality control and optimization to ensure the percentage of patients who see improved quality of life and reduced symptomatology is high. This can also on a disorder-level be measured by the outcomes of extra mortality compared to the overall populace mortality that patients with schizophrenia and bipolar may face. On the other hand, disorders such as substance abuse and addiction may have numerous phased indicators such as completion of addiction treatment programs, overall decreased consumption across substance abusers due to treatment, degree of remission and abstinence compared to readmission, and relapse or presence of drug abuse. Tracking these measures on a holistic view can provide indications to the patient's progress longitudinally, identify triggers, and provide support from a multidimensional approach. Most of the target performances for such indicators are focused on having no harmful behaviors at all.

The increasing prioritization toward ensuring improved quality is clear. Initiatives such as the Care Under Pressure (CUP3) realist evaluation study protocol that focus on the collaboration of purposely chosen NHS trusts in the United Kingdom to create an evidence-based implementation toolkit for all NHS trusts to decrease HCP mental health burden and corresponding deterioration witnessed across the medical workforce exemplify strategies in place for quality mental health services. This is a direct example of optimizing resource allocation and usage by incorporating services of staff and considering environmental shifts such as how this was an ongoing concern, only furthered by the COVID-19 pandemic. Similarly, there are also skill-based or competency-focused indicators for the workforce such as the presence of lifelong learning programs for mental health professionals to ensure they participate in staying up to date and eventually lead up to participation in a qualitative and measured educational system. On the patient side, the evaluation of user interviews and concerns via qualitative as well as quantitative questionnaires and interviews can significantly support quality optimization. Indicators such as the average patient satisfaction rating, records of previous patient experiences, the patient's access to their medical information and knowledge of their rights, the number of patients leaving with a discharge or information note, and the number of patients that use the suggestions/concerns box. The performance targets would include maximizing average patient satisfaction, minimizing negative experiences, improving patients' knowledge of their rights, ensuring all patients leave with a discharge note, and minimizing patient complaints.

Overall, quality optimization methods focus on the use of data to drive monitoring and improvement of quality healthcare, strategic plans and economic evaluation of service introductions, and patient-focused indicators to improve the existing medical infrastructure and utilization with key priorities being effectiveness, accessibility, and appropriateness.

7.18 **Quality optimization in investigational medical product development and deployment**

An investigational medical product (IMP) is defined as "a medicinal product which is being tested or used as a reference, including as a placebo, in a clinical trial' as per Regulation (EU) No. 536/2014 Article 2 (5)." This documentation also mentions that such products when given a marketing authorization constitute IMPs when utilized for testing, as a reference license drug for dissolution or generic testing or placebo within a clinical trial. The European Medicines Agency (EMA) is a decentralized scientific agency for the European Union (EU) and is one of the key constituents of the regulatory framework that exists in the region. The regulatory body has functions of guarding and encouraging public and animal health via assessment and supervision of medicines for human and veterinary usage and marketing of any medicine for the EU is dependent on the scientific evaluation of the parameters of quality, safety, and efficacy stated by EMA. These medicines then receive marketing authorization from the European Commission, one of the many bodies that the EMA links with to achieve better health for those in the EU.

The EMA also issues guidelines in terms of what is required for quality documentation concerning biological investigational medicinal products that are being used in clinical trials which outline the description and composition of the IMP, the specifications for pharmaceutical development and manufacture as well as control of excipients and the IMP itself. Additionally, they provide details regarding the expected reference standards or materials, the containers' closure system, and requirements of stability for IMPs. The guidelines also inform the reader regarding the quality of authorized, unmodified biological test and comparator products as well as modified authorized biological comparators in clinical trials. On the other hand, information regarding the chemical and pharmaceutical quality in terms of placebo products employed for clinical trials and any changes to IMP or auxiliary medicinal products with a requirement to request a substantial modification to the investigational medicinal product dossier (IMPD). An IMPD is essentially the collation of data collection relevant to the specific clinical trial during the time of submission for the clinical trial application. If, however, the active substance that is to be studied has been authorized as part of a finished product within the region or ICH regions, the applicant can refer to the existing valid marketing authorization and depending on the type of product it is, further information may then be mandatory.

Given the numerous variables and considerations that must be accounted for during clinical development such as the number of product variants and impurities related to processes with unpredictable safety and efficacies, it is no surprise that ensuring the quality of medicinal processes has its challenges. These issues can often be traced to the mechanism of action of the product being investigated and how it reacts with the immune system. To support the marketing authorization application of IMPs, numerous clinical trials and products from various reiterations of manufacturing may be started to get clinical data; the guidelines serve as quality assurance or provide standards for the IMP within a certain clinical trial as opposed to the overarching developmental strategy for a product to be developed and launched.

Additionally, these guidelines can have more requirements based on the complexity or novelty of a certain drug that is to be manufactured and state the responsibility of the applicant to ensure that participants within clinical trials remain safe and get access to a high-quality IMP that is appropriately developed. In addition, to EMA guidelines, manufacturers also must account for compliance with good manufacturing practices (GMP) for their products.

The first requirement by the EMA is regarding the provision of general information related to the drug (including nomenclature, structure, and general properties) and the manufacturer. In the case of an active substance, details regarding nomenclature are in reference to the active substance, and any recommended international nonproprietary name (INN), pharmacopeial name, proprietary name, and company code among other details must be provided. Similarly, the predicted structure of the substance including its higher-order structure, sequences, and masses of molecules must be incorporated. Additionally, the relevant physicochemical and relevant properties of the active substance should be given such as biological impact as per expected outcomes and the mechanism of action expected. Lastly, the manufacturer's details inclusive of sites of production or manufacture, batch testing, and release sites must also be mentioned in the documentation. In case of testing an IMP, the qualitative and quantitative composition should be mentioned, which includes a short statement or table of the dosage form, its composition (a list of all constituents of the dosage form and the amount each accounts for per unit), what each constituent does, and reference to the quality standards such as manufacturer requirements. Additionally, a description of the diluent utilized and the plan for type of storage methods for dosage form as well as any supplementary diluent or devices. During early pharmaceutical development, the extra information that could be documented would include elaboration regarding the formulation itself and explaining the use of any novel forms or excipients, if employed. If the products need extra preparation steps such as rebuilding, diluting, or mixing, the results and methods of conducting those processes with the proposed materials must be summarized within a clinical protocol. A key consideration when developing a formulation is its compatibility with the chosen storage or preservation format in a way that prevents reactions or degradation from occurring, and to minimize the risks for participants, sometimes minimal effective doses may be employed for first-in-human (FIH) studies.

The second quality requirement for testing IMPs is surrounding elaboration of the manufacturing process used and the controls within the process. This requirement ensures that any changes in the process such as formulation or dosage form compared to previously conducted trials are described and justifiably explain why these changes must occur; this allows for an appropriate safety evaluation for patients of any potential repercussions. The parameters that are then assessed due to formulation-based modulations are quality, safety, clinical features, dosing changes, and stability of the product. Information regarding the manufacturer (name, address, responsibilities) and each site for manufacture, test, and batch release must be incorporated, and in the case of multiple manufacturers, responsibilities and accountability must be made clear. Additionally, the formula used for the batches that are to be employed in the clinical trial must be mentioned, which is inclusive of each component, batch size, or the range of batch sizes being utilized. In describing the manufacturing process and its controls, a flow chart with every step, detailing each parameter and testing process within each step of manufacturing should be outlined. With safety as the key priority, control strategies that emphasize in-process controls (IPCs) and acceptance criteria must be described; whereas, for some IPCs, only monitoring may be acceptable. The details remain reiterative in terms of reviewing acceptance criteria and providing information regarding IPCs as it is generated. Novel technologies employed or nonstandardized manufacturing processes must be elaborated upon for validation of processes such as in the case of monoclonal antibodies for oncology products or recombinant proteins for major diseases such as diabetes, heart failure, and multiple sclerosis. When failures or inadequacies occur during manufacturing, reprocessing may be conducted but only for specific steps such as refiltration and only in cases where it is appropriately justifiable to do so.

Critical steps and intermediates are then subject to control within the manufacturing process with tests and acceptance criteria per step provided, and these may be limited during earlier stages of clinical development, that is, during Phases 1 and 2. In the case of holds put on process intermediates, the length of the hold and the conditions for storage must be detailed and evaluated as valid based on physiochemical, biological, and microbiological parameters. Similarly, to sterilize the product by filtration, there must be mention of the maximum acceptable bioburden before the filtration takes place, and in most cases, the standard is NMT 10 CFU/100 mL with any lower volumes used in testing being justified by writing.

Processes must be validated when employing aseptic processing or lyophilization and must be of the same quality standards as for the fully authorized product for marketing with EudraLex Vol. 4, Annex 13 in consideration. The priority of product safety remains the same across the overall process and is reflected in the details on the same parameter within the dossier, for instance, related to bioburden and media fill runs.

To control the excipients, specifications must either be reflective of those used by an EU Member State, USP (United States Pharmacopoeia), or JP (Japanese Pharmacopoeia); whereas, if this is not the case or an excipient is noncompendial in nature, in-house standards are described. Furthermore, analytical methodologies are described. Additionally, the nature of the excipient in terms of whether it originates from humans or animals has to be provided for safety evaluation from a sourcing, test, and virology perspective to minimize risks of zoonosis via animal agents in human or veterinary medicinal products must be documented for evaluated. In the case of plasma derivatives or human albumin usage, safety information and evaluation must be followed as per guidance unless it is a constituent in a previously authorized product in which case this can be mentioned. Similarly, to novel products, novel excipients being used for the first time or via a new route must provide significant safety data with manufacturing details, characterizations, and controls.

On the other hand, to control the investigational medicinal product specifications must be mentioned with testing employed, and what products are accepted for the batch or batches that are to be employed in the clinical trial, thereby allowing for quality control. The acceptance criteria for IMP must consider safety and developmental stage as they are decided upon a limited number of development batches and those used across studies (clinical and nonclinical), which may be refined as the studies progress. Analytical methodologies and upper and lower bounds for content and biological activity can optimize the selection of appropriate dosing. The tests for the parameters required are as follows:

(1) Mandatory
  a. Content
  b. Identity
  c. Purity
(2) Sterile Products
  a. Sterility
  b. Endotoxins
(3) Biological Activity (unless proven otherwise)

Across testing including postactive substance specification, upper bounds for impurities must be in place to avoid AEs that undergo ongoing calibration and optimization. The impurities that may be seen as additional or products of degradation must be listed and quantified. It is key to note that as there is an increase in data collected and the clinical trials progress, changes may be required to parameters and thus ongoing review is a key part of quality management to reflect the learnings of generated data.

Validation and description of analytical methodologies should be detailed with analysis of real batch data for quality assessments to support specifications with quantitative data. For preliminary testing during the early stages, there may be lesser data for specific batches that have been produced and their test findings must be provided from clinical and nonclinical studies and those that are going to be employed within the clinical trial itself whereas, products that have been manufactured and have historical data, certain batches that represent performance and quality may be provided. The batches must be identifiable by a specific batch number, size, manufacturing site and date, methods of control, acceptance criteria, and results with the usage of respective batches. This information should incorporate confirmation of whether represented batches will be employed during trials or whether additional in-progress batches are planned for usage.

The quality seen in the IMP specifications must be offered in accordance with details of the active substance, and here the priority would be on stability attributes with an explanation of the acceptance criteria mentioned. Additionally, the characterization features regarding the reference standard must also be provided, as necessary.

Lastly, containment systems and stability must be examined and controlled. There are often two types of packaging on medicine: Primary and Secondary Packaging. In the case of an oral tablet, for example, the primary packaging that is going to be used in a clinical trial must be defined. On the other hand, if a product is packaged in a novel device for administration or if noncompendial materials are employed, explanation and conditions must be described. In case a medicinal product is utilized in conjunction with a medical device and the main mechanism of action is due to the medicinal product, the conjunction of the two products is then regulated by the medicines legislation and a CE mark would not be necessary during development. In the case where a route of administration presents a risk of interaction between the product and the container it is in, more data may be required for submission. The regulation that must be considered during the marketing authorization approval for this is article 117 of Regulation (EU) 2017/745. For stability, the stability protocol, findings, shelf-life, and extension of shelf-life data as well as commitment and postapproval extension must be detailed. The reason stability studies are conducted is to ensure that the IMP is stable when it is stored, and the data should validate that it will be stable from release to patient administration.

As mentioned previously, there may be changes in the IMP over time and these changes must be documented per product at their relevant site and be continuously updated as development progresses to be able to track each previous version. A change in this case, which complies with Clinical Trials Regulation (CTR), would be a significant alteration, a change in who or how a trial is being supervised, and a nonsignificant alteration that does not constitute the previous categories. When a modification comes into effect during a new clinical trial, there must be notification provided as a supplement to the application being sent. For ongoing trials, submissions regarding substantial alterations become mandatory.

In terms of deployment, there are three main models within the EU that are utilized, which are as follows:

(1) Investigative site-to-participant wherein an IMP is shipped from a clinical trial site or its respective pharmacy to a participant's address. This model has minimal regulatory-based hurdles; however, there is an associated workload for workers on site.

(2) Central pharmacy or pharmacy depot-to-participant model is when the IMP is sent from a centralized pharmacy depot that has facilities for distribution linked to a pharmacist as opposed to the clinical trial site's pharmacy. In the case of there being multiple sites for clinical trials, one site's pharmacy can become the centralized pharmacy that sends the IMP to trial participants within or across borders. This model decreases financial burden and facilitates direct-to-participant sending with specific stability requirements but may not be acceptable to all EU country regulatory bodies and there is a greater distance between the sender and receiver in this process.

(3) Local pharmacy-to-participant model is when the participant picks up the IMP or an authorized representative from a local pharmacy which is not the clinical trial site and this allows for low-intervention trials with an authorized IMP however, local pharmacists get a higher workload.

There is also a sponsor-to-participant model wherein the IMP is sent from the private firm's depot or via an outsourced manufacturing site, wholesaler, or distributor with no pharmacist-participant interaction; however, this has not been significantly seen or present in the EU.

Overall, the information for IMPs emphasizes safety and focuses on minimizing risk while taking into account various factors such as the nature of the drug, the stage of clinical development, the relevant patient population being targeted, the type and degree of the disorder, as well as the study design and length of the clinical trials in place. These tested IMPs must then undergo evaluation for authorization as per a submitted marketing authorization dossier and the approval decision itself per country may be influenced by multiple variables but rests on some key parameters: quality, efficacy, safety, and provision of net positive advantages as compared to the risk profile for patient populations.

7.19 Quality methods in medical device development and deployment

An article by Mckinsey reported that the medical device industry has expended greatly over time with global sales increasing up to $380 billion in 2006. The market size was valued at $519.29 billion in 2022 with projections of growth at around 535.12 billion US dollars this year and 799.67 billion US dollars by 2030, at a rate of 5.9% compound annual growth rate (CAGR). Despite growth, quality maintenance is a major challenge with studies showing that half of the FDA inspections conducted between the years 2010 and 2015 showed noncompliance across quality systems. The study conducted by Mckinsey also found that the direct costs of quality within the industry translated to 6.8%–9.4% of overall sales with direct costs of ensuring the quality (activities such as prevention, appraisal, quality control, and audit) were 2%–2.5% of sales, remediation costs of 0.4%–0.7% of sales and internal or externals failures rendering 2.1% and 0.4%–1.6% of sales, respectively. Additionally, external quality failures including recalls or actions by regulatory bodies also add on another 1.9%–2.5% of sales. The study also found that enhancing quality could recoup costs to around 1.6%–3.0% of industry sales. Evidently, quality has a major role to play in terms of both, economic benefits, compliance, and overall improved medical device development. Certain major activities that form the basis of enhancing quality are robust product and process controls, standardized quality systems, and a strong cultural emphasis on quality.

In the United Kingdom, NHS AI and Digital Regulations Service for health and social care has a pathway for medical device development and deployment that incorporates quality management and control aspects. The first step for medical device development is identifying whether the proposed technology is included within the umbrella of medical devices. As summarized by the UK Medical Device Regulations 2002, a medical device is defined as "*any instrument, apparatus, appliance, software, material or other article, whether used on its own or in combination as a supplement to any accessories including the software intended by its manufacturer to be used specifically for diagnosis or therapeutic purposes or both and necessary for its proper application, which is intended by the manufacturer to be used for human beings for the purpose of diagnosis, prevention, treatment or alleviation of disease or injury and handicap or investigation, replacement or modification of the anatomy, or of a physiological process, or control of conception.*" It must not gain its main purpose and associated outcome via pharmacological, immunological, or metabolic methods even if those are involved or supporting. These may be employed for the administration of a medicinal product such as an autoinjector or electrical stimulus such as in the case of a DBS device. A medical device may also incorporate a pharmacological substance which when used solely would act as medicine and is meant to have an impact on the human body without the device. It is key to note that with the sheer advancement in technology, software applications may also be part of the medical device umbrella and are determined to be one if the software is not incorporated in a device, is a computer program or a functional document with a medical purpose and does not qualify as an in vitro diagnostic (IVD).

After defining a proposed technology as a medical device, the medical device is then classified as per its risk assessment and this is where controls are placed, that is, the higher the risk of a device, the more stringent the control on its use is to ensure human safety.

There are four classes in medical devices: Class 1 (low risk), Class 2a (medium risk), Class 2b (medium risk) and Class 3 (high risk).

This classification is based on the proposed use case as per stated classification guidance and legislative factors which must be mentioned across every label and all registration-based activities. These classifications also tell the creator or manufacturer what regulatory proceedings to follow, what data and evidence needs to be shown over the product lifecycle, and what type of assessment (self or via an authorized body) the device must go under to meet the legislative criteria and the ways to conform via UK MDR 2002, which may not apply to all risk classes.

The classification is based on set rules that are to be compared against, that is, the UK MDR 2002, and upon matching the applicable rules and following the implementation as per the classification annex should allow for appropriate classification. This is crucial for innovators as incorrect classification can severely impact the pipeline of perceived milestones to launch a medical device and lead to both economic as well as image-based negative repercussions. On the other hand, if there are alterations made to the medical device itself, that could also modify its risk classification over time, and this must be under review continually across development.

The next step is building a value proposition for the technology across health and social setting markets and then supporting the claims with evidence is key to technology approval and uptake. If these claims cannot be substantiated, uptake by the market remains unlikely thus, information regarding what the purpose of the technology is, who it is intended to support, how it does so, and why key stakeholders including users/patient groups and healthcare services may accrue benefit from it is crucial. In doing so, one must conduct competitive intelligence activities, compare the proposed technology to the standard of care, and evaluate whether the proposed technology can either enhance patient health outcomes or reduce costs and resources in some way. Conducting feasibility assessments for the proposed data collection, having a clear purpose statement to qualify the medical device and associated classification, testing the device by incorporating HCP and user feedback to ensure it is meeting needs optimally, and developing a long-term evidence-generation strategy as per frameworks provided by NICE place the medical device in a strong place early on.

The innovator must have an intended purpose statement as it outlines the user of the medical device, its mechanism of action, and the ideal environment of use as well as its placement in the overarching medical system, its classification as a medical device further stratified by risk, and subsequent evidence generation required. During the conception, the purpose statement and value proposition must then be aligned to follow appropriate regulations. Quality control methods in the next steps surround compliance and legislation wherein the technology is a medical device, an active implantable medical device, or an in vitro diagnostic, all of which have separate requirements to get a UK Conformity Assessed (UKCA) mark. The UKCA marking denotes conformity with the necessary requirements to be sold or marketed in the United Kingdom. Based on the medical device requirements, documentation must be collected and stored to align with the risk classification and conformity route chosen. In alignment with the creation of this pipeline, the corresponding medical device assessment be accounted for with lower-risk devices being self-certifiable and higher-risk devices being approved by an authorizing body.

After the planning stages, it is legally mandatory to incorporate a quality management system (QMS), and it is characterized by internal processes and frameworks to ensure strong documentation management, monitoring of key decisions, and straightforward pathways for sign-off. A QMS comprises processes and documents, including policies, SOPs, and records, which outline objectives, methods, and outcomes of activities. Such management systems can decrease production, deployment, and surveillance-related risks, and innovators may also be held to provide evidence of certification by an authorized body to meet quality standards such as those in ISO 13485 requirements. ISO 13485 defines the requirements for creating and maintaining QMSs for medical devices, essential for meeting the UK Medical Device Regulations 2002 (UK MDR 2002). ISO 13485 certification involves auditing by an approved body and regular maintenance and auditing of the QMS throughout the device lifecycle. Upon reviewing the ISO standards, management systems must be implemented, which combine various attributes that address numerous needs and have some core features such as evidence collection, storage, and audit capabilities. External consultancies may be hired for the implementation of such systems and changes in management must be done carefully in the initial stages with appropriate system management through the product lifecycle. The scope of the QMS may vary based on the specific activities during the device's life-cycle, and it must be defined and audited accordingly. Key considerations of implementing QMS are ensuring training on correct usage, appropriate uptake by users, and establishing a culture that is quality-centric to integrate it across the organization as it must be well set up and certified before the completion of device development—which must all be conducted and implemented for a high-quality product.

After doing so, it is key to plan evidence generation to ensure the development of a medical device that is high quality by ensuring parameters of safety, clinical efficacy, and accessibility via cost-effectiveness. By planning early to select appropriate study designs that can support maximization of evidence utility for approval, aligning purpose statements to necessary compliance for medical device regulation, continuously keeping evidence updated, getting research-related approvals, employing guidelines by NICE and digital technology assessment criteria, as well as being mindful of resource allocation are all effective ways of ensuring development of a high-quality product. This evidence, partly overlapping with that required for a UKCA mark, should focus on relative effectiveness compared to current standard care. Developers need to ensure their studies accurately reflect clinical practice, including appropriate patient populations and testing sites. Long-term follow-up is crucial for capturing relevant outcomes, especially for technologies targeting patient survival or disease progression. Developers must consider the type of evidence required by adopters, health technology assessors, and regulators at each stage of the technology's lifecycle. This includes proof-of-concept studies during conceptualization, validation studies and clinical investigations during development, and real-world evidence studies postmarket. The study's design, execution, and validity are critically appraised using tools like the Cochrane risk-of-bias tool. The evaluation design should also balance the effectiveness of data collection methods with the time and resources available. Cost-effectiveness evidence varies depending on the technology's performance relative to current practice, requiring analyses like cost-consequence or cost-utility analysis. The increasing emphasis on quality in technological development is evident through the initiative of AI-Airlock being implemented by the Medicines and Healthcare Products Regulatory Agency (MHRA), which will enable a regulator-monitored online space for innovators to create robust data, plan novel technologies, and deploy appropriately.

This is followed by gaining clarity on the pathways to NICE health technology assessment (HTA), which is a form of quality optimization as it involves early planning and evaluation of the technology based on specific programs such as for diagnostics, medical technologies, technology appraisal, and interventional procedures. The NHS provides an NHS Innovation Service that also allows for a NICE evaluation upon which further development can take place.

One of the main concerns in developing a medical technology is the prioritization of high-quality data sets for training, testing, and validation as well as its ability to be applicable to the population of interest and the market. In digital health technology development, NICE advocates for a comprehensive approach to data quality. Essential aspects include ensuring data representativeness for the target health and social care population and specific technology applications, such as image quality in imaging tools. Training and validation data sets must be relevant, diverse, and applicable to real-world settings, emphasizing the generalizability of findings to the broader population and clinical practice. The integrity of these data sets is rigorously assessed for accuracy and consistency. External validation, ethical considerations, and equity are crucial to prevent biases and ensure fairness. Additionally, the data-labeling process incorporates quality management to mitigate AI bias within technologies.

High-quality medical devices, however, are not just limited to practical performance or device performance but must also demonstrate clinical performance. Such measures are captured within a Clinical Evaluation Report (CER), which supports the innovator to meet the essential requirements of the UK Medical Devices Regulations and obtain a UKCA mark. The CER, a living document maintained throughout the device's lifecycle, must include evidence showing that the benefits of the device outweigh its risks. This involves a structured clinical evaluation process, including scientific, analytical, and clinical validation. Key methods for meeting these requirements include conducting a literature review to define the "state of the art," in-house testing, prospective premarket trials, and postmarket clinical follow-up studies. The complexity of the CER depends on the device and its intended use, necessitating a clear intended use statement to identify evidence requirements. The CER must be periodically reviewed and updated to reflect changes in the state of the art and new evidence related to the device. Guidance from the International Medical Device Regulators Forum and MEDDEV can support the clinical evaluation process.

It is key to note that for medical devices that do require a UKCA mark, a clinical investigation may be necessary to demonstrate safety and performance. This investigation, a type of prospective clinical trial, is essential for devices without a UKCA mark and is conducted under normal conditions within the intended use. Clinical data can be sourced from scientific literature or from clinical data of equivalent compliant devices, demonstrating clinical, technical, and biological equivalency. This approach can save time and avoid redundant investigations. However, for AI-driven digital technology, clinical data from equivalent devices may not suffice due to variations in training data, necessitating a specific clinical investigation. Approvals from the MHRA and the Health Research Authority (HRA) are required, including ethical opinion from a Research Ethics Committee. The MHRA assessment process takes up to 60 days, and HRA approval around 40 days. Noncompliance or failure to conduct a necessary clinical investigation could lead to compliance issues, delays, or legal penalties.

In regard to the adoption of the technology, there are two key aspects: ensuring patient needs are captured and met and compliance with NHS Digital clinical risk safety standards. Developers must meet DCB0129, which ensures the creation of a clinical risk-management system (includes clinical risk-management governance, activities, and competency) and associated risk analysis to place their product on the market. Meeting risk-management requirements for medical devices ISO 14971:2019 sets the standards for risk-management systems in medical devices, aligning with the UK Medical Devices Regulations 2002 (UK MDR 2002) and the QMS standards, ISO 13485. This standard is essential for developers to evaluate risks associated with processes, device components, or scenarios. It encompasses clinical safety, data and information governance, cybersecurity, and medical device safety. Risk management involves identifying, analyzing, and quantifying risks, mitigating unacceptable risks, and justifying residual risks. Developers must adopt a risk-based approach in their assessments and design decisions, ensuring that the overall device risks are outweighed by the expected benefits. The results of these analyses must then be provided to the adopter. Complying with DCB0129, ISO 14971, and digital technology assessment criteria (DTAC) to ensure best practices have been employed on a national baseline requirement. Abiding by technical standards ensures the reliability and quality of technology, incorporates compliance costs within the budget, and stays updated with changing standards and regulations.

It is key to note that screening services and relevant digital technologies may have more stringent and higher barriers to entry due to different standards as various patient populations may employ such services and go through the UK National Screening Committee (UK NSC) and developers must consider clinical impact, ethical considerations, and usability across populations. The Ionizing Radiation (Medical Exposure) Regulations is a vital compliance aspect that must be carefully considered and used by trianed personnel.

To gain the UKCA mark and put the product on the market, the documents that are pertinent to every requirement as identified by classification and pathway selected for the medical device must be compiled as evidence of meeting all requirements. This documentation stems from the QMS in place, which can show proof of processes, risk management, device design and development, and clinical assessment, and upon passing the assessment, a certificate is given to the innovator so they can place the UKCA mark on the technology. Then an identification number of the approved body is also added to the device and then the device and developer or innovator can be registered with the MHRA. Noncompliance can result in legal penalties, emphasizing the importance of adhering to these standards and controls for quality and safety.

In terms of deployment for medical devices, the devices may require direct-to-consumer advertising as well as marketing to adopters which may consist of commissioners. They are also subject to laws that mandate postmarket surveillance that could be tracked to better understand long-term outcomes by way of a QMS gathering feedback loops. This would allow, any recalls, if required, and promptly alarming any safety concerns. In case an adverse event due to a medical device causing an unexpected side effect or issues arise, this must be reported to the MHRA via portal called MORE. These events must then be compiled into documentation alongside the remedial strategies adopted by the developer.

7.20 Quality control and assurance in digital technology development and deployment

In recent years, the NHS England and the UK government have reiterated their vision for a technologically adept future and its potential to transform healthcare including health education, as we know it. With the UK Digital Strategy emphasizing the United Kingdom's role as a Global Science and Tech Superpower and the HRA providing guidance for data-driven technologies to be integrated within health and social care systems, the need to ensure high-quality digital technology development and deployment is not just inevitable but will also act as fundamental building blocks of these systems for current patient populations and future generations.

Digital health incorporates a relatively wide spectrum of technologies such as mobile health via smart devices, software applications, and wearable devices; health information technology; provision of telehealth services such as remote GPs; and personalized healthcare. A similarly encompassing definition is provided by the National Institute of Health and Care Research (NIHR) with the benefits of employing digital health being its capabilities to enhance availability or accessibility to the user or patient 24/7 and from any geographical location thereby reducing hospital commute or otherwise, costs of medical care and encouraging patient autonomy for their personal health management.

As per the NHS HRA, there are certain legal stipulations and guidance provided for innovators who are developing, deploying, and tracking the progress of digital technologies that are data-driven in nature, that is, their functions involve data collection, utilization, and analysis to support users and patient care or the healthcare system and key stakeholders within it. The development of a digital technology can be bifurcated into four stages:

(1) Studying proof of concept: During the predeployment phase, the innovator must test and create support evidence to ensure the viability of their data-driven technology (whether it be an idea or a design). Some quality assurance methodologies and standards to be abided by during this phase include using anonymized or constructed data to maximize patient data security and reduce consent barriers. The UK GDPR laws also mandate the employment of the necessary amount of data for any given use and that data must be protected by strict access rights and audits of trails from the beginning. In terms of anonymization, pseudonyms are not considered strong enough and proof of efficacy regarding anonymization must abide by the Information Commissioner's Office (ICO) guidelines, remaining consistent even when data is moved. Regarding data sharing, especially with sensitive patient data, if it has to be released anywhere out of the team that is directly responsible for the patient, there must be consent for this.

(2) Testing in the care environment: It is also crucial to test the technology's safety and efficacy within a live care setting before deployment within the overall medical or social architecture it is intended for. An example of such trials was conducted in 2022 wherein NHS Digital was testing wireless technologies to develop real-time online diagnosis and referrals via a mobile health unit intended for high-risk populations that may be rendered vulnerable due to lower socioeconomic status. In these trials, HCPs had access to an application known as eObs (short for eObservations) wherein handheld tools were employed to update health records online while doing patient observations in real time. When piloting novel technologies, quality is ensured by following NICE evidence standards. The NICE real-world evidence framework, DECIDE-AI guidelines, and evidence standard frameworks support planning, implementing, and documenting of pilot studies appropriately. Standards 10 to 13 focus on the specification of the technology's value proposition, currently employed or proposed pathway for approval and evaluation of health, resource and economic costs as well as benefits. Outcomes are measured as per standards 14 and 15 which emphasis on data collection to show the technology's effectiveness and patient experience with the proposed technology. Standards 17 and 18 require assessments regarding changes seen in terms of efficiency, operations, and financial impacts of introducing proposed technology via budget impact or cost-effective analysis, respectively. Standards 19 and 20 discuss descriptions needed from deployment plans such as communication strategies, consent, and provision of training.

(3) Providing direct care: Direct care is defined as *"consisting of medical, social benefit public health activities to do with preventing, diagnosing or treating disorders and improving patient wellbeing by reduced symptomatology, better functioning, and assertion regarding high-quality care* via *auditing activities, adverse event management and reporting, and representative inclusion of patient feedback regarding the technology."* When deploying the technology for direct care to support the user, compliance surrounding data processing including confidentiality and data protection laws including Articles 6 and 9 of GDPR must be abided by.

(4) Evaluating the service and conducting postmarket surveillance: In the postmarket phase, adopters will focus on how well the technology integrates into the existing frameworks and medical architecture and this may require technology compatibility testing. This involves taking into account the data type involved by the digital technology, personnel with access rights, infrastructure, and processes in place for data collection, storage, and sharing and associated safety measures. During the compatibility testing, the confidential data may be processed in one of the three following ways:

   i. Already be compatible with existing infrastructure and would not need to process the data; therefore, approval will not be necessary, however, strict data measures must be in place

   ii. Processed by someone in the direct care team, when data has not been shared, explicit consent nor NHS Act 2006, section 251 is needed

iii. Section 251 is requested and an application to the Confidential Advisory Group (CAG) is submitted for data sharing unless explicit consent is obtained. This may usually occur in the case of changes needing to be made by a technical team or developer outside the direct carers of the patient.

In terms of common laws, all phases other than when the technology is used for direct care require either explicit consent by the patient or support of Section 251 if sensitive health data are being employed; whereas, in terms of data protection, GDPR Articles 6 and 9 remain mandated across all stages. On the other hand, research approvals are solely limited to predeployment, that is, proof-of-concept studies and testing in care environments.

In terms of ensuring quality, there is a checklist that asks questions such as whether the development and deployment of a technology are considered as part of the research, if there are the correct approvals for the proposed research to be conducted, whether the technology is a medical device, and if so, has the relevant authority been notified. Additionally, questions that ensure a CE or UKCA mark is present with the manufacturer if it is necessary, the conformation of the proposed tool to NICE standards, NHS Digital Clinical Risk Management standards, Deployment of Health IT Systems standards, and Guide to Good Practice for Digital and Data-Driven Health Technologies. All these questions are important to developing and deploying an appropriate, high-quality digital technology and must be reiteratively monitored as development and the product's lifecycle progresses as changes can lead to the implementation of new pipelines by the developers being necessary or different legislation or pathways to be considered for redeployment.

A major consideration in the tools that are in development today, especially in the healthcare and medical field, is the health data being utilized due to its sensitivity and thus, the associated legislation that regulates its appropriate usage. There are two data types—personal (identifiable to the patient or deidentified but can be reidentified) and nonpersonal data (anonymized data that cannot be reidentified). The main legal frameworks that have to be considered that are involved with data-driven technologies are the UK General Data Protection Regulation (UK GDPR) and the Data Protection Act 2018. The UK GDPR regulates aspects of data processing such as how lawful it is, how fair the data is, how much transparency is provided, whether the data is minimized as it is to be, how accurate it is, and who is accountable or liable for the data. It also specifies legal conditions for how to process personal data such as requiring explicit consent for sensitive information such as health data. In addition to the GDPR, the Data Protection Act 2018 has provisions specific to the United Kingdom regarding data processing, patient or individual rights, and punishments for noncompliance. The three other main factors for consideration of data are as follows:

(1) Confidentiality: Patient confidentiality is legally mandated and any personal data that can be tracked back to the person has to comply with confidentiality requirements.

(2) Consent: Explicit or implied consent is present as per the stage of deployment in question however, for any use case outside of direct care, consent has to be received from the individuals regarding the use of their data (unless exempt in specific cases).

(3) Ethics: Outside of the bounds of solely legal compliance, ensuring respectful treatment of patients, their privacy, obtaining informed consent, and conducting fair risk—benefit evaluations of the technology are best practices that both, researchers and innovators, must follow.

To optimize the quality of digital technologies, the technologies must show meet safety and quality standards with the patient population or relevant user's acceptability in mind. Providing value via the technology across or within a clinical pathway with repercussions of introduction must be at the center of initiating development. Additionally, factors such as environmental sustainability, health inequity, and bias minimization may also be considered to ensure accessibility of the technology. Best practices across stages start with compliant data and are maintained across the product lifecycle by continuous evaluation and clear systemic processes. Additionally, performance must be tested across settings to generate evidence, and associated value analyses such as budget impact or cost-effectiveness must be conducted. Lastly, meeting compliance requirements for deployment and placing effective processes for HCP or patient testing and consent from patients is necessary for the success of digital technology. Over time, the focus on quality and appropriate deployment can render ease of scalability, and thus, the overall impact of the introduced digital technology.

7.21 Managing quality protocols for mental healthcare populations

Three factors are crucial to effective healthcare systems that serve the needs of patient populations: quality, accessibility, and affordability. In terms of mental healthcare, effective psychological interventions are available for use across various mental health disorders; however, there remains a gap in accessibility of the treatments from a patient perspective. As many people suffering from mental illness do not have access to these treatments, there has been an increasing focus on improving the distribution and implementation of these effective interventions. Strategies that have been recommended to enhance the implementation of these treatments include the usage of standardized protocols, practical methods or principles, and national guidance or policies. One way of systematizing care would be to minimize differences in terms of practice and care provided. This could be an economical method for any healthcare system as the use of evidence-based clinical care protocols could continuously improve quality. Evidence-based protocols can support guiding clinicians in regard to carrying out diagnostic tests, prescriptions, and referrals as well as preventing negligence or medical mistreatment in the grand scheme of concerns. This is demonstrable by the Never Events Publication by the NHS that reported 295 serious, preventable patient safety events that ideally should not occur if healthcare professionals applied national guidance and safety recommendations.

In 1996, the WHO published a report called diagnostic and management guidelines for mental disorders in primary care, which outlined how to diagnose based on patient's presenting symptoms, diagnostic features, details on differential diagnosis per disease and how to manage disease based on essential information for caregivers, counseling of the patient and caregivers, notes regarding medication, and any specialist consultation that may be required to provide a general template of the clinical protocol. Globally, it is also common for there to be the presence of national strategies and frameworks per country that discuss or prioritize mental health (e.g.,—the National Service Framework for NHS in the United Kingdom, National Safety and Quality Digital Mental Health Standards in Australia). True impact lies in the successful implementation of such evidence-based treatment protocols, and outlined guidelines for mental health are crucial on a population level. Research conducted by Kendall and Frank focused on the role that flexibility or adaptability within reliable protocols plays in personalizing patient needs and improving healthcare outcomes. Additionally, use of frameworks such as the Consolidated Framework for Implementation Research (CFIR) can be utilized to implement evidence-based treatments effectively and improve accessibility of these treatments. For instance, the CFIR includes the intervention itself, outer and inner settings (i.e., features outside the firm and organization utilizing the intervention), individual (includes features of people involved in the execution), and procedures being implemented (e.g., organization). Based on findings by Damschroder in 2009 [116], the procedures or interventions have "core" pieces that are immovable with "adaptable" peripheries that can be modulated to tailor interventions for specified contexts and mental health settings.

Another study conducted on the implementation and adherence to evidence-based protocols for the use of psychotherapy in depression from the point of view of Dutch specialty mental healthcare therapists found that adapting treatment protocols or usage of medication is a common practice even in the case of research trials with the variance between changes made being heterogenous. Additionally, factors that interplay to impact adherence to evidence-based protocols include the mental health personnel's training and supervision or management style, their experience with the disorder, and intrapersonal characteristics of the mental healthcare specialist as well as the patient. In terms of the environment of operations, the organizational culture and adaptability impact whether therapists have or feel a perceived sense of autonomy in prescribing treatments or interventions and further altering them for personalization. In terms of cultures identified across organizations, authors identified three types of environments characterized by the degrees of flexibility and social control or standardization of care as follows:

i. Rigid culture with standardized mental healthcare programs

These environments increase the adherence conducted by therapists with minimal space for changes to be made, and although such environments support in consistency toward protocols, there may be minimal personalization of care in a patient-centric manner, which may lead to treatment-based delays due to bureaucracy or strict processes.

ii. Adaptable culture with shared vision and room for discussion

Therapists described these environments optimistically as they offer flexibility while retaining a cohesive shared vision and allow space for discussion regarding the best use of existing protocols and proposed alterations

iii. Highly adaptable culture with minimal social control

Such environments enhance therapists' autonomy within the organization to execute new workflows and frequencies of treatment or therapy; however, this may lead to high variance between patients in the organization based on the mental healthcare personnel and may render treatments that are less focused or standardized due to lack of structure or supervision and monitoring of healthcare professionals.

Often a major debate against the use of protocols within mental health is surrounding the large volume of protocols to be learned by the mental health personnel who require regular updates based on how patients with similar symptomatology, but varying diagnoses may present; however, the number of evidence-based protocols is not that high. In fact, there is significant overlap across protocols, and these can be traced with basic knowledge of the theory and principles underlying protocols alongside practical experience of how to adapt them for patients. Additionally, successful protocols are not as rigid and can account for the individualized needs of patients while still being valid in the integrity of symptoms being measured. However, a protocol is only good if effective in nature, and measuring a protocol's effectiveness requires evaluation. It is crucial to see if protocols are evaluated at more than one location by more than one principal investigator with real cases and blind, rigorous assessment of outcomes. This information in the case of quality protocols being employed that are evidence based also enables the therapist to reassure the patient of intervention therapy, for instance, EMDR therapy has shown 84%–100% rates of success across studies in patients with trauma based on a single major event with percentages being related to the severity of trauma and number of sessions undergone by the patient. The structured and adaptable nature of a well-written protocol can enable better decision making for healthcare personnel to decide on treatment strategies and decrease overall confusion making it a valuable tool to have in a mental healthcare professional's arsenal. Furthermore, protocols can be adapted to diverse backgrounds and clinical backgrounds to broaden their applicability and contribute to more efficient therapy, thereby potentially reducing the number of sessions offered and offering principle-driven approaches to address patient challenges. Overall, quality protocols serve the function of improving the quality and effectiveness of psychological treatments.

7.22 Quality optimization in complex intervention development and deployment

Mental health issues are complex in nature and characterized by varying severity, individual presentation, and comorbidity among other facts of which common issues across healthcare conditions are comorbidities, burden of intervention, concerns surrounding combinatorial interventions, and social inequalities. To address mental health issues from an evidence-based perspective, the intervention itself must be complex due to its multiple interrelated constituents, and due to these complexities, there are resulting variances in implementation. An intervention may be categorized as complex based on the core properties of the intervention itself, the behaviors that are being addressed, the number of people, settings, or levels being addressed, or the flexibility the intervention itself allows. To support standardization, in 2021, the Medical Research Council and the National Institute of Health Research have provided a new guidance framework to support the process of intervention development and deployment, which includes the various stages of research and development from conception to monitoring and execution on a population level. They have bifurcated complex intervention research into the following phases:

i. Developing or identifying an intervention

Either researchers create a novel intervention or alter an existing intervention for a novel use case based on a literature review or the problem itself. Alternatively, the researcher may select an intervention that already exists via policy or practice and conduct an evaluability assessment.

This stage involves conceptualization and initial design, involving tailoring existing interventions for new settings or patient population, or analyzing interventions from policy or practical initiatives. Also, during this stage, the researcher must discern the aspects of the intervention that require modifications and that must remain consistent for use in diverse use cases. The goal of this stage is to ensure the integrity of intervention in terms of basic mechanisms while customizing it for varied populations and outcomes.

ii. Assessing the viability or feasibility of the proposed intervention and evaluation design

Researchers must assess the viability and acceptability of the intervention and evaluate the design to decide whether the intervention should progress to the next stage of development. During this stage, the researcher evaluates factors such as recruitment, data collection, retention of participants, and study outcomes, which are all key to the intervention and assessment stage. Feasibility studies followed by evaluability allow to validate the intervention's viability for effectiveness and cost-efficient evaluation. Additionally, economic analysis is conducted to determine the intervention's effectiveness before deciding to progress the intervention.

iii. Assessment and evaluation of the intervention

Researchers must evaluate an intervention using the most appropriate methodology to address research questions. This stage evaluates applicability by exploring topics such as the intervention's larger effects, how it functions within its application environment, its role in systemic transformation, and its contribution to informed decision making. Collaborating with stakeholders, evaluators identify critical outcomes, incorporating a variety of outcomes into their analysis. Researchers may use a mixed-methods approach of research and evaluations to gain a sense of metrics such as patient adherence, disruptive capabilities, and mechanisms as well as quantify the impact of context on intervention itself.

iv. Intervention implementation

This stage is ensuring systemic effort is made in increasing impact and patient uptake or adherence to the novel and successfully developed innovation/intervention. Here the researchers contemplate how the intervention will be launched to ensure it remains effective in the overall architecture of the medical system, which includes focusing on implementation-related outcomes, examining the components of implementation strategy, and identifying the environmental aspects that may impact the intervention. Remaining adaptable and having early engagement with stakeholders and economic factors can significantly influence the feasibility, launch, and outcomes of the intervention.

All four phases have some common aspects such as considering the context, developing, testing, or retesting the program, engaging involved parties, identifying ambiguities, refining the intervention, and exploring the economic considerations.

It is key to note that within each phrase from 1 through 4, there are six key elements that are considered: how the intervention interacts with its settings or context, what the underlying program theory is, how diverse perspectives from numerous stakeholders can be incorporated within the research, the key ambiguities, how intervention can be refined, and what the comparative resource or outcome aftermath of the intervention looks like. Answering these questions across each stage allows researchers to make decisions regarding the progress of the research itself, that is, the intervention gets developed into the next stage, the intervention is refined in a preceding stage, a stage is repeated for validity or reliability, or the research is halted completely.

The new framework supports a shift in paradigm for hyper focus on efficacy toward how an intervention may be more accepted, better implemented, cost-effective, more scalable, and transferable across settings. Additionally, it views research from four lenses: efficacy, effectiveness, theory based, and systems perspectives.

When taking an efficacy perspective, the intervention is likely to be tested in ideal conditions to optimize for internal validity and provide as accurately as possible the impact of the intervention so the researcher can understand what effect size the intervention is leading to on intended outcomes in experimental environments. Whereas, from an effectiveness lens, the intervention is tested against the existing standard of care with results that help decide whether the novel, proposed solution is better for the health outcome compared to the current one and shines a light on the intervention in real-world settings. On a more discriminative lens, the theory-based perspective allows researchers to bifurcate between the various settings and is focused on the "why" behind identified variations, which can improve our theoretical understanding of underlying mechanisms as well as contexts. Using a theory-based approach also allows for the identification of critical success factors for the implementation beyond efficacy. Lastly, there is a systems approach that alludes to how the overall medical architecture and intervention work together and views the intervention as a disruptive technology to an ongoing system to understand the interplay of the intervention itself, the system, and the population among other factors.

In terms of developing and deploying a complex intervention for quality optimization adaptably, the BounceBack project from 2016 serves as a noteworthy case. This initiative, a collaborative effort between a mental health charity, academia, and GP practices, aimed to revolutionize mental healthcare in primary settings. The project initially encountered significant implementation challenges due to stakeholders' limited understanding of the new care model. Addressing these issues involved employing the Normalization Process Theory to refine and adapt the intervention, emphasizing development through implementation. The project's moderate success highlighted key lessons, including the necessity of comprehensive stakeholder engagement, treating new services as integral to systemic change, and the critical need for continual investment and flexibility to adapt to changing circumstances.

Similarly, another complex intervention as noted in 2018 was the Cardiovascular (CV) Toolkit project exemplifies a multifaceted approach to healthcare improvement, utilizing a variety of strategies across different stages. This project employed the Replicating Effective Program (REP) framework, strategically deploying interventions in phases from initial setup to long-term maintenance. The process involved a systematic mapping of each strategy, identifying its role, timing, participants, and expected outcomes. The results demonstrated a strategic timing of these interventions, with early phases focusing on stakeholder relationships and training, while later stages concentrated on communication and feedback mechanisms. This approach underscores the need for a comprehensive, multilevel strategy in complex interventions, ensuring thorough evaluation and practical implementation.

One way the REP framework could be adopted could be as a use case for mental health as opposed to cardiovascular, which may be summarized as follows: In the preconditions phase of developing mental health interventions, the primary goal would be to lay the groundwork for new initiatives. This may involve assessing existing practices, identifying care gaps, engaging with stakeholders like healthcare providers, patients, and community leaders, and performing needs assessments to fully grasp the current state of mental healthcare and prepare for change. Following this, the preimplementation phase would focus on developing and customizing interventions to meet community-specific needs, which includes training healthcare providers in new mental health practices, creating resources and materials, and conducting pilot tests in select environments. This would ensure that healthcare providers are well-prepared, resources are in place, and the intervention is set for wider application. As the intervention rolls out in the implementation phase, the aim would be to broadly deploy it across varied settings, while continuously monitoring its implementation, offering ongoing training and support, and actively involving the community. This phase services to ensure that any new mental health practices are effectively adopted in diverse settings with consistent support and program fidelity. Finally, in the maintenance and evolution phase, the objective would be to sustain and evolve the intervention. Regular evaluations are conducted, feedback is gathered, and the intervention is adapted and improved as needed, with policies established for long-term implementation. The desired outcome is for the intervention to become an enduring and evolving component of mental healthcare, responsive to changing needs over time.

Clearly, following systematic frameworks and guidance and proper execution can support maintaining high-quality services across phases of complex intervention development and deployment; however, it is crucial to note that the way high-quality interventions manifest themselves relies heavily on the underlying fabric of the medical system these interventions are to be embedded in. A study conducted in 2018 within the primary care settings to explore complex interventions to deliver mental health in India highlighted the sheer treatment gaps that exist within LMICS regarding the integration of mental healthcare services and how introducing a new implementation approach known as "design-focused implementation" which may be better employable in low-resource systems. In this case study, The PRIME (Program for Improving Mental Health Care) project in India focused on addressing three key mental health conditions—depression, alcohol use disorder, and psychosis—within the framework of the health system, covering community, primary care, and district hospital levels. The initiative's goal was to seamlessly incorporate mental health services into the existing healthcare infrastructure, prioritizing disorders identified as critical by the World Health Organization's mhGAP program. To achieve this, the project developed and assessed mental healthcare plans (MHCPs) at various organizational levels within the health system, starting in one district and eventually expanding to others. The MHCP in India was structured into two primary components: enabling and service delivery packages. The enabling packages, comprising program management, capacity building, and community mobilization, laid the groundwork necessary for effective service delivery. Meanwhile, the service delivery packages were directed toward raising awareness, facilitating diagnosis, providing treatment, and supporting recovery from mental health issues.

In summary, it is imperative that interventions are tailored to meet the specific challenges and requirements of individual countries. This approach should concentrate on developing robust health systems, diminishing disparities in care, and fostering the generation of substantial evidence supporting the integration of mental health services within primary and maternal healthcare environments. Such a focused strategy ensures that the unique context of each country is addressed, promoting equitable and effective mental healthcare tailored to the diverse needs of their populations.

7.23 Quality control and assurance procedures in the development and deployment of novel therapeutics

The need to address the previously discussed challenges faced by those with mental illnesses regarding the accessibility of appropriate treatments in specific, evidence-based psychological treatments (EBPTs), has given rise to the genesis of novel therapeutic manuals. The American Psychiatry Association (APA) defines manualized therapy, also known as manual-assisted therapy or manual-based therapy, as interventions that are performed based on specific guidelines for administration to maximize the probability of therapy being conducted consistently across settings, therapists, and clients. Given the high prevalence of mental illness and inaccessibility to EBPTs that show great evidence for use in treatment as single or adjunctive treatments, it is imperative to investigate further development and deployment of novel therapeutic manuals. The rationale behind employing a protocolized manual lies in the fact that they are often pretested in clinical trials therefore, it is likely that if followed appropriately and accurately the positive effects or outcomes witnessed in trials may be replicated in real-world settings. This is furthered by the use of multisite trials to ensure reproducibility and there are more methods to measure uptake, viability, and reliability by using therapy-based milestones and progress tracking by use of participant records and ranking of manuals as objective tools based on existing rating scales. An example of where protocolized manuals are used is in the case of CBT. CBT is defined as a form of psychotherapy that combines theories on cognition and learning with treatment techniques stemming from both, cognitive and behavior therapy. The underlying principle for this treatment is the belief that all three, cognitive, emotional, and behavioral aspects of a human are functionally interlinked with positive treatment outcomes being focused on recognizing and altering the patient's maladaptive cognitions or behaviors via cognitive restructuring and behavioral techniques. Such manualized therapies have been utilized across contexts such as schizophrenia, psychosis, mood disorders, substance use disorders, social anxiety disorders, and dementia.

In the case of schizophrenia, a manualized group therapy was developed by Dr. Rodrigue to improve medication management and patient satisfaction given the perceived imbalance between patient and physician autonomies as a result of stigma and dependence on pharmacological interventions that may exist due to this mental illness thereby, allowing a shifted focus for the patient to choose their preferred tools of medical management as per their treatment goals and personal needs. The employed intervention, also known as the Medication Management and Satisfaction Program, consisted of a group facilitator manual and materials for group members, guest speaker, and recovery-orientation assessors. The main factors identified to be key to the clinical practice of developing such a program were found to be as follows: the degree to which the practicing organization supports the use of the recovery model underlying the program as opposed to a strictly medical model, the language used by the healthcare personnel to deliver the program appropriately in a manner that encourages recovery of the patient and destigmatizes their self-perception. Similarly, clinical trials focused on the deployment side of manualized therapies for psychosis have shown a manualized treatment protocol that has exhibited positive clinical outcomes when delivered in a routine clinical mental health treatment setting such as reduced adverse symptomatology and decreased likelihood of high-risk patients to transition to psychosis. The general model of the protocol contains an underlying fabric that consists of specific principles and values such as being collaborative and problem-orientated in a way that normalizes or validates the person's presentation which are overlaid by technical elements such as milestones and change strategies that include evaluating appraisals, cognitions, cognitive and behavioral responses while maintaining active engagement and using homework or tasks between sessions supported by an empirically tested cognitive model. These protocols are then bifurcated into phases such as assessment and engagement to identify challenges and ideal treatment outcomes. Change strategies could then be employed as agreed upon by the person which can include normalization, situational assessment and judgment, coping mechanisms, role play or skill building, and evidence-based analysis.

A study by Harvey and Gumport identified barriers that exist on a treatment level as challenges in identifying an appropriate EBPT due to the lack of a unified source for their identification, current EBPTs requiring improvement through enhanced innovation, and the problem of overavailability of empirically supported treatment options that could be replaced either by providing more methods to deliver the treatments or through replacement with treatments that are transdiagnostic and modularized.

An example wherein manualized treatments have been employed is in the case of mood disorders including depression. In fact, for mood disorders, there have even been explorations toward more unified protocols for transdiagnostic treatment of affective disorders in this research including anxiety and depression. A systematic review found that a unified protocol was effective in targeting the origins of disorders thereby decreasing symptomatology seen in comorbidity with significant alteration of large overall effect size seen across populations from children and adolescents to adults. Another use of manualized therapy has been in the case of group therapy. A study by Fox and colleagues conducted in 2021 tested the feasibility of a standardized group manual in a university healthcare setting wherein, they found that the introduction of the standardized manual was associated with improvements in patient outcomes related to decreased fear and higher compassion predictive of improvements in psychological distress levels. However, all of these findings considered the need to identify the measures that exist to ensure that manuals are developed and maintained as high-quality tools in mental illness are ever growing. An ongoing study by Creed and team that began in 2022 is looking to evaluate the quality of EBPTs such as CBT to treat mental illness in a scalable manner by creating AI-based technologies that are cost-effective to allow for training of mental health personnel in and supervision of utilization of EBPTs. The tool being created will offer HIPAA-compliant, cloud-based software to record, share, and evaluate the quality of therapy sessions and incorporate AI-generated measures for CBT. Similarly, Flemotomos and team proposed a BERT (bidirectional encoder representation from transformers)-based model that can enable quality assurance for CBT sessions by providing automated scoring by classifying therapy sessions based on global scores as per the Cognitive Therapy Rating Scale (CTRS), a commonly employed measure. Given that the model is trained on multiple tasks for enhanced interpretability and utilization of available therapy metadata, there is scope for its improvement and further clinical translation as a digital tool for QA.

A crucial consideration that remains constant in the use of even manualized treatments and protocols is the idea that the medical professional, mental health personnel, or psychotherapist conducting the sessions and their perceptions surrounding patient care and procedures used are significant. A study exploring CBT therapists and their perceptions surrounding practicing CBT found that incorporating discoveries from research into clinical use rendered that treatment protocols be used with patients. Additionally, though CBT trainers educate trainees regarding how crucial evidence-based clinical practice is and prescribe associated skills, the responsibility to have proper clinical conduct and stay up to date regarding evidence-based guidelines or apply the scientist-practitioner methodology also lies with the therapists themselves. By using competency assessments within CBT across real and artificial settings as well as utilizing validated and reliable measures, quality assurance of CBT can be made routine in healthcare structures. The current gap is focused on quality assurance not being a top-tier priority in clinical care, potentially due to its demand for resources or lack of incentivization. Additionally, there is still a lack of confirmation in terms of translation of manual-based treatments which may offer research-based benefits but was found to have shown similar efficacy to nonmanualized treatment as per a systematic review of six studies by Truijens and team.

Current NICE guidelines for CBT for psychosis (CBTp) in treatment for schizophrenia assess the CBT and clinical care as per the Donabedian framework, which include:

- Ensuring structures such as local services are available for CBTp use for those living with schizophrenia and psychosis based on local data collection.

- The process examines quality based on accessibility or the number of people that are provided the service, that is, proportions of adults with psychosis or schizophrenia who receive CBTp.
- The evaluation of outcomes focuses on the relapse rates seen in adults who have schizophrenia and psychosis.
- Similar quality measures and standards are also placed for treatments across mental illnesses such as depression and generalized anxiety disorder.

The Improved Access to Psychological Manual outlines the NICE-recommended psychological interventions for low- and high-intensity interventions across disorders including depression and generalized anxiety disorder. Current NICE guidelines for depression in adults recommend the use of psychological and psychosocial treatment manuals that guide the form, duration, and termination of utilized interventions as well as consideration of competence frameworks that stem from treatment manuals that enable supporting effective training, delivery, and supervision of the same. The selected treatment manuals are created from those used in trials that provided findings for the efficacy of the treatments within NICE guidelines.

Additionally, the quality guidelines also outline how various stakeholders are involved and impacted by these guidelines. For instance, service providers such as general practitioners and community-based mental health providers are to make sure there are systems intact for adults with psychosis or schizophrenia who could benefit from CBTp services as well as provision of the appropriate training for HCPs in CBTp. On the other hand, HCPs then offer the CBTp sessions to the receivers of such services, that is, adults with psychosis or schizophrenia presentation. The commissioners such as local authority groups and the NHS England commissioning group commission CBTp services and make sure referral pathways exist for patients to be linked to appropriate services. As previously discussed, such standards are focused on ideally providing high-quality, accessible, and affordable treatments however, with a dearth of studies on the subject, the evidence suggests that quality assurance and control measures or standards are within their primary stages of evolution and much work must be established within this field to ensure optimization of these three levers.

7.24 **Future directions**

To guarantee the provision of superior mental health and neuropsychiatric support, it is vital to implement rigorous quality assurance and control measures throughout the patient journey. This includes critical points such as when HCPs employ standardized protocols for therapy and treatment of illnesses. Additionally, there should be a robust system for monitoring both the quality of therapy sessions and the adherence to these protocols. Such meticulous oversight ensures that every phase of patient care meets the highest standards, thereby enhancing the efficacy of treatments and ensuring optimal patient outcomes. This approach not only fortifies the reliability of mental health services but also instills confidence in patients about the care they receive.

Similarly, stakeholders must be held accountable to ensure quality is at the center of their vested interests when providing healthcare services to such populations on a systemic level. This prioritization is exemplified in the case of Mental Health Commissions by providing a systematic analysis to provide incentivization across the organization. For instance, the National Quality Framework for Mental Health Services of Ireland has emphasized the need to ensure high quality across the following themes (of which themes 2, 3, 4, 5, and 7 are directly relevant):

(1) Leadership and Governance
(2) Needs of the Service Users
    i. Prioritizes the needs of the patient and associated caretakers to make sure service is tailored to the needs of individuals or groups in a multidisciplinary manner to address acute or episodic and prolonged disease
(3) Holistic Service
    ii. Places focus on equality across the mental health system to encourage prevention and recovery to provide an assimilated service that is optimized in terms of entry and termination of services and appropriately responsive as well as accessible
(4) Equal, Inclusive, and Diverse Service
    iii. Highlights quality in terms of ensuring an inclusive and diverse mental health structure that encourages inclusion and awareness regarding social determinants of health and employs a trauma-informed approach to healthcare
(5) Recovery
    iv. Takes into account patient autonomy, these services underline advocating for the receiver to feel included and the treatment to focus on their fortes as individuals to accomplish treatment goals
(6) Care Planning
(7) Provision of Services
    v. Ensure high quality via good governance and appropriate resource allocation such as adequate services, upskilling of staff, and enrichment of environments to emphasize recovery for patients
(8) Connected Service

In both manualized treatments and complex interventions, it is imperative to sustain a focus on quality, ensuring that these interventions are inclusive, patient-centric, and uniformly integrated within the mental health framework. This commitment to quality is essential for delivering seamless and accessible services. Such an approach not only respects the diverse needs of patients but also facilitates the delivery of care that is both effective and attuned to the unique circumstances of each individual. By prioritizing inclusivity and patient-centeredness, mental health services can become more responsive and equitable, ultimately enhancing the overall effectiveness and reach of mental healthcare.

References

[1] Freemon FR. Galen's ideas on neurological function. J Hist Neurosci October, 1994; 3(4):263−71. https://doi.org/10.1080/09647049409525619. PMID: 11618827.

[2] Hansotia P. A neurologist looks at mind and brain: "the enchanted loom". Clin Med Res October, 2003;1(4):327−32. https://doi.org/10.3121/cmr.1.4.327. PMID: 15931326; PMCID: PMC1069062.

[3] Fischbach GD. Mind and brain. Sci Am 1992;267:48−57.

[4] Hansotia PL. Persistent vegetative state. Review and report of electrodiagnostic studies in eight cases. Arch Neurol 1985;42:1048−52.

[5] Agrawal N, Faruqui R, Bodani M, editors. Oxford textbook of neuropsychiatry, Oxford textbooks in psychiatry. Oxford: Oxford Academic; 2020. https://doi.org/10.1093/med/9780198757139.001.0001. 1 Aug. 2020, [Accessed 6 December 2023].

[6] Schwartz JM, Begley S, editors. Neuroplasticity and the power of mental force. New York: Harper Collins; 2002 [The mind and the brain].

[7] Hassan A, Okun MS. Emerging subspecialties in neurology: deep brain stimulation and electrical neuro-network modulation. Neurology January 29, 2013;80(5): e47−50. https://doi.org/10.1212/WNL.0b013e31827f0f91.

[8] Schiefer TK, Matsumoto JY, Lee KH. Moving forward: advances in the treatment of movement disorders with deep brain stimulation. Front Integr Neurosci 2011;5:1−16.

[9] Obeso JA, Rodriguez-Oroz MC, Rodriguez M, et al. Pathophysiologic basis of surgery for Parkinson's disease. Neurology 2000;55(12 Suppl. 6). S7−S12.

[10] Perez DL, Keshavan MS, Scharf JM, Boes AD, Price BH. Bridging the great divide: what can neurology learn from psychiatry? J Neuropsychiat Clin Neurosci 2018; 30(4):271−8. https://doi.org/10.1176/appi.neuropsych.

[11] Cunningham MG, Goldstein M, Katz D, et al. Coalescence of psychiatry, neurology, and neuropsychology: from theory to practice. Harv Rev Psychiatr 2006;14:127−40.

[12] Silbersweig D. Integrating models of neurologic and psychiatric disease. JAMA Neurol 2017;74:759−60.

[13] Heckers S. Project for a scientific psychiatry: neuroscience literacy. JAMA Psychiatr 2017;74:315.

[14] Lyketsos CG, Lopez O, Jones B, Fitzpatrick AL, Breitner J, DeKosky S. Prevalence of neuropsychiatric symptoms in dementia and mild cognitive impairment: results from the cardiovascular health study. JAMA September 25, 2002;288(12):1475−83. https://doi.org/10.1001/jama.288.12.1475.

[15] Van Dam D, Vermeiren Y, Dekker AD, Naudé PJ, Deyn PP. Neuropsychiatric disturbances in Alzheimer's disease: what have we learned from neuropathological studies? Curr Alzheimer Res 2016;13(10):1145−64. https://doi.org/10.2174/1567205013666160502123607.

[16] Najjar S, Pearlman DM, Alper K, Najjar A, Devinsky O. Neuroinflammation and psychiatric illness. J Neuroinflammation 2013;10:43.

[17] Bozyczko-Coyne D, O'Kane TM, Wu ZL, Dobrzanski P, Murthy S, Vaught JL, et al. CEP-1347/KT-7515, an inhibitor of SAPK/JNK pathway activation, promotes survival and blocks multiple events associated with Abeta-induced cortical neuron apoptosis. J Neurochem 2001;77:849−63.

[18] Donev R, Kolev M, Millet B, Thome J. Neuronal death in Alzheimer's disease and therapeutic opportunities. J Cell Mol Med 2009;13:4329−48.

[19] Mucke L, Masliah E, Yu GQ, Mallory M, Rockenstein EM, Tatsuno G, et al. High-level neuronal expression of abeta 1-42 in wild-type human amyloid protein precursor transgenic mice: synaptotoxicity without plaque formation. J Neurosci 2000;20: 4050−8.

[20] Heneka MT, Carson MJ, El Khoury J, Landreth GE, Brosseron F, Feinstein DL, et al. Neuroinflammation in Alzheimer's disease. Lancet Neurol 2015;14:388−405.

[21] National Institute for Health and Care Excellence [NICE] (2013).

[22] American Psychiatric Association. Diagnostic and statistical manual of mental disorders. 5th ed. 2022. https://doi.org/10.1176/appi.books.9780890425787. textrev.

[23] Khoury B, Kogan C, Daouk S. International classification of diseases 11th edition (ICD-11). In: Encyclopedia of personality and individual differences. Cham: Springer International Publishing; 2020. p. 2350−5.

[24] Ma C, Wang Z, Li C, Lu J, Long J, Li R, Zhao M. The clinical consistency and utility of ICD-11 diagnostic guidelines for gaming disorder: a field study among the Chinese population. Front Psychiatr 2021;12:781992.

[25] Dalgleish T, Black M, Johnston D, Bevan A. Transdiagnostic approaches to mental health problems: current status and future directions. J Consult Clin Psychol 2020; 88(3):179.

[26] Bach B, First MB. Application of the ICD-11 classification of personality disorders. BMC Psychiatr 2018;18:351. https://doi.org/10.1186/s12888-018-1908-3.

[27] Gautam R, Sharma M. Prevalence and diagnosis of neurological disorders using different deep learning techniques: a meta-analysis. J Med Syst 2020;44:49. https://doi.org/10.1007/s10916-019-1519-7.

[28] Schläpfer TE, Bewernick BH. Deep brain stimulation for psychiatric disorders — state of the art. In: Advances and technical standards in neurosurgery. Advances and technical standards in neurosurgery, vol. 34. Vienna: Springer; 2009. https://doi.org/10.1007/978-3-211-78741-0_2.

[29] Parsa M, Rad HY, Vaezi H, Hossein-Zadeh G-A, Setarehdan SK, Rostami R, et al. EEG-based classification of individuals with neuropsychiatric disorders using deep neural networks: a systematic review of current status and future directions. In: Computer methods and programs in biomedicine; 2023. https://doi.org/10.1016/J.CMPB.2023.107683.

[30] Vieira S, Pinaya WH, Mechelli A. Using deep learning to investigate the neuroimaging correlates of psychiatric and neurological disorders: methods and applications. Neurosci Biobehav Rev 2017;74:58−75.

[31] Gaebel W. Status of psychotic disorders in ICD-11. Schizophr Bull 2012;38(5):895−8. https://doi.org/10.1093/schbul/sbs104. Erratum in: Schizophr Bull. 2012 Nov;38(6): 1336. PMID: 22987845; PMCID: PMC3446222.

[32] Insel T, Cuthbert B, Garvey M, Heinssen R, Pine DS, Quinn K, Wang P. Research domain criteria (RDoC): toward a new classification framework for research on mental disorders. Am J Psychiatr 2010;167(7):748−51.

[33] World Health Organization. Basic documents. 46th ed. Geneva: World Health Organization; 2007.

[34] International Advisory Group for the Revision of ICD-10 Mental and Behavioural Disorders A conceptual framework for the revision of the ICD-10 classification of mental and behavioural disorders. World Psychiatr 2011;10:86−92.

[35] Jablensky A. The diagnostic concept of schizophrenia: its history, evolution, and future prospects. Dialogues Clin Neurosci 2010;12(3):271−87. https://doi.org/10.31887/DCNS.2010.12.3/ajablensky. PMID: 20954425; PMCID: PMC3181977.

[36] Keller WR, Fischer BA, Carpenter Jr WT. Revisiting the diagnosis of schizophrenia: where have we been and where are we going? CNS Neurosci Ther 2011;17:83−8.

[37] Gaebel W, Stricker J, Kerst A. Changes from ICD-10 to ICD-11 and future directions in psychiatric classification dialogues. Clin Neurosci 2020;22(1):7−15. https://doi.org/10.31887/DCNS.2020.22.1/wgaebel. PMID: 32699501; PMCID: PMC7365296.

[38] Reed GM, First MB, Kogan CS, et al. Innovations and changes in the ICD-11 classification of mental, behavioural and neurodevelopmental disorders. World Psychiatr 2019;18(1):3−19.

[39] Aarseth E, Bean AM, Boonen H, et al. Scholars' open debate paper on the world health organization ICD-11 gaming disorder proposal. J Behav Addict 2017;6(3):267−70.

[40] Lebeau RT, Glenn DE, Hanover LN, Beesdo-Baum K, Wittchen HU, Craske MG. A dimensional approach to measuring anxiety for DSM-5. Int J Meth Psychiatr Res 2012;21(4):258−72. https://doi.org/10.1002/mpr.1369. Epub 2012 Nov 13. PMID: 23148016; PMCID: PMC6878356.

[41] Pemberton R, Tyszkiewicz MDF. Factors contributing to depressive mood states in everyday life: a systematic review. J Affect Disord 2016;200:103−10.

[42] Simon GE, Bauer MS, Ludman EJ, Operskalski BH, Unutzer J. Mood symptoms, functional impairment, and disability in people with bipolar disorder: specific effects of mania and depression. J Clin Psychiatr 2007;68(8):1237−45.

[43] Cassidy F, Forest K, Murry E, Carroll BJ. A factor analysis of the signs and symptoms of mania. Arch Gen Psychiatr 1998;55(1):27−32.

[44] Schrijvers D, Hulstijn W, Sabbe BG. Psychomotor symptoms in depression: a diagnostic, pathophysiological and therapeutic tool. J Affect Disord 2008;109(1−2):1−20.

[45] García-Mieres H, Lundin NB, Minor KS, Dimaggio G, Popolo R, Cheli S, et al. A cognitive model of diminished expression in schizophrenia: the interface of metacognition, cognitive symptoms and language disturbances. J Psychiatr Res 2020; 131:169−76.

[46] Contreras JA, Goñi J, Risacher SL, Sporns O, Saykin AJ. The structural and functional connectome and prediction of risk for cognitive impairment in older adults. Curr Behav Neurosci Rep 2015;2:234−45.

[47] Findley LJ, Barth JT, Powers DC, Wilhoit SC, Boyd DG, Suratt PM. Cognitive impairment in patients with obstructive sleep apnea and associated hypoxemia. Chest 1986; 90(5):686−90.

[48] Buckley PF, Miller BJ, Lehrer DS, Castle DJ. Psychiatric comorbidities and schizophrenia. Schizophr Bull 2009;35(2):383−402. https://doi.org/10.1093/schbul/sbn135.

[49] Habtewold TD, Tiles-Sar N, Liemburg EJ, et al. Six-year trajectories and associated factors of positive and negative symptoms in schizophrenia patients, siblings, and controls: genetic risk and outcome of psychosis (GROUP) study. Sci Rep 2023;13:9391. https://doi.org/10.1038/s41598-023-36235-9.

[50] Vyas NS, Patel NH, Puri BK. Neurobiology and phenotypic expression in early onset schizophrenia. Early Intervent psychiat 2011;5(1):3−14.

[51] Abashkin DA, Kurishev AO, Karpov DS, Golimbet VE. Cellular models in schizophrenia research. Int J Mol Sci 2021;22(16):8518. https://doi.org/10.3390/ijms22168518.

[52] Huizink AC, Robles de Medina PG, Mulder EJ, Visser GH, Buitelaar JK. Stress during pregnancy is associated with developmental outcome in infancy. J Child Psychol Psychiatry 2003;44(6):810−8.

[53] Escudero I, Johnstone M. Genetics of schizophrenia. Curr Psychiatr Rep 2014;16:1−6. https://doi.org/10.1007/s11920-014-0502-8.

[54] Guan J, Cai JJ, Ji G, Sham PC. Commonality in dysregulated expression of gene sets in cortical brains of individuals with autism, schizophrenia, and bipolar disorder. Transl Psychiatr 2019;9:1−15. https://doi.org/10.1038/s41398-019-0488-4.

[55] Pardiñas AF, Holmans P, Pocklington AJ, Escott-Price V, Ripke S, Carrera N, et al. Common schizophrenia alleles are enriched in mutation-intolerant genes and in regions under strong background selection. Nat Genet 2018;50:381−9. https://doi.org/10.1038/s41588-018-0059-2.

[56] oszła O, Targowska-Duda KM, Kedzierska E, Kaczor AA. In vitro and in vivo models for the investigation of potential drugs against schizophrenia. Biomolecules 2020;10: 160. https://doi.org/10.3390/biom10010160.

[57] Pezzini F, Bettinetti L, Di Leva F, Bianchi M, Zoratti E, Carrozzo R, et al. Transcriptomic profiling discloses molecular and cellular events related to neuronal differentiation in SH-SY5Y neuroblastoma cells. Cell Mol Neurobiol 2017;37:665−82. https://doi.org/10.1007/s10571-016-0403-y.

[58] Zhuo C, Zhang Q, Wang L, Ma X, Li R, Ping J, Jiang D. Insulin resistance/diabetes and schizophrenia: potential shared genetic factors and implications for better management of patients with schizophrenia. CNS Drug 2023:1−12.

[59] Ayora M, Fraguas D, Abregú-Crespo R, et al. Leukocyte telomere length in patients with schizophrenia and related disorders: a meta-analysis of case-control studies. Mol Psychiatr 2022;27:2968−75. https://doi.org/10.1038/s41380-022-01541-7.

[60] Solana C, Pereira D, Tarazona R. Early senescence and leukocyte telomere shortening in schizophrenia: a role for cytomegalovirus infection? Brain Sci 2018;8(10):188. https://doi.org/10.3390/brainsci810018.

[61] Zampieri E, Bellani M, Crespo-Facorro B, Brambilla P. Basal ganglia anatomy and schizophrenia: the role of antipsychotic treatment. Epidemiol Psychiatr Sci 2014; 23(4):333−6. https://doi.org/10.1017/S204579601400064X.

[62] Najjar S, Pahlajani S, De Sanctis V, Stern JN, Najjar A, Chong D. Neurovascular unit dysfunction and blood−brain barrier hyperpermeability contribute to schizophrenia neurobiology: a theoretical integration of clinical and experimental evidence. Front Psychiatr 2017;8:83.

[63] Goldwaser EL, Swanson RL, Arroyo EJ, Venkataraman V, Kosciuk MC, Nagele RG, Acharya NK. A preliminary report: the Hippocampus and surrounding temporal cortex of patients with schizophrenia have impaired blood-brain barrier. Front Hum Neurosci 2022;16:836980.

[64] Hertzberg L, Nicola Maggio, Muler I, Yitzhaky A, Majer M, Haroutunian V, et al. Comprehensive gene expression analysis detects global reduction of proteasome subunits in schizophrenia. Schizophr Bull 2021;47(3):785−95. https://doi.org/10.1093/schbul/sbaa160.

[65] Jiang S, Huang H, Zhou J, et al. Progressive trajectories of schizophrenia across symptoms, genes, and the brain. BMC Med 2023;21:237. https://doi.org/10.1186/s12916-023-02935-2.

[66] Speers LJ, Bilkey DK. Disorganization of oscillatory activity in animal models of schizophrenia. Front Neural Circ 2021;15:741767.

[67] Hemsley DR. What have cognitive deficits to do with schizophrenic symptoms? Br J Psychiatr 1977;130(2):167−73.

[68] Scheff TJ. Schizophrenia as ideology. Schizophr Bull 1970;1(2):15.

[69] Torous J, Roberts LW. The ethical use of mobile health technology in clinical psychiatry. J Nerv Ment Dis 2017;205(1):4−8.

[70] Aschauer D, Rumpel S. The sensory neocortex and associative memory. In: Clark RE, Martin S, editors. Behavioral neuroscience of learning and memory. Current topics in behavioral neurosciences, vol. 37. Cham: Springer; 2016. https://doi.org/10.1007/7854_2016_453.

[71] Wright A. Chap. 9: higher cortical functions: association and executive processing. 2015.

[72] Cannon TD. How schizophrenia develops: cognitive and brain mechanisms underlying onset of psychosis. Trend Cognit Sci 2015;19(12):744−56.

[73] Ermakov EA, Dmitrieva EM, Parshukova DA, Kazantseva DV, Vasilieva AR, Smirnova LP. Oxidative stress-related mechanisms in schizophrenia pathogenesis and new treatment perspectives. Oxid Med Cell Longev 2021:2021.

[74] Arnsten AF, Woo E, Yang S, Wang M, Datta D. Unusual molecular regulation of dorso-lateral prefrontal cortex layer III synapses increases vulnerability to genetic and environmental insults in Schizophrenia. Biol Psychiatr 2022;92(6):480−90.

[75] Adell A. Brain NMDA receptors in schizophrenia and depression. Biomolecules 2020; 10(6):947. https://doi.org/10.3390/biom10060947.

[76] Robert V, Cassim S, Chevaleyre V, et al. Hippocampal area CA2: properties and contribution to hippocampal function. Cell Tissue Res 2018;373:525−40. https://doi.org/10.1007/s00441-017-2769-7.

[77] Chopra S, Segal A, Oldham S, et al. Network-based spreading of gray matter changes across different stages of psychosis. JAMA Psychiatr 2023;80(12):1246−57. https://doi.org/10.1001/jamapsychiatry.2023.3293.

[78] Uscătescu LC, Kronbichler L, Stelzig-Schöler R, Pearce BG, Said-Yürekli S, Reich LA, Kronbichler M. Effective connectivity of the hippocampus can differentiate patients with schizophrenia from healthy controls: a spectral DCM approach. Brain Topogr 2021;34:762−78.

[79] Uscătescu LC, Kronbichler L, Stelzig-Schöler R, et al. Effective connectivity of the Hippocampus can differentiate patients with schizophrenia from healthy controls: a spectral DCM approach. Brain Topogr 2021;34(6):762−78. https://doi.org/10.1007/s10548-021-00868-8. PMID: 34482503; PMCID: PMC8556208.

[80] Boyer P, Phillips JL, Rousseau FL, Ilivitsky S. Hippocampal abnormalities and memory deficits: new evidence of a strong pathophysiological link in schizophrenia. Brain Res Rev 2007;54:92−112. https://doi.org/10.1016/j.brainresrev.2006.12.008.

[81] Uscătescu LC, Said-Yürekli S, Kronbichler L, et al. Reduced intrinsic neural time-scales in schizophrenia along posterior parietal and occipital areas. NPJ Schizophr 2021;7:55. https://doi.org/10.1038/s41537-021-00184-x.

[82] Spijker J, Claes S. Mood disorders in the DSM-5. Tijdschr Psychiatr 2014;56(3): 173−6.

[83] Kurumaji A. The trends of mood disorders in ICD-11: bipolar and depressive disorders. Seishin Shinkeigaku Zasshi 2013;115(1):60−8.

[84] Palma-Gudiel H, Córdova-Palomera A, Navarro V, Fañanás L. Twin study designs as a tool to identify new candidate genes for depression: a systematic review of DNA methylation studies. Neurosci Biobehav Rev 2020;112:345−52.

[85] Quello SB, Brady KT, Sonne SC. Mood disorders and substance use disorder: a complex comorbidity. Sci Pract Perspect December 2005;3(1):13−21. https://doi.org/10.1151/spp053113.

[86] Correll CU, Smith CW, Auther AM, McLaughlin D, Shah M, Foley C, et al. Predictors of remission, schizophrenia, and bipolar disorder in adolescents with brief psychotic disorder or psychotic disorder not otherwise specified considered at very high risk for schizophrenia. J Child Adolesc Psychopharmacol October 2008;18(5):475−90. https://doi.org/10.1089/cap.2007.110.

[87] Abdel-Baki A, Letourneau G, Morin C, Ng A. Resumption of work or studies after first-episode psychosis: the impact of vocational case management. Early Intervent Psychiat 2013;7(4):391−8. PubMed.

[88] Abramowitz JS, Foa EB, Franklin ME. Exposure and ritual prevention for obsessive−compulsive disorder: effects of intensive versus twice-weekly sessions. J Consult Clin Psychol 2003;71(2):394−8 [PubMed].

[89] Acarturk C, Smit F, de Graaf R, van Straten A, ten Have M, Cuijpers P. Incidence of social phobia and identification of its risk indicators: a model for prevention. Acta Psychiatr Scand 2009;119(1):62−70.

[90] Stein DJ, Szatmari P, Gaebel W, et al. Mental, behavioral and neurodevelopmental disorders in the ICD-11: an international perspective on key changes and controversies. BMC Med 2020;18:21. https://doi.org/10.1186/s12916-020-1495-2.

[91] Lohoff FW. Overview of the genetics of major depressive disorder. Curr Psychiatr Rep December, 2010;12(6):539−46. https://doi.org/10.1007/s11920-010-0150-6. PMID: 20848240.

[92] Tsuang MT, Taylor L, Faraone SV. An overview of the genetics of psychotic mood disorders. J Psychiatr Res 2004;38:3−15.

[93] Prathikanti S, Weinberger DR. Psychiatric genetics − the new era: genetic research and some clinical implications. Br Med Bull 2005;73−74(1):107−22. https://doi.org/10.1093/bmb/ldh055.

[94] Priess-Groben HA, Hyde JS. 5-HTTLPR X stress in adolescent depression: moderation by MAOA and gender. J Abnorm Child Psychol 2013;41:281−94. https://doi.org/10.1007/s10802-012-9672-1.

[95] Fergusson DM, Horwood LJ, Miller AL, Kennedy MA. Life stress, 5-HTTLPR and mental disorder: findings from a 30-year longitudinal study. Br J Psychiatr 2011;198(2):129−35. https://doi.org/10.1192/bjp.bp.110.085993.

[96] Zammit S, Owen MJ. Stressful life events, 5-HTT genotype and risk of depression. Br J Psychiat 2006;188(3):199−201. https://doi.org/10.1192/bjp.bp.105.020644.

[97] Iurescia S, Seripa D, Rinaldi M. Role of the 5-HTTLPR and SNP promoter polymorphisms on serotonin transporter gene expression: a closer look at genetic architecture and in vitro functional studies of common and uncommon allelic variants. Mol Neurobiol 2016;53:5510−26. https://doi.org/10.1007/s12035-015-9409-6.

[98] Lozano AM, Lipsman N. Probing and regulating dysfunctional circuits using deep brain stimulation. Neuron 2013;77:406−24.

[99]   Lipsman N, et al. Subcallosal cingulate deep brain stimulation for treatment-refractory anorexia nervosa: a phase 1 pilot trial. Lancet 2013;381.

[100]   Ballanger B, et al. Cerebral blood flow changes induced by pedunculopontine nucleus stimulation in patients with advanced Parkinson's disease: a [(15)O] H2O PET study. Hum Brain Mapp 2009;30:3901—9.

[101]   Bucher D, Goaillard JM. Beyond faithful conduction: short-term dynamics, neuromodulation, and long-term regulation of spike propagation in the axon. Prog Neurobiol 2011;94:307—46.

[102]   Lindner B, Gangloff D, Longtin A, Lewis JE. Broadband coding with dynamic synapses. J Neurosci 2009;29:2076—88.

[103]   Wagle Shukla A, Okun MS. Surgical treatment of Parkinson's disease: patients, targets, devices, and approaches. Neurotherapeutics 2014;11(1):47—59. pmid: 24198187; PubMed Central PMCID: PMC3899492.

[104]   Rhew H-G, Jeong J, Fredenburg JA, Dodani S, Patil PG, Flynn MP. A fully self-contained logarithmic closed-loop deep brain stimulation SoC with wireless telemetry and wireless power management. IEEE J Solid State Circ 2014;49.

[105]   Rosin B, Slovik M, Mitelman R, Rivlin-Etzion M, Haber SN, Israel Z, et al. Closed-loop deep brain stimulation is superior in ameliorating parkinsonism. Neuron 2011;72: 370—84. https://doi.org/10.1016/j.neuron.2011.08.023.

[105a] Zhang ZH, Jhaveri DJ, Marshall VM, Bauer DC, Edson J, et al. A comparative study of techniques for differential expression analysis on RNA-Seq data. PLoS One 2014;9(8): e103207. https://doi.org/10.1371/journal.pone.0103207.

[106]   Lozano AM, Giacobbe P, Hamani C, Rizvi SJ, Kennedy SH, Kolivakis TT, et al. A multicenter pilot study of subcallosal cingulate area deep brain stimulation for treatment-resistant depression. J Neurosurg 2012;116:315—22. https://doi.org/ 10.3171/2011.10.JNS102122.

[107]   e Koning PP, Figee M, van den Munckhof P, Schuurman PR, Denys D. Current status of deep brain stimulation for obsessive-compulsive disorder: a clinical review of different targets. Curr Psychiatr Rep 2011;13:274—82. https://doi.org/10.1007/ s11920-011-0200-8.

[108]   Hen P-C, Lal A, editors. Detachable ultrasonic enabled inserter for neural probe insertion using biodissolvable polyethylene glycol. Solid-State Sensors, Actuators and Microsystems (TRANSDUCERS), 2015 Transducers-2015 18th International Conference on. IEEE; 2015.

[108a] Rhew E, Piro JS, Goolkasian P, Cosentino P. The effects of a growth mindset on self-efficacy and motivation. Cogent Education 2018;5(1):1492337. https://doi.org/ 10.1080/2331186X.2018.1492337.

[109]   Rebello TJ, Keeley JW, Kogan CS, Sharan P, Matsumoto C, Kuligyna M, Reed GM. Anxiety and fear-related disorders in the ICD-11: results from a global case-controlled field study. Arch Med Res 2019;50(8):490—501.

[110]   Gallo KP, Thompson-Hollands J, Pincus DB, Barlow DH. Anxiety disorders. Handbook of psychology. 2nd ed. 2012. p. 8.

[111]   Ratan Y, Rajput A, Maleysm S, Pareek A, Jain V, Pareek A, et al. An insight into cellular and molecular mechanisms underlying the pathogenesis of neurodegeneration in Alzheimer's disease. Biomedicines 2023;11:1398. https://doi.org/10.3390/ biomedicines11051398.

[112]   Steward A, Biel D, Dewenter A, et al. ApoE4 and connectivity-mediated spreading of tau pathology at lower amyloid levels. JAMA Neurol 2023;80(12):1295—306. https:// doi.org/10.1001/jamaneurol.2023.4038.

[113] Rothoerl RD, Woertgen C, Brawanski A. The determination of the impact of age on neurological outcome after severe brain trauma. J Neurosurg Sci 2003;47(3):129−33.

[114] Yarascavitch BA, Koumaras GM, Sugar AW, Farquhar DR, Kaddoura IL. Dental students' perceptions of oral and maxillofacial surgery as a specialty. J Oral Maxillofacial Surg 2012;70(12):2806−12. https://doi.org/10.1016/j.joms.2012.06.019.

[115] Samartzis D, Talias MA. A cost utility analysis of surgical versus non-surgical treatment of lumbar disc herniation. Int Orthopaed 2002;26(6):359−63. https://doi.org/10.1007/s00264-002-0391-7.

[116] Damschroder LJ, Aron DC, Keith RE, Kirsh SR, Alexander JA, Lowery JC. Fostering implementation of health services research findings into practice: a consolidated framework for advancing implementation science. Implement Sci. 2009;4:50. https://doi.org/10.1186/1748-5908-4-50.

Further reading

[1] Lohoff FW, Berrettini WH. Genetics of mood disorders. In: Charney DS, editor. Neurobiology of mental illness. New York: Oxford University Press; 2008. p. 1504.

[2] Ullerton J, Cubin M, Tiwari H, et al. Linkage analysis of extremely discordant and concordant sibling pairs identifies quantitative-trait loci that influence variation in the human personality trait neuroticism. Am J Hum Genet 2003;72:879−90.

[3] Uher R, McGuffin P. The moderation by the serotonin transporter gene of environmental adversity in the etiology of depression: 2009 update. Mol Psychiatr 2010;15:18−22.

[4] Doré V, Krishnadas N, Bourgeat P, et al. Relationship between amyloid and tau levels and its impact on tau spreading. Eur J Nucl Med Mol Imag 2021;48:2225−32. https://doi.org/10.1007/s00259-021-05191-9.

Clinical and translational radiology

Abstract

Medical imaging is a method used to visualize the structure and function of organs and tissue composition of the human body, which can be conducted for clinical and research practices. The use of radiation is not limited to radiological procedures alone, as such a common term used within clinical medicine is *Imaging*. Imaging is a high-risk area within clinical medicine that is reliant on multiple technologies and significantly legislated.

Keywords: Biomarkers; Diagnostic radiology; Dosimetry; Functional imaging; Imaging; MRI; Nuclear medicine; PET/CT, CT and X-ray; Radiotracers; Radiology; Translational research.

Key messages

- Imaging is a vital component of clinical and research practice
- Advancement of medicine has a codependent relationship with imaging
- Quality control processes are an integral part of quality assurance programs when performing imaging procedures while remaining safe
- Quality assurance within imaging occurs at every stage: from setting up an imaging protocol through scanning patients to reading and completion of the radiology report
- Clinical radiation and medical physics expertise are crucial to assess and ensure risks are reduced and safety rules are considered and implemented by the clinical team linked to exposure to ionizing radiation.

8.1 Background

8.1.1 Historical background

Medical imaging is a method used to visualize the structure and function of organs and tissue composition of the human body, which can be conducted for clinical and research practices. The use of radiation is not limited to Radiological procedures alone, as such a common term used within clinical medicine is *Imaging*. Imaging is a high-risk area within clinical medicine that is reliant on multiple technologies and significantly legislated.

Historically, medical diagnosis was primarily dependent upon clinical presentations and any observations doctors noticed during a first-hand examination. The

Quality Assurance Management. https://doi.org/10.1016/B978-0-12-822732-9.00005-9

oldest medical tests date back to Egyptian and Mesopotamian times of 400 BCE where urine and saliva were used to measure issues with the digestive track, spleen, liver, and circulation [1]. Hippocrates promoted the mind and sense as diagnostic tools around 300 BCE where he setup diagnostic protocols for testing patients' urine by way of observing the color. Hereditary links with disease were also recorded by Hippocrates [2]. By the 19th century, X-rays and microscopes were in use to diagnose and treat illnesses. In the 1850s, tools such as stethoscopes, laryngoscopes, and ophthalmoscopes were in use. This paved the way for the development of a variety of tests such as microscopy, bacteriology, and chemical tests. During these renaissance years, Wilhelm Conrad Roentgen discovered X-rays while experimenting with cathode ray tubes. Roentgen's wife Bertha and her hand is considered as the first X-ray image. This image demonstrated X-rays are absorbed by the bones in comparison to the soft and fatty tissue to produce a clear image that can assist with diagnosing and any ongoing treatment. Discovering X-rays gave rise to the field of Radiography and Roentgen received the Nobel Prize in 1901. The military was one of the most prominent industries to adopt X-ray technology to assess battlefield injuries during World War I. Marie Curie furthered the use of X-rays when she drove a truck around the French battlefields with an X-ray machine. Radiologists refer to X-rays often as "plane films" that were commonly used to determine chest abnormalities and bone fractures. Further advancement led to the development of fluoroscopy, which led to radiologists providing insightful details into esophageal cancers and ulcers. Fluoroscopy also led to the development of angiography (Fig. 8.1) [3].

Fluoroscopy was quickly developed into computed tomography (CT), which is the most commonly used imaging technique for diagnosing diseases in the 21st century. Italian radiologist, Alessandro Vallebona, developed tomography, which in its conventional form, used simultaneously moving X-rays and a detector. Conventional tomography evolved although it remained ineffective for imaging soft tissue and the whole body [4]. Approximately 76 years later, CT was developed using radiographic projections using multiple angles using a mathematical model resulting in a two-dimensional (2D) image. Sir Godfrey Hounsfield invented the first CT scanner at EMI research laboratories in 1967, and the first patient was scanned on October 1, 1971. Alan M. Cormack and Hounsfield received the Novel Prize in 1979 for developing *computer-assisted tomography* [5]. Modern-day CT is able to display images with a soft tissue contrast again with anatomical details. The 2D images were created in large volumes across healthcare systems by the early 1980s and a variety of scanning technologies are available in the 21st century. Technological advancements have made CT provide high-quality images at reduced radiation doses and smaller slice thicknesses. The slice thickness of the images is now as thin as a fraction of a millimeter assisting with using improved reconstruction techniques [6].

Magnetic resonance imaging (MRI) has a complex developmental history. Felix Bloch and Edward Purcell simultaneously and independently developed the concept of nuclear magnetic resonance (NMR). This discovery led to the joint Nobel Prize in Physics in 1952 [5]. In 1973, Paul Lauterbur published the first NMR images that led to the Nobel Prize in Physiology and Medicine in 2003. MRI is based on different

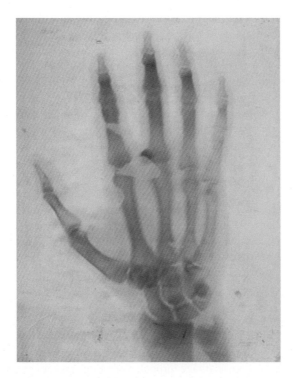

FIGURE 8.1

X-ray 1897: Hand radiograph of Sebastian Gilbert Scott (sometime BIR Hon Treasurer).

principles in comparison to CT where a magnet is used to produce a strong fixed magnetic field around the whole body of the patient. The excited protons eventually reach a resting state that is captured and mapped into an image.

Ultrasound (US) is another imaging technology that was developed by a number of scientists and physicians in the 20th century although the backdrop began in the 1700s by Lazzaro Spallanzani. The initial hypothesis of the use of bats to navigate sound was proposed by Spallanzani [7]. This step was furthered by Jean-Daniel Colladon in 1826 where he calculated the speed of sound of water to be 1482 m/s [8]. Then, the Doppler effect was proposed in 1842 by Christian Doppler, which assisted in the understanding of blood flow [9]. The Curie brothers then discovered Piezo-electric crystal vibrations that have an alternating current, which was the principle for developing ultrasound transducers [9]. In 1958, Ian Donald, a Gynecologist used US to examine the pelvis and fetus [10].

Another aspect of medical imaging is the use of radioactive tracers to develop functional images. This subfield of imaging is referred to as nuclear medicine. Sensors to detect the radioactive emission of tracers using single-photo-emission computed tomography (SPECT) and positron emission tomography (PET) use a morphological scanning approach. In 1961, James Robertson developed the first single-plane PET scanner at the Brookhaven National Laboratory. This was furthered with the combining of functional and morphological imaging with the first hybrid imaging method, PET-CT. PET-CT was proposed by Ronald Nutt and David Townsend and the first clinical scan was performed in 1998 [11]. Functional metabolic imaging was the next advancement in hybrid imaging, where PET-MRI has become part of clinical and research practices in the 21st century.

Interventional medical imaging is another facet of imaging that was developed with catheter angiography in the early 1900s. Egas Moniz, a Portuguese Neurologist performed the first cerebral angiography in 1927 and was awarded the Nobel Prize in Medicine in 1949 [11]. The first cardiac angiography was performed in 1929 by Werner Forssmann when he used the catheter in his own arm vein and heart. He shared the Nobel Prize in 1956 in Medicine alongside Andre F. Cournand and Dickinson W. Richards, as pioneers of cardiac catheterization [12]. Catheter angiography has advanced to diagnose and treat most cardiovascular emergencies including tumor ablations and occlusion of active arterial hemorrhage in trauma patients. Other image-guided procedures included biopsy and invasive procedures for draining abscesses and tissue ablation using real-time image use in surgical procedures. A few ablation techniques include cryoablation, radiofrequency ablation, and stereotactic laser ablation.

High-intensity focused ultrasound (HIFU) is another imaging method that was founded in 1942. HIFU was proposed by Lynn and colleagues to be used as a real-time imaging approach that uses an external beam to target tissues or organs, as needed. HIFU procedures damage through cavitation and irreversible coagulation necrosis [8]. MR-guided ultrasound (MRGFUS) is another successful image-guided approach to treat medication-resistant Parkinson's disease [13]. MRGFUS is also used to ablate uterine fibroids, bone metastases, and prostate cancer.

The use of quality assurance methods in the context of imaging is a complex area and requires careful consideration, in particular, based on clinical and research imaging modalities as well as all its' adjunct applications.

8.1.2 Radiation biology

Radiation biology is a vital component of imaging especially from a translational perspective as it is necessary to understand the impact of ionizing radiation on biological systems. Radiation biology is a multidisciplinary field that encompasses various areas of knowledge, including cell biology, chemistry, radiation physics, human physiology, radiation safety, epidemiology, biostatistics, and toxicology. It's important to recognize that information in this field is continually evolving as we gain a deeper understanding of how ionizing radiation interacts with cells. Delving into radiation biology can be complex, and this article provides only a basic overview of the subject. It's essential to acknowledge that this overview only scratches the surface of the extensive information available in the field of radiation biology.

Basic radiation biology concepts were initially reported by Bergonie and Tribondeau in 1906, suggesting cells that are immature and undifferentiated could be more radiosensitive. The theory suggested, actively dividing cells such as the stomach mucosa, basal layer of skin and stem cells could respond to radiation by cell injury or premature death. Cells mature and differentiate differently, and some, such as neurons could be more radioresistant [14]. This original theory has evolved considerably, including with the use of terms such as *radioresponsive* which assists in the use of radiation within radiological practices [15]. Ionizing radiation can induce two general types of biological effects: deterministic effects and stochastic effects. Stochastic effects are those whose frequency in the exposed population is directly proportional to the dose received, with no threshold. In other words, any level of radiation exposure, no matter how low, carries a probability of causing these effects. Stochastic effects are often associated with the risk of cancer induction and genetic mutations. Deterministic effects are dependent on the dose of radiation, and they typically have a threshold. These effects are characterized by increasing severity with increasing dose. Deterministic effects are often the result of cell killing. In organs and tissues with a continuous process of cell loss and replacement, a slight increase in cell loss due to radiation exposure can be compensated for by an increased replacement rate. However, at higher radiation doses, there may be a reduction in the function of that particular tissue or organ. Deterministic effects are associated with the severity of the exposure, while stochastic effects are associated with the probability of occurrence and can manifest even at low doses.

Radiation biology influenced the development of radiation oncology as a medical discipline in the United States can be traced back to 1956 when the first patient was treated with a linear accelerator by Henry Kaplan. This marked the beginning of radiation therapy as a maturing field in medical science. The development of technology, particularly the repurposing of radar systems from World War II, led to the creation of compact linear accelerators designed for patient care. By the 1960s, linear accelerator technology had advanced to the point where daily treatments could be reliably and consistently administered. As a result, both academic centers and community hospitals were able to acquire this equipment for patient care. During this period, as radiation oncology continued to evolve, medical professionals in the field began collaborating to share patient treatment strategies and develop treatment protocols. These collaborations involved regular meetings to review protocol progress and plan for future trials. While these commitments were initially informal, their potential to advance clinical care was recognized. Subsequently, the National Cancer Institute (NCI) recognized the value of collaboration in advancing cancer treatment. Over the years, a network of cooperative groups was established to create protocols for clinical trials, collect data, assess outcomes, and contribute to the standardization and improvement of clinical care in radiation oncology. This collaborative approach has played a significant role in the development and progress of radiation therapy as a medical specialty.

As the field of radiation biology furthered, experiments with fruit flies and mice were conducted to demonstrate ionizing radiation can induce mutations in offspring, but these mutations are not unique to radiation exposure and can also occur naturally. Additionally, the research demonstrates that the impact of ionizing radiation depends on both the total dose and the rate of exposure. A higher dose administered over a short period is more harmful than the same dose spread out over a longer duration [16]. The interaction of radiation with cells is a probabilistic event, and cellular repair mechanisms often prevent permanent damage from occurring. Energy deposition in a cell from radiation happens very rapidly, typically within 10-18 s, in a random manner. These interactions occur at the cellular level and can affect the entire organ or system. Notably, there is no distinct cellular damage exclusive to radiation, as similar damage can result from chemical, heat, or physical factors. Following radiation exposure, there is a latent period before any visible effects appear, which can range from decades for low radiation doses to minutes or hours for high exposure. These fundamental principles underpin the field of radiation biology [17].

Direct interaction between ionizing radiation and a cell's macromolecules (such as proteins or DNA) can have various effects, including cell death or DNA mutation. Studies indicate that double-stranded DNA is more resilient to damage than single-stranded DNA. Interestingly, some cells behave as if they have single-stranded, non-paired chromosomes and are more sensitive to radiation. Different types of direct hits can occur, and the nature of the damage determines whether the cell can repair itself. If a direct hit leads to a complete break in the DNA or other permanent damage, the cell either dies immediately or will eventually die. Humans have numerous cells, and cell replacement through mitosis is a continuous process to replace dying cells. Radiation effects become evident when this cell replacement system is compromised, which typically occurs at higher radiation doses [18]. Radiosensitivity varies between actively dividing cells and nondividing cells. The cell cycle consists of four phases: M Phase (cell division), G1 Phase (preparation for DNA replication), S Phase (DNA replication), and G2 Phase (preparation for mitosis). Among these, M Phase, characterized by condensed and paired chromosomes, is the most radiosensitive. This phase has a higher concentration of DNA in one area, making it more susceptible to radiation damage. Additionally, cancer cells, which have increased chromatin and rapid mitotic rates, tend to be more radiosensitive than normal cells due to these factors [19].

Indirect cellular interaction with radiation happens when radiation energy interacts with cellular water instead of the cell's macromolecules. This interaction leads to the hydrolysis of water, producing a hydrogen molecule and a hydroxyl (free radical) molecule. When two hydroxyl molecules recombine, they create hydrogen peroxide, which is highly unstable in the cell. This unstable form can turn into a stable organic hydrogen peroxide molecule by combining with organic compounds within the cell. This process can lead to the loss of essential enzymes in the cell, potentially resulting in cell death or future mutations [18]. Antioxidants have garnered significant attention due to their ability to block the recombination of hydroxyl (free radicals) into hydrogen peroxide during indirect radiation interactions within cells. By preventing the formation of stable organic hydrogen peroxide compounds, antioxidants serve as a defense mechanism the body employs to protect against the harmful effects of radiation exposure at the cellular level. This property is one of the reasons antioxidants have received considerable research and publicity as potential agents for cancer prevention [20].

The nomenclature of ionizing radiation includes nonparticulate and particulate, which could transfer energy to the substance. Nonparticulate form include Gamma and X-rays while particulate includes Alpha and Beta particles, Protons, and Neutrons. In the presence of high incoming radiation, the ejection of electrons from atoms is referred to as ionization. Electromagnetic radiation is a type of light energy that comprises a spectrum from long wavelengths including television and radio and electric power sources that may emit visible and ultraviolet light. The opposite end of the spectrum comprises shorter wavelengths such as radar, microwaves, and infrared radiation. The particulate type of radiation comprises subatomic particles that are neutral or charges that could be of considerable mass. Different types of radiation penetrate at varying depths. For example, almost all types of ionizing radiation can be stopped by dense material than water or tissue within the human body. Hence, X-rays and Gama rays are more penetrable than Alpha or Beta particles [21]. Cellular injury following ionizing radiation exposure can occur through three main mechanisms:

1. **Division Delay**: This involves a dose-dependent delay in cell division. After exposure to radiation, cells experience a delay in mitotic division, which may vary depending on the radiation dose. In some cases, mitotic division eventually returns to near-normal levels for reasons that are not entirely understood. This effect is typically observed at doses greater than 0.5 Gy (50 rads) and up to around 3 Gy (300 rads). It represents the initial observable impact of ionizing radiation exposure
2. **Reproductive Failure**: Reproductive failure occurs when cells are unable to complete mitosis, either immediately or after one or more generations. Radiation exposure can disrupt the normal cell division process, leading to reproductive failure, which may result in cell death
3. **Interphase Death**: Interphase death is a relatively prompt form of cell death caused by the apoptosis mechanism. This mechanism is most commonly observed in lymphocytes, but some cancer cells may also undergo apoptosis in response to radiation exposure

Notably, at radiation doses exceeding 3 Gy (300 rads), the mitotic rate does not recover, and cell division may never occur, ultimately leading to cell death. Reproductive failure of a cell is dose-dependent. Below or at 1.5 Gy (150 rads), it is random and nonlinear, meaning it occurs sporadically and is not directly proportional to the dose. However, above 1.5 Gy (150 rads), it becomes linear and nonrandom, meaning as the dose increases, so does the likelihood of reproductive failure. In the case of interphase death, cell demise can occur many generations after initial radiation exposure. This phenomenon may be due to natural aging processes in cells (apoptosis) or alterations in critical cell replication mechanisms. The occurrence of interphase death depends on the cell type affected and the dose received. Generally, rapidly dividing and undifferentiated cells are more prone to interphase death at lower doses compared to nondividing, differentiated cells. Importantly, any of these forms of cellular injury can result from either direct or indirect interactions of radiation with cells [18]. These aspects are vital to understand especially within the context of QA as the findings of any experiments need to be reliable. The common approach to ensure quality assurance would be to follow a strict protocol which includes quality control processes and the repetition of the experiments using the same methods. If there are variations to the findings, often there are acceptable thresholds that many researchers use. These may often require additional validation protocols to establish appropriate metrics where the thresholds could be described well. Anomaly detection is another QC measure within the context of radiation biology which is accepted.

8.1.2.1 Dose response models

There is a variety of theoretical dose-response models that can be used to explain the effects of radiation exposure. These models offer different perspectives on how organisms respond to radiation. A few common models include the following:

1. Linear-No Threshold (LNT): This model suggests that any level of radiation exposure, even background radiation, is harmful
2. Linear-Threshold: This model posits that harm from radiation begins at a certain threshold level, meaning exposures below this threshold are considered safe
3. Linear-Quadratic: This model involves a more complex relationship between radiation dose and response, taking into account both linear and quadratic components

These dose-response models are used in radiation biology to estimate the effects of high-dose radiation exposure and extrapolate these effects to the low-dose range, which is less reliably understood or detected. The models offer different viewpoints on radiation's potential risks and benefits.

8.1.2.2 Linear no-threshold model

Another aspect of this would be to use a linear-no threshold dose-response model in relation to carcinogens like benzene, asbestos, and high-dose radiation across various industries. This model suggests that any exposure, no matter how small, can potentially induce cancer. However, clinical effects are generally not observed below a certain threshold, approximately 0.5 Gy (50 rads) in the case of radiation. The linear-no threshold model is employed for regulatory purposes whenever a known carcinogenic substance is present, with an emphasis on caution and the "as low as reasonably achievable" (ALARA) principle. At higher doses, radiation exposure can lead to clinical symptoms and is clearly a carcinogen, particularly associated with leukemia, although cancer causation is often the result of multiple factors.

8.1.2.3 Linear threshold-model

The linear-threshold dose-response model involves a known threshold below which no effects are observed, and as the dose increases beyond the threshold, the effects increase linearly. This model is practical since it aligns with the generally accepted view that clinical effects from radiation exposure are not seen at or below 0.5 Gy (50 rads). In 1996, the Health Physics Society released a position statement on low-level radiation, indicating that quantitative estimation of health risks should not be performed below an individual dose of 0.05 Sv (5 rem) in 1 year or a lifetime dose of 0.1 Sv (10 rem) in addition to background radiation. Below 0.1 Sv (10 rem), the statement suggests that the risks of health effects are either too small to be observed or nonexistent, favoring a linear-threshold dose-response model with a threshold of 0.1 Sv (10 rems).

8.1.2.4 Linear quadratic model

The linear-quadratic dose-response model is employed to describe the human response to radiation exposure. In this model, the response to low levels of radiation is linear, while higher doses exhibit a quadratic relationship. Importantly, this model does not incorporate a threshold, meaning that even low levels of radiation exposure can have an effect. In the context of cell survival theories, the linear-quadratic dose-response model is utilized to represent the multiple target/single hit theory. This theory provides a useful explanation for how human cells react to ionizing radiation exposure.

The text emphasizes the importance of understanding that the dose of a substance determines whether it acts as a poison or a remedy, echoing Paracelsus' famous quote. It is generally observed that as the dose increases, the response becomes more toxic, highlighting that excessive amounts of anything can be harmful. In the context of radiation, dose-response models vary depending on the specific analysis. While some evidence suggests the possibility of a threshold for radiation exposure, which would support the linear-threshold dose-response model, it's crucial to remember that models for radiation at lower levels are based on extrapolations from high-dose data and remain theoretical rather than proven. The Nuclear Regulatory Commission (NRC) only accepts the linear-no threshold dose-response model, which implies that any level of radiation exposure carries the potential for cancer induction.

8.1.2.5 Radiation exposure; stochastic versus nonstochastic effects

Stochastic effects are random in nature and are associated with diseases that could result from exposure to various xenobiotics or carcinogens. In the context of cancer, it's challenging to attribute a specific cancer case to a particular exposure due to the long latency period (around 20 years) between exposure and manifestation. Chronic low-dose radiation exposure is considered stochastic, and at diagnostic levels, the odds of any effect occurring are extremely low and unpredictable. Radiation risks from diagnostic imaging and hereditary effects are also seen as stochastic. Nonstochastic effects are specific and predictable outcomes of radiation exposure that occur at certain doses and dose rates. These effects can vary from blood and chromosome aberrations to radiation sickness and, in extreme cases, even death. The severity of nonstochastic effects depends on factors such as the dose, dose rate, the individual's age, immune capacity, and the type of radiation. For gamma and X-ray radiation, exposure is measured in Grays and Sieverts (rads and rems) in an equivalent manner, but this equivalence does not hold for neutron radiation or when the quality factor exceeds one in the conversion between rads and rems. Some examples of nonstochastic effects include hematologic syndrome (pancytopenia), erythema (skin redness), gastrointestinal (GI) syndrome (radiation sickness), and central nervous system (CNS) syndrome. These effects are highly predictable and directly related to radiation exposure [18].

8.1.2.6 Radiation effects

Acute ionizing radiation exposure is considered harmless at background or diagnostic levels. However, at high-dose levels, it becomes nonstochastic and harmful. Typically, at or above around 0.5 Gy (50 rads), acute radiation effects are predictable and follow a linear pattern. While some chromosome aberrations may be visible under a microscope at doses below 0.5 Gy (50 rads), no clinical symptoms have been observed from these abnormalities. Nevertheless, this observation can serve as a bioassay technique for detecting radiation exposure many years after an acute exposure event. In radiation therapy, acute nonstochastic effects of radiation exposure can result in conditions like radiation fibrosis in the lung when normal lung tissue is exposed to radiation. Similar effects can also occur in the kidney, brain, and spinal cord. These nonstochastic effects are well-understood, and guidelines in radiotherapy are established to prevent exceeding specific dose thresholds to avoid causing tissue injuries. These guidelines are crucial for ensuring the safety and effectiveness of radiation therapy. Chronic effects of ionizing radiation exposure are primarily stochastic in nature, with the primary concern being the potential induction of cancer. However, noncancerous effects are also possible, such as cataract formation in the eye. The likelihood of cataracts occurring as a chronic stochastic effect increases with higher radiation doses. Specifically, radiation doses ranging from 500 to 800 R directed at the lens of the eye can lead to cataract formation. At lower doses, the damage may resemble senile cataracts but is less severe. Another potential chronic stochastic effect is the shortening of the lifespan. Although conclusive evidence is lacking, some literature theorizes this possibility as a consequence of chronic radiation exposure Leukemia is considered a stochastic effect of chronic radiation exposure, and there is an association with doses as low as 50–100 cGy (50–100 rads) [22]. Between 100 and 500 cGy (100–500 rads), there is a linear correlation between radiation dose and the incidence of leukemia. Data suggests that the incidence of leukemia increases at a rate of 1–2 cases per million per year per cGy (1 rad) of exposure. Moreover, there is an average latency period of approximately 14 years from radiation exposure to the onset of leukemia. Additionally, higher doses of ionizing radiation have been associated with an increased risk of other cancers, including those affecting the thyroid, bones, lungs, and various other organs.

Radiation biology has also supported the identification of highly sensitive subgroups. Among these subgroups, two groups of individuals with genetic or chromosomal defects have been identified as having heightened sensitivities to various forms of ionizing radiation. Ataxia-Telangiectasia (AT) is a rare inherited disorder, occurring in approximately 2 to 3 out of every 100,000 live births. It is characterized by symptoms such as a staggering gait (ataxia), bloodshot eyes (conjunctival telangiectasia), chromosomal breakage when their fibroblasts are cultured, and a significantly increased risk of developing lymphoma. Notably, when patients with AT receive conventional doses of X-rays to treat their lymphoma, they often experience a severe and potentially lethal acute radiation reaction. This extreme sensitivity to radiation in AT patients is attributed to the inability of their cells to repair DNA damage caused by ionizing radiation. Further studies have been conducted to explore the possibility of other diseases with DNA repair capacity defects that might influence radiosensitivity. While some impairment of fibroblast survival in culture after gamma irradiation was identified in five rare single-gene disorders, it did not reach the same level of sensitivity observed in AT homozygotes. In contrast, individuals who were AT heterozygous had normal test results, suggesting that their DNA repair capabilities were not significantly compromised (Paterson et al., 1984). These findings highlight the increased radiosensitivity of individuals with AT and shed light on the role of DNA repair mechanisms in determining sensitivity to ionizing radiation in specific genetic conditions.

8.1.3 Introduction to clinical radiology

The notions of the X-ray beam also led to the development of mammography where the high-resolution allowed physicians to diagnose and monitor breast cancers. Medical imaging transcended to hybrid-imaging methods and the use of radioactive compounds to improve the images obtained to analyze diseases. Hybrid imaging techniques include the combining of established modalities of CT, PET, MRI, and SPECT) (Fig. 8.2) [23]. Healthcare practices mostly use ionizing and nonionizing imaging techniques. These techniques are vital for diagnosing, managing, and treating a variety of diseases such as Trauma, Neurological, Gynecological, and Cardiovascular conditions. A commonly used radioactive compound is Technetium 99m to determine bone tumors. This approach is referred to as nuclear bone scans and is a key part of cancer imaging [24].

Advancements in imaging in the United Kingdom evolved with the restructuring and accreditation of academic radiology by the Royal College of Radiologists (RCR) [1]. Their aim was to increase the number of research active radiologists and the quality of imaging research. The National Institute of Health Research (NIHR) in the United Kingdom reported 250 studies between 2017 and 2018 alone used imaging as a primary or secondary outcome in studies. In addition, the NIHR clinical research network in the United Kingdom typically supports approximately 2000 studies annually where is an important facet. This work combined with the training programs provided by the RCR allowed the NIHR to award 54 fellows in imaging research in a range of clinical disciplines within 2016 alone. The basic task of diagnostic radiology is to provide the best possible in well-structured

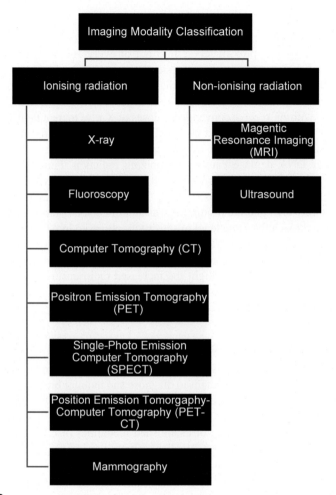

FIGURE 8.2

Schematic representation of imaging modalities based on the type of radiation used. The ionising radiation modalities use X-rays, gamma rays and positrons; the nonionizing imaging modalities use radio and ultrasound electromagnetic waves.

imaging data format to help Radiologists, Radionuclide Radiologists and clinical researchers to unveil anatomical details and/or ongoing physiological or pathophysiological processes within patient's body in the form of using ionizing and nonionizing radiation techniques.

Success stories of medical imaging has advanced further over the centuries, and these have covered both technological, digital and image reporting methods. Regardless of the modalities used, images have been digitalized and made available using workstations for Radiologists to complete the required clinical as well as research reports, where applicable. The use of digital images have meant that plane films have been replaced as the primary method paving the way to multiplanar image reconstruction. As of the early 2000s, radiology is mostly filmless globally, thereby making remote interpretation of images a reality. This has been a vital component for conducting global clinical trials.

Including imaging in studies can present some specific design and statistical challenges. To address this, the NIHR developed a statistics imaging group that assists researcher discuss methods to overcome the challenges. However, it is vital to recognize that the involvement of Radiologists and Radionuclide Radiologists as well as Medical Physicists cannot be considered as an option. Clinical trial steering committees could also provide independent advice and oversight to the conduct of studies where imaging is used as a core component. This is particularly important when using Radiology and Molecular imaging data within a single study as the nuances of the data and its' interpretation require careful consideration. This further purport the requirement for quality assurance for affirming the findings and the implications to clinical and healthcare practice.

Being a multidisciplinary field, Radiology and Nuclear Medicine routine practice, heavily involve Technologists, Radiographers, Medical Physicists and Nurses. The clinical workflow requires specialized input from all these professional groups. Technologists and Nurses duties focus mainly on patient preparation, scanning, data management, daily quality controls of basic equipment, and interactions with other medical departments and wards; a good example is the administration of radionuclide therapies often carried-out in purpose-built rooms in the oncology wards, especially in the case of inpatients.

On the other hand, medical physicists are clinical scientists (registered with a specialized medical physics board; the health care Professions Council (HCPC) in the United Kingdom; board certified clinical physicists with the American Board of Medical Physics (ABMP) in the United States; the Canadian College of Physicists in Medicine COMP board in Canada, etc). Their main duties consist of providing scientific and technical support to imaging, nonimaging procedures as well as radionuclide therapy procedures (procurement, technical specification, commissioning, acceptance tests, and regular control tests). The other facet of their duties consists of training junior staff and carry-out primary research and contribute to secondary research projects and large clinical trials (such as, development, validation nonstandard imaging protocols, performance of specific quality controls as required for clinical trials quality check and assessment of radiation doses as described later in this chapter). It is of relevance to mention that medical physicists are instrumental in the introduction and assessment of new imaging technologies; a good example in recent years is the deployment of artificial intelligence techniques into Radiology and Nuclear Medicine practice as described and the end of the chapter. It is worth emphasizing that all three professional categories, in addition to Clinical Radiologists, Radionuclide Radiologists and Managers play a crucial role in the local quality assurance program, including its the development, implementation, monitoring, surveys, regular review and update based on most recent guidelines, best code of practice and relevant regulations.

One of the core principles of providing diagnostic and therapeutic efficacy date is to keep-up with the *"as low as reasonably achievable"* (ALARA) principle that consists of delivering the lowest possible amount of radiation doses to patients. This becomes one of the primary aims of QA within imaging. There are a variety of QA programs at institutional and department levels to ensure optimal and effective use radiological images at any stage of disease. Fundamentally, imaging QA programs involve several aspects [2] such as:

(a) Compliance with legal requirements using quality control (QC) processes to advance investigations using imaging protocol methods such as X-rays, CT, MRI, Ultrasound, SPECT/CT, PET/CT and PET/MR scans.
(b) Effective use of QC processes to maintain optimal imaging equipment performance and increase confidence in reporting scans; hence maximize outcomes.
(c) QC processes and QA guidelines for radiation protection and safety of areas where equipment is installed
(d) Optimal use of equipment to achieve required levels of performance.
(e) Demand and capacity modeling of human resources in Diagnostic Radiology
(f) Image quality-driven rejection analysis
(g) Dose monitoring and compliance with radiation protection of patients' annual occupational dose limits.

Radiology and Nuclear medicine (NM) further divide the risk of exposure and standards required for quality insurance. One of the main differences across NM modalities in comparison to radiology provides a unique minimally-invasive functional information of the human body, hence the term functional imaging. As the imaging process involves the use of radiolabeed pharmaceuticals (called often radiopharmaceuticals or radiotracers) to study the function of cells, the term Molecular Imaging is also used [3]. The procedures involve both imaging and nonimaging equipment where radiation emissions and their detection is measured to the best possible accuracy. Two key principles in QA linked to Nuclear Medicine equipment is as follows.

(a) Gamma cameras (GC), also known as single-photon emission computed tomography (SPECT)
(b) PET scanner

Both SPECT and PET combined with state-of-the-art data acquisition and image reconstruction software provide two-dimensional (2D) and three-dimensional (3D) images based on the distribution of radiolabeed pharmaceuticals in the body.

Quality control tools within nuclear medicine include pocket dosimeters, radiation survey meters, well counters, dose calibrators, and radioactive contamination surveys. This formulates part of the ongoing governance and legislative measures for using radiation-based imaging as a noninvasive tool in clinical practice. To maintain compliance, these devices' performance is checked at multiple time intervals and findings recorded and audited as part of routine independent oversight programs. Most QC processes are recommended by third-party vendors for instruments used within Radiology and Nuclear Medicine modalities based on the specifications of international regulatory bodies such as the National Electrical Manufacturing Association (NEMA) [4], American Association of Physicists in Medicine (AAPM) [5], Society of Nuclear Medicine and Molecular Imaging (SNMMI) [6], and European Association of Nuclear Medicine (EANM) [7].

Modern day radiology has the potential to become part of point-of-care testing for both communicable and noncommunicable diseases with the use of teleradiology with primary and secondary reads.

8.1.3.1 End-to-end quality assurance

End-to-end (E2E) quality assurance tests are used to validate patient treatment processes in external radiotherapy. The tests are conducted in 3D for accuracy and use Fricke-Xylenol orange-Gelatin (FXG) gel dosimeter and a dual-wavelength reading method. The Vista16 optical CT scanner (ModusQA) is utilized for these tests, which cover three treatment techniques in stereotactic radiotherapy using Novalis (Varian) and CyberKnife (Accuray) linear accelerators [25].

Stereotactic radiotherapy is a widely used treatment technique for the past 2 decades, delivering high doses to small tumor volumes while sparing healthy tissues. It involves dynamic methods like volumetric-modulated arc therapy (VMAT) with automatic processes, which can increase the risk of missing the target or causing dose errors. Therefore, regular and tailored quality assurance tests are essential. E2E tests are among the QA methods that verify and validate the entire patient treatment process, from imaging to treatment delivery using anthropomorphic phantoms, with a focus on detecting dose and spatial errors. Ideally, QA tests in stereotactic radiotherapy should involve measuring 3D dose distributions with high spatial precision. However, the dosimeters commonly used in clinical practice, such as ion chambers and radiochromic films, are not well-suited for this purpose because they only capture point or 2D dose information. Even when 3D detector arrays are used, they often require interpolation calculations to generate 3D dose distributions, which can result in lower spatial resolution. Gel dosimeters show promise for conducting the QA tests in stereotactic radiotherapy because they can accurately measure 3D dose distributions with a high level of spatial detail. Over the past decade, numerous studies have explored the use of dosimetric gels, including Fricke-based gels, polymer gels, and PRESAGE [26], in the implementation of 3D E2E QA tests. These studies have also investigated various readout techniques, such as MRI, optical CT, and X-ray CT, to analyze the gel dosimeter data effectively [27].

In a recent study by Rousseau et al. in 2022, a novel dosimetric approach was developed to achieve accurate 3D dose measurements with high spatial resolution and a linear dose-response [28]. This method was designed to cover a dose range relevant to stereotactic and dynamic radiotherapy treatments, ranging from 0.25 to 10 Gy. The technique used a FXG gel and a unique dual-wavelength reading method implemented on the cone-beam Vista16 optical CT scanner (ModusQA, London, Ontario, Canada. This reading method allowed for the simultaneous scanning of low and high doses within a single dosimeter by utilizing two distinct light sources, one at 590 nm for low doses and another at 633 nm for high doses. This is an improvement over previous FXG gel dosimeters, which could only read doses below 4 Gy with a single scan at 590 nm. The new dosimetric method was thoroughly characterized and validated for absolute dose profile measurements, particularly in the context of small-field dosimetry [29]. Rousseau and colleagues conducted another E2E quality assurance study to implement this dosimetric method on Novalis True-Beam STx (Varian) and CyberKnife M6 (Accuracy) accelerators using anthropomorphic head phantoms. The researchers also used additional measurements using Razor Nano Chamber (IBA) and EBT3 Gafchromic films (Ashland) at the isocenters and slices involved with treatment plans delivered on the Novalis accelerator to compare the findings to those of the gel method. By assessing the performance of its method and validity, this quality assurance method could be implemented when performing radiotherapy [30]. The study evaluated the results using 3D local gamma-index analyses with a 2% dose difference and a 2 mm distance-to-agreement criteria, with a 10% dose cut-off. The gamma passing rates exceeded 95% for all three applications, indicating good agreement between gel measurements and radiation treatment planning. Point dose differences between gel measurements and treatment planning in the high-dose region for both QA tests on the Novalis accelerator were below 2.3%. However, for the CyberKnife QA test, the point dose differences were around 4%, leading to the conclusion that only the E2E QA tests conducted on the Novalis accelerator were validated. Additionally, point and 2D dose measurements obtained using ion chambers and radiochromic films were consistent with the results from gel dosimetry, confirming the robustness of the dosimetric method used in the study. The method demonstrated excellent dosimetric accuracy with 3D absolute dose measurements and an associated uncertainty of 2%

However, some areas for improvement were identified. The dual-wavelength reading method on the CT scanner was noted to be time-consuming and requires optimization for practical use. Additionally, an artifact observed in the convex organ at risk (OAR) region in one of the quality assurance tests needs further investigation, potentially involving a study of the physical models used in the CT reconstruction of gel measurements.

8.1.4 Translational imaging

Translational imaging is the developmental arm of clinical imagining where the advancement of radiological and nuclear medicine practices are developed, both from a biomedical, technological, and application perspective. These approaches often start in vitro and scale up commonly part of a translational pipeline where findings from animal models are translated to humans by way of evaluation and validation. The current drug discovery process primarily relies on empirically selecting potential drug candidates by screening compound libraries based on specific target ideas. These candidates then undergo thorough safety and efficacy testing, both in vitro and in vivo, during the preclinical phase. This data is essential for progressing these candidates to clinical trials. Unfortunately, it's not uncommon for issues with the chosen compounds to surface later in the development process or even after final drug approval, leading to significant resource wastage. The primary culprit behind these issues is often compound toxicity, which tends to go unnoticed during the early stages of drug discovery. Minimally invasive in vivo imaging techniques like MRI, PET, CT, and SPECT hold the potential to revolutionize translational toxicology. These methods offer unique capabilities by providing repeated and detailed information about target organs and systems within the same subject with minimal disruption [31]. This enhanced ability increases the statistical reliability of measurements and reduces the need for a large number of animals to achieve high sensitivity, surpassing the limitations of current techniques. Moreover, in vivo imaging often offers insights that are difficult or impossible to obtain through other means. Assessing toxicity using imaging is valuable not only in drug discovery but also for evaluating the potential impact of environmental and other toxic substances on public health [32].

Translational research has gained popularity within the biomedical community, particularly at the National Institutes of Health (NIH) and the National Institute of Health Research (NIHR), in the United States (US) and the United Kingdom, respectively. The NIH and NIHR understand the importance of translational research in imaging given its ability to bridge knowledge and practice gaps by way of basic science discoveries and their application in clinical settings. The NIH's Roadmap for Medical Research, introduced in 2003, focuses on three key trends: developing new methods for understanding complex biological systems, fostering interdisciplinary research teams, and improving clinical and translational research. Several initiatives have emerged to support translational research in radiology, including Institutional Clinical and Translational Science Awards (CTSA), the NIH Rapid Access to Interventional Development Pilot Program, and the National Center for Biomedical Computing. Translational research, as defined by Lean et al. involves a process that goes from evidence-based medicine to sustainable solutions for public health problems. This process consists of three phases.

- Exploration and development of potential treatments through basic laboratory research, including safety and efficacy testing
- Assessment of how these findings apply to routine clinical practice
- Collecting information to transform effective tools discovered in phase 2 research into sustainable solutions and evidence-based policies

In the context of imaging research, these phases involve developing more sensitive and specific imaging techniques or disease markers, assessing their performance in clinical practice, and further investigating these techniques at an epidemiological level to influence and improve the standard of care in imaging. To fully harness the potential of translational imaging in drug development and make medicines safer and more cost-effective, a systematic approach is required to qualify these biomarkers with regulatory authorities, ensuring their standardized and widespread use. As part of the assessment for widespread, rigorous QC and QA procedures are a requirement.

8.1.4.1 In vivo imaging

In vivo imaging has the potential to revolutionize translational toxicology in the field of drug discovery. This encompasses various imaging techniques like MRI, PET, and CT. These imaging methods offer the advantage of providing minimally invasive biomarkers, which are crucial for safety assessment and decision-making during drug development. There are two types of biomarkers used in this context: nonspecific and specific. Nonspecific biomarkers, such as MRI relaxometry, CT density, or PET 18F-fluoro-2-deoxy-D-glucose, are well-suited for general toxicology studies in preclinical and clinical settings. Specific biomarkers, like many PET and single photon emission tomography ligands, are particularly valuable for understanding the mechanisms of toxicity or unintended interactions with specific targets. However, the use of these biomarkers is currently inconsistent, driven more by scientific interest and availability than by their utility. In vivo toxicity testing of new drug candidates begins early in the drug development process, often during the lead optimization stage. This involves conducting small-scale studies to determine dose ranges and maximum tolerated doses. The data from these studies are then used to design preclinical toxicity assessments, which help determine dosages for initial human trials and subsequent clinical phases. In vivo imaging techniques, such as MRI, PET, SPECT, and CT, offer a promising solution as translational assays. These techniques operate on similar physical and biological principles in both animals and humans. For example, MRI uses strong magnetic fields and radiofrequency pulses to generate images of biological tissues, making it a minimally invasive imaging modality. PET and SPECT are highly sensitive devices that detect positrons and gamma rays emitted by radiolabeled molecules injected into living tissue. Common isotopes like 99mTc, 123I (SPECT), and 18F, 11C, and 68Ga (PET) are used in trace amounts, with short half-lives, making these modalities minimally invasive as well. CT employs X-rays to obtain multiple transmission projections of an object, which are then reconstructed into 3D images using specialized algorithms. At the preclinical stage, the gold standard for assessing toxicity is often the microscopic examination of histological samples, a practice that is challenging to replicate in clinical settings. Therefore, there is a need for surrogate safety endpoints, or biomarkers, to continue monitoring toxicity throughout clinical development and after drug approval. Ideally, these biomarkers should be "translational," meaning they can be measured consistently in both preclinical and clinical studies.

8.1.4.2 Imaging biomarkers for drug discovery

An imaging biomarker is a measurable characteristic or feature obtained through medical imaging techniques that provide information about a biological process, disease, or the effects of treatment. These biomarkers are typically derived from various imaging modalities such as MRI, PET, CT, SPECT, ultrasound, and others. Imaging biomarkers play a crucial role in medical research, drug development, and clinical practice for several reasons:

- **Early Detection and Diagnosis**: They can help identify diseases or abnormalities at an early stage when they may not be visible through other means, allowing for earlier intervention and treatment
- **Disease Monitoring**: Imaging biomarkers can track disease progression or treatment response over time, enabling physicians to adjust treatment plans as needed
- **Treatment Evaluation**: They can assess the effectiveness of therapeutic interventions, aiding in the decision-making process for treatment continuation or modification
- **Patient Stratification**: Imaging biomarkers can be used to categorize patients into subgroups based on disease characteristics, helping to personalize treatment approaches
- **Drug Development**: In pharmaceutical research, imaging biomarkers can serve as endpoints in clinical trials, allowing researchers to assess a drug's impact on a specific biological process or target

Examples of imaging biomarkers include:

- **Tumor size and volume**: Used to assess the response of cancerous tumors to treatment
- **Cerebral blood flow**: Used in neurological research and for diagnosing conditions like stroke
- **Amyloid plaque deposition**: An indicator of Alzheimer's disease
- **Glucose uptake**: Used in PET scans to detect areas of high metabolic activity, such as in cancer cells
- **Perfusion imaging**: Used to assess blood flow in tissues or organs

Imaging biomarkers can be categorized into two types: general and specific. General Biomarkers: These provide nonspecific information about a wide range of potential adverse reactions to a toxic substance, without delving into the detailed mechanisms of toxicity. General biomarkers are valuable for initial screening, determining maximum tolerated doses, establishing dose ranges, and assessing dose-response relationships during lead optimization and preclinical toxicity testing. They encompass both structural and functional biomarkers, measuring aspects such as anatomical and morphological features, tissue composition, and overall cellular health (e.g., tissue cellularity, density, microstructure, necrosis, apoptosis, edema, and energy metabolism). Specific Biomarkers: These are typically functional biomarkers that offer insights into established metabolic or physiological pathways that may be impacted by a substance or when assurance of the safety of a particular target is required. Specific biomarkers include ligands labeled with radionuclides or contrast media used in imaging techniques like PET, SPECT, MRI, or CT. Magnetic resonance spectroscopy is also a part of this category. Specific biomarkers are particularly valuable for understanding the mechanisms of toxicity, identifying unwanted target interactions, and gaining insights into potential human toxicity based on preclinical data. It's important to note that the term "biomarker" is used broadly in this review to refer to any measurement of a relevant biological parameter. However, according to major regulatory agencies, biomarkers must undergo a rigorous qualification process to establish their properties, including sensitivity and specificity, as well as define their context of use to become valid tools in drug development. Unfortunately, as of the present time, there are no qualified imaging safety biomarkers listed by the US Food and Drug Administration (FDA) or other regulatory bodies. This underscores the need for further research and qualification efforts to establish robust imaging biomarkers for assessing drug safety during development [33].

Using in vivo imaging to measure morphological endpoints is a fundamental approach in toxicity testing. It involves assessing anatomical changes in the body, often with a focus on the brain [34]. For instance, MRI has been used to detect brain morphological changes in cases of arsenic, cadmium, copper, and lead poisoning in both clinical and preclinical studies. In rats, chronic administration of olanzapine resulted in a decrease in brain cortex volume, while guinea pigs exposed to chlorpyrifos during pregnancy had smaller brains than control subjects. Children undergoing combined antileukemic treatment with methotrexate and radiotherapy exhibited decreased gray matter volumes in the brain. Additionally, acute glyphosate intoxication led to hippocampal atrophy. While many of these studies have employed MRI due to its excellent soft tissue contrast and ability to distinguish between brain gray and white matter, there are limitations. MRI may have lower resolution compared to CT, is susceptible to motion artifacts, requires complex image analysis, and necessitates a baseline scan for reliable change detection. Furthermore, detectable morphological changes are believed to occur later in the toxicity process and may not possess sufficient predictive power for early detection [35–37].

Imaging biomarkers that reflect changes in tissue composition and microstructure are typically measured using MRI (proton relaxation and water diffusion) or CT (tissue density). These biomarkers, while not specific, can detect alterations in tissue even if the exact cause of the change isn't clear. For instance, various factors like water concentration, blood flow, temperature, and cellularity can influence proton relaxation parameters and water diffusion characteristics. Within toxicological research, it's often valuable to identify any deviation from the normal state, even if the cause is not specific. One example is the apparent transverse relaxation time (T2) of water protons, which tends to remain stable in the brain under normal conditions. This stability allows for the relatively straightforward measurement of T2 with precision through quantitative T2 mapping. This technique has been used to assess the neurotoxicity of various substances in rats, such as kainic acid, hexachlorophene, 3-nitropropionic acid, trimethyl tin, pyrithiamine, and others. A simpler method involves measuring relative changes in T2-weighted MRI signals, which has been widely employed to detect neurotoxicity in response to substances like pilocarpine, N-methyl-D-aspartate, and diisopropylfluorophosphate in preclinical studies. T2-weighted MRI is also commonly used in clinical settings to diagnose neurotoxic incidents resulting from prescribed medications, environmental exposures, or accidental contact with toxic substances, as evidenced in numerous case reports. T2 MRI has found applications beyond the CNS as well. For instance, it has been used to detect paracetamol-induced liver injury in rats, with quantitative T2 mapping proving more effective than qualitative T2-weighted imaging in identifying hepatotoxicity. Additionally, MRI T2/T1 imaging and parametric mapping have served as sensitive indicators of cardiotoxicity during anthracycline chemotherapy and fluorouracil treatment in clinical cases [38−41].

Another set of biomarkers that can only be measured by MRI involves parameters related to water diffusivity. These are assessed using techniques such as diffusion-weighted imaging (DWI), diffusion tensor imaging (DTI), and diffusion kurtosis imaging. These parameters are valuable indicators of changes in water content and distribution within tissues, including phenomena like oedema, tissue cellularity, cellular or membrane alterations, the presence and damage of fibers or other structures that restrict water diffusion, the status of ionic pumps in cell membranes, and other factors that affect water micromotion [35]. In preclinical studies, changes in water diffusion in the brain have been observed in response to substances like diisopropylfluorophosphate, 3-nitropropionic acid, prenatal exposure to cocaine, and chlorpyrifos. Nonhuman primate studies have shown alterations in certain brain DTI parameters after chronic administration of domoic acid and in acute toxicity induced by 1-methyl-4-phenyl-1,2,3,6-tetrahydropyridine. In clinical settings, DWI/DTI/diffusion kurtosis imaging has been used to diagnose and study the neurotoxic effects of substances such as carbon monoxide, methotrexate, and copper. Several clinical reports highlight the utility of DWI in detecting brain oedema. However, it's important to note that diffusion MRI can be sensitive to subject motion, making it more commonly used for brain applications where motion artifacts can be better controlled. CT, on the other hand, provides information about tissue density based on X-ray attenuation, which can change in response to toxicity. For example, brain CT scans of carbon monoxide poisoning patients have shown decreased image density in areas like the globus pallidus, correlating with delayed encephalopathy. In contrast, amiodarone-induced liver toxicity has been manifested as increased image density on CT scans. It's worth mentioning that CT is the most invasive imaging technique among those discussed, primarily due to its use of ionizing radiation. Concerns about radiation exposure are especially relevant in preclinical imaging when higher resolution is required, as it necessitates increased radiation exposure. CT also lacks the soft tissue contrast provided by MRI and can be prone to artifacts caused by bones. However, it is often used in combination with low-resolution PET scans to provide transmission correction and anatomical localization of the signal [42−45]. This category of biomarkers involves measurements that assess the general functional state of target tissues or organs, including factors like energy metabolism or mechanical performance (especially in the case of the heart). MRI and, particularly, PET and SPECT are imaging techniques well-suited for providing this type of information. MRI is commonly used to assess cardiac function by measuring heart chamber volumes during peak systole and diastole, allowing for the calculation of parameters like left ventricle ejection fraction. For instance, doxorubicin cardiotoxicity significantly affected left ventricle ejection fraction in pigs. Similarly, breast cancer patients treated with trastuzumab and anthracyclines experienced decreased left and right ventricle ejection fractions, highlighting the clinical utility of MRI. PET and SPECT, on the other hand, rely on radiolabeled ligands to assess organ or tissue health. When probing general health, glucose uptake markers like 18F-fluoro-2-deoxy-D-glucose (FDG) are commonly used. In preclinical studies, the neurotoxic substance MK-801 caused increased FDG uptake in specific brain regions of rats. Conversely, chemotherapy-induced neurotoxicity was associated with reduced brain FDG uptake in mice and rats, along with altered uptake patterns in pediatric patients. Furthermore, doxorubicin-induced cardiotoxicity was characterized by increased FDG uptake in the hearts of both mice and patients. It's important to note that the baseline state of these functional biomarkers is less stable than that of structural biomarkers. It can vary depending on an individual's fitness and nutritional status, often necessitating a separate baseline scan and careful consideration during measurements [46–49].

Several imaging approaches can be employed to investigate specific biochemical pathways or tissue and organ functions related to toxicological manifestations. Here are some notable techniques and examples.

1. **Dynamic Contrast-Enhanced (DCE) MRI**: DCE MRI involves the use of fast T1-weighted MRI to monitor rapid changes in tissue image intensity following the injection of an MRI contrast agent, such as gadolinium-diethylenetriamine pentaacetate chelate. It can quantify the transfer rates of contrast agents between different tissue compartments. DCE MRI has been used to measure blood-brain barrier permeability, which was impaired in cases of pilocarpine-induced status epilepticus in rats. A similar approach using radiolabeled compounds like 99mTc and 68Ga has been employed with PET and SPECT to assess blood-brain barrier function [42].

2. **Arterial Spin Labeling MRI**: This technique allows for noninvasive quantification of organ perfusion by labeling arterial blood water as an endogenous contrast agent. It was used to detect decreased cerebral perfusion in rats after olanzapine treatment

3. **Magnetic Resonance Spectroscopy (MRS)**: MRS is a unique MRI technique that can quantitatively measure intrinsic biochemical compounds in living tissues. For example, MRS has been used to measure lactate concentrations in the brain, which correlated with domoic acid-induced tremors in nonhuman primates. It has also been employed to quantify gamma-aminobutyric acid levels in the brains of welders exposed to manganese

4. **PET and SPECT Imaging**: Various PET and SPECT isotopes and ligands have been used to probe metabolic and functional pathways of toxicity. Examples include the use of PET ligands to study dopamine transport and presynaptic function in nonhuman primates exposed to toxins, assess cardiac mitochondrial function impairment by doxorubicin, and investigate brain microglia activation in a mouse model of temporal lobe epilepsy. Additionally, PET imaging has been used to explore histone deacetylase activity affected by chemotherapy-induced neurotoxicity in mice.

The use of specific biomarkers through these imaging techniques is typically based on prior knowledge of the potential mechanisms of toxicity. It is particularly valuable when general preclinical screening has already identified toxicity or when monitoring specific targets during clinical trials is necessary. These techniques provide insights into the functional and biochemical changes occurring within the body in response to toxic substances or treatments [33].

8.1.4.3 Intraoperative imaging biomarkers

Fluorescence-guided surgery (FGS) is a powerful intraoperative imaging technique used in oncologic surgery to enhance the identification and removal of cancerous tissues. It relies on the use of contrast agents that emit signals in the near-infrared (NIR) spectral range (750−900 nm) to improve image contrast and sensitivity. These contrast agents can passively accumulate in tumors or be actively targeted to them. In 2021, the FDA approved the first receptor-targeted FGS agent called Cytalux (pafolacianine) for detecting folate receptor-positive ovarian cancer during surgery. Clinical trials showed that using this agent with NIR fluorescence imaging helped identify lesions that were not visible under white light inspection or by palpation. Ongoing trials are exploring the potential expanded use of pafolacianine in lung cancer and other types of cancers. Clinical development of novel FGS agents often involves using targeting moieties with known in vivo properties to reduce risk. Therapeutic antibodies are commonly repurposed for FGS due to their established tumor-targeting capabilities and minimal impact on binding specificity and biodistribution when conjugated with fluorescent dyes. Low molecular weight agents, such as peptides and small molecules, are another class of targeting moieties with high binding affinity. They are rapidly cleared from the body and are well-suited for surgical workflows and clinical imaging at lower total doses compared to antibodies. An alternative strategy for developing FGS agents is to use clinically approved radiopharmaceuticals as model systems. Radiopharmaceuticals have been designed with high target selectivity for diagnostic purposes. These agents can be adapted for FGS by incorporating a fluorescent analog. Since the biodistribution of radiopharmaceuticals is already known through noninvasive PET imaging, it becomes possible to approximate the on-target and off-target uptake of the fluorescent analogue. This approach offers potential translational efficiency in developing new FGS agents, Overall, FGS is a promising technique that combines imaging and surgery to improve the precision of cancer removal, and ongoing research is expanding its applications and capabilities.

Another approach is the use of PET imaging techniques utilize the positron-emitting radionuclide gallium-68 (68Ga) and have established a robust radiochemistry and imaging infrastructure. This infrastructure was initially developed during the clinical translation of radiolabeled somatostatin analogs, such as 68Ga-DOTA-TATE and 68Ga-DOTA-TOC, which gained FDA approval in 2016 and 2019, respectively. These radiopharmaceuticals revolutionized tumor imaging for their respective diseases. One significant advancement in PET imaging involves prostate cancer, where 68Ga-PSMA-11 was the first prostate-specific membrane antigen

(PSMA)-targeted radiopharmaceutical tested in humans in 2011 and gained FDA approval in 2020. PSMA is highly expressed in prostate cancer cells, making it an attractive biomarker for targeted probe development. Over the last decade, several high-affinity PSMA-directed small molecules (analogous ligands) have been used to develop radiopharmaceuticals for PET imaging and tumor-targeted radionuclide therapy. These agents have urea-based motifs that facilitate internalization and retention within tumors. They also maintain their targeting properties after conjugation to various linkers, chelating agents, and radionuclides. In addition to PET imaging, efforts have been made to develop fluorescent counterparts of these PSMA-targeted agents for potential use in intraoperative imaging. For example, one study conjugated the NIR dye S0456 to a PSMA ligand known as DUPA, creating a promising agent named OTL78. This agent demonstrated high-affinity, PSMA-dependent binding in cells, excellent image contrast in animal models, and the potential for complete cancer cell removal. It is currently being evaluated in clinical studies. Another study aimed to improve the in vivo performance of a PSMA-targeted FGS agent called YC-27 by systematically testing 10 novel agents in animal models. The study highlighted the importance of linker selection on pharmacokinetics and concluded that certain agents may be more effective for specific types of cancer surgery. Overall, these advancements in PET imaging and the development of corresponding fluorescent agents hold great promise for improving cancer diagnosis and surgical interventions.

In addition to purely fluorescent probes, PSMA analogs have been dual-labeled with radionuclides to enable multimodal imaging. This approach allows for both nuclear and optical imaging with a single agent, offering the advantages of quantitative biodistribution measurement and cross-validation of fluorescence readouts in cell and animal experiments. Several multimodal compounds have been tested in patients with prostate cancer. One study labeled the urea-based PSMA inhibitor ACUPA with fluorine-18 (18F) for nuclear imaging and Cy3 for intraoperative optical imaging. The results consistently demonstrated high specificity for PSMA-positive tumors with both modalities, and the agent was well-tolerated in human studies. However, limitations of Cy3 as a fluorophore required optical imaging to be performed at the back table rather than in the intraoperative setting.

Another strategy involved converting two well-established PSMA-targeting compounds into multimodal counterparts with various fluorophores. Dye conjugation did not alter the favorable pharmacokinetics and tumor uptake characteristics of the parent radiotracers. The most promising multimodal analogue, referred to as 68Ga-PSMA-914, was evaluated in patients with high-risk prostate cancer and demonstrated clear tumor uptake on PET, along with intraoperative tumor visualization by NIRF imaging that guided resection. Additionally, the clinically approved Theranostics PSMA-targeting agent PSMA-617 was fluorescently labeled with IRDye800CW, showing similar PSMA-specific uptake to its parent radiopharmaceutical. Various bioconjugation strategies have been employed to synthesize multimodal PSMA analogs, including N-hydroxysuccinimide (NHS) chemistry, strain-promoted azide—alkyne cycloaddition (SPAAC or "click chemistry"), and the use of specific PSMA-targeting scaffolds like Oxalyldiaminopropionic acid-urea (ODAP-Urea). These approaches have resulted in the development of promising contrast agents for multimodal imaging, demonstrating high specificity and tumor contrast. Overall, these studies show the potential of multimodal PSMA analogs for improving the accuracy of prostate cancer imaging and guiding surgical interventions.

Another agent FGS agent is SSTR2 (Somatostatin Receptor Subtype 2). This is a cell membrane-localized G protein-coupled receptor that is commonly overexpressed in well-differentiated gastroentero-pancreatic neuroendocrine tumors (GEP-NETs). For many years, high-affinity SSTR2 agonists have been used as primary therapies to reduce hormone secretion in GEP-NETs. Recently, these agonists have been employed as ^{68}Ga-DOTA -DOTA-TOC) and for delivering cytotoxic radionuclides in peptide-receptor radionuclide therapy (PRRT). To leverage the excellent targeting properties and biodistribution of radiolabeled somatostatin analogs for real-time intraoperative guidance, researchers converted the clinically approved PET agent v-TOC into a multimodal fluorescent analog known as 68/67Ga-MMC(IR800)-TOC. They achieved this conversion by replacing the standard chelator DOTA with a "radioactive linker" called multimodality chelator (MMC), which allowed for radiolabeling and fluorescence imaging with IRDye800CW (abbreviated as IR800). This approach reduced steric interference on the binding region of the peptide and had minimal impact on the binding properties, including potency and selectivity. While MMC(IR800)-TOC exhibited high-affinity binding in cell studies and animal xenograft models, the addition of the dye prolonged blood circulation time and resulted in significant background signal in primary sites of GEP-NET surgery, such as the pancreas and small intestine. To address this issue, the researchers replaced IR800 with a zwitterionic dye called FNIR-Tag, leading to the development of a second-generation compound, MMC(FNIR-Tag)-TOC. In comprehensive studies that utilized both fluorescent and radioactive readouts in cells and animal models, MMC(FNIR-Tag)-TOC demonstrated superior targeting specificity and clearance. This improvement allowed for excellent tumor contrast as early as 3 h postinjection in surgically relevant tissues. Additionally, the researchers successfully demonstrated the translational potential of their fluorescent agent by using it to ex vivo stain human GEP-NET tissues. Overall, this research highlighted the feasibility of converting an SSTR2-targeted radiotracer into a multimodal fluorescent agent and underscored how the physiochemical properties of the fluorophore can impact pharmacokinetics and image contrast. Heing-Becker and colleagues developed a multimodal agent targeting SSTR2 in gastroenteropancreatic neuroendocrine tumors (GEP-NETs). Their approach involved modifying the structure of ^{68}Ga-DOTA-TATE by introducing the dye indocarbocyanine (ICC) as a linker between the targeting moiety (TATE) and the chelator (DOTA). The resulting compound, named 68Ga-DOTA-ICC-TATE, was subjected to in vitro analysis using both fluorescence and radioactive modalities. Their findings indicated that ^{68}Ga-DOTA-ICC-TATE possessed a low nanomolar binding affinity for SSTR2, which was comparable to that of ^{68}Ga-DOTA-TATE. This demonstrated that the close proximity of the dye and the pharmacophore did not negatively impact the peptide's binding properties. PET imaging performed 48 min after injection of ^{68}Ga-DOTA TA-ICC-TATE showed specific uptake in receptor-positive tumors, consistent with results obtained through; ex vivo tissue quantification and fluorescence microscopy. However, there was also noticeable off-target binding observed, suggesting that further optimization of the agent might be beneficial to enhance its specificity.

The potential clinical impact of using validated radiopharmaceutical counterparts in FGS is evident. However, preoperative confirmation of specific molecular targets, such as SSTR2 expression in gastroenteropancreatic neuroendocrine tumors (GEP-NETs) via PET scans with agents like ^{68}Ga-DOTA -TATE, can improve patient selection for intraoperative FGS with a corresponding fluorescent agent. The advantages of using multimodal agents, which combine both radioisotopes and fluorescent labels, are emphasized. Such agents can help identify the location and extent of primary tumors, detect multifocal lesions, and assess potential metastases, ultimately improving surgical outcomes. The passage cites examples of successful multimodal approaches in other medical contexts, such as clear cell renal cell carcinoma and gliomas. Additionally, the passage mentions the option of coadministering the FGS agent with the parent radiopharmaceutical to enable gamma probe detection for tumors in deep locations. However, it notes that using two single-labeled agents with different targeting and pharmacokinetics properties may lead to confounding results.

Another useful example is the use of imaging to promote best practices in dermatology. The development of artificial intelligence (AI) algorithms in dermatology, particularly for the classification of skin lesions using photographic images. It emphasizes the importance of optimizing the process of acquiring clinical and dermoscopic images for training and testing these AI algorithms. Key considerations for acquiring high-quality clinical and dermoscopic images for dermatology AI research include [50–60].

1. **Choice of Device**: Researchers should consider what type of device will be used to capture images, such as smartphone cameras or specialized dermoscopy attachments. The selection should align with clinical practice or the intended use setting of the AI algorithm

2. **Consistent Lighting and Distance**: During image capture, maintaining consistent lighting conditions and distance from the lesions (e.g., 6 inches) is crucial. Consistency helps ensure that the images are of high quality and free from artifacts

3. **Diversity and Representation**: Efforts should be made to include images of skin of color to improve diversity and representation in the training and testing datasets. Following best practices for capturing high-quality clinical photographs of patients with dark skin is essential

4. **Lesion Marking**: It's common practice to mark lesions with surgical skin markers or include a ruler in clinical photography and dermoscopy. However, these markings can introduce artifacts that interfere with AI classification.

Therefore, researchers may consider capturing images for AI analysis before marking the skin

5. **Standardization and Training**: Standardizing equipment, training the clinical team, and implementing quality improvement processes are essential for consistent data acquisition. However, complete elimination of variability should be avoided to ensure AI algorithms can handle noisy and nonstandardized data

The labeling of clinical images for use in machine learning, particularly for skin cancer research, and highlights the challenges and considerations involved in the labeling process. Key points regarding image labeling for machine learning in dermatology include.

- **Gold Standard Labeling for Malignant Lesions**: Histopathological diagnosis from a biopsy is considered the gold standard for labeling malignant lesions due to its lower error rate
- **Labeling Benign and Non-Biopsied Images**: For benign and nonbiopsy-verified images, labeling can be based on consensus among dermatologists or the lack of lesion stability over time. These images may not have histopathological confirmation
- **Label Noise and Inter-Observer Variability**: Even histopathology-based labels can introduce noise, especially for diagnoses like melanoma, where inter-observer agreement may be poor. This highlights the challenge of establishing a definitive gold standard
- **Availability of Clinical Labels**: Clinical impressions documented in electronic medical records provide valuable labels for lesion images, especially for non-biopsied or archived images. These labels may not have histopathological confirmation but are more readily available
- **Justification for Labeling Methods**: It's essential to provide a clear justification for the chosen method(s) of image labeling to address potential label noise and systematic errors when training neural networks
- **Collection of Race and Ethnicity Data**: Understanding the demographics of the dataset is crucial to assess algorithm generalizability and potential biases. Collecting race, ethnicity, and skin tone data, along with a description of how this data was collected, can help evaluate model performance
- **Fitzpatrick Photo Type and Skin Tone**: While the Fitzpatrick photo type scale is commonly used to label skin tone, it has limitations and does not capture the full range of human skin tones. Race, ethnicity, and objective color measurements should be considered for more accurate skin tone characterization
- **Objective Color Measurement**: When collecting data prospectively, objective methods like colorimeters or spectrophotometers can be used to measure color characteristics more precisely

The accurate labeling of clinical images for machine learning in dermatology is crucial for training and evaluating algorithms. It involves considering the gold standard for labeling, addressing label noise, and documenting patient demographics such as race, ethnicity, and skin tone to ensure algorithm generalizability and fairness. The importance of a robust data preparation and curation pipeline in translational AI dermatology research is crucial and key quality control considerations and recommendations for executing successful clinical data collection in this field is as follows:

- **Structured, Annotated, De-identified Datasets**: Ideal datasets for AI algorithm development should be structured, fully annotated, deidentified, and ethically approved with minimal noise. This ensures that the data is well-suited for specific machine learning tasks
- **Communication Between Clinical and Technical Teams**: Regular communication between the clinical team responsible for assessing, photographing, and collecting lesion data and the technical team using the dataset for algorithm development is essential. This communication helps define data fields and types and consider hypotheses to be tested
- **Statistical and Quality Tests**: Periodic statistical and quality tests should be conducted by both teams to identify underlying data distributions or biases, ensuring data quality
- **Data Storage Infrastructure**: Planning a solid infrastructure to store large volumes of machine learning data is crucial. An intermediary data housing or entry platform is recommended to structure data into a machine-readable format
- **Design Considerations for Data Storage**: When designing data storage infrastructure, consider data security and compliance, controlled access for authorized personnel, unique patient identifiers with options to remove identifiers, clear indication of lesions linked to the same patient, standardized data field names and functionality for identifying missing or incorrect information and conducting regular QC checks.
- **On-Premise versus Cloud-Based Storage**: Decide where the data will be stored, whether on-premise (secure but limited sharing) or on a cloud-based server (more flexible but potentially costly). Consider data privacy and security
- **Data Sharing**: For deidentified data, explore options for data sharing, such as public data repositories like the International Skin Imaging Collaboration
- **Future-Proofing Data Curation**: While AI algorithms may evolve, the types of curated data will likely remain relevant. Establishing a solid foundational infrastructure for data curation ensures the training of robust and generalizable models

The need for careful planning and standardization in the image acquisition process to facilitate the development and evaluation of AI algorithms in dermatology. Researchers should consider various factors, including device choice, lighting conditions, diversity in datasets, and the impact of lesion markings on image quality. Balancing standardization with the ability to handle real-world variability is also crucial for the scalability and effectiveness of AI algorithms in clinical practice.

8.1.4.4 Translational cardio-oncology imaging

Cardio-oncology is an emerging field that combines cardiovascular medicine, hematology, and oncology. With improved cancer patient survival rates, there is a growing awareness of cardiac complications resulting from anticancer therapies. Cancer survivors experiencing cardiovascular side effects not only face increased cardiac risk but also reduced progression-free and overall survival. Therefore, identifying at-risk patients early and diagnosing cardiotoxic events promptly can optimize outcomes after cancer treatment. Cardiovascular imaging, including established methods and emerging specialized techniques, can play a crucial role in a cardio-oncological surveillance strategy, helping select appropriate cardioprotective strategies. In cardio-oncology patients, cardiovascular changes can arise from underlying diseases like cardiac hypertrophy or accompanying amyloidosis, as well as from cardiotoxic therapies, such as cardiac atrophy in those undergoing anthracycline treatments. Established methods like echocardiography, conventional cardiac magnetic resonance imaging (cMRI), and PET-tracer-based imaging can detect specific tissue characteristics associated with these changes. However, these alterations often represent advanced stages of cancer or anticancer therapy-related toxicities, and they may signify late and potentially irreversible cardiovascular damage. Therefore, there is a growing interest in early detection methods that assess cellular functional parameters like cardiac metabolism, inflammation, cellular activation, and vascularization to identify cardiac damage at its onset.

For example, 3D Transethoracic echo-cardiography also known as an echo is the most commonly used imaging technique in cardio-oncology due to its widespread availability, cost-effectiveness, and excellent safety record. It plays a pivotal role in detecting chemotherapy-related cardiac dysfunction (CTRCD) by assessing left ventricular systolic function (LV) and measuring the LV ejection fraction (LVEF). Research has shown that most CTRCD associated with anthracycline therapy occurs within a year of treatment, allowing for early detection using echo. In the case of HER2-related CTRCD, echo is also crucial for early detection, with echo assessments performed every 3 months during treatment. Traditionally, two-dimensional (2D) LVEF has been the go-to measure of cardiac function before, during, and after cancer therapy, as well as in cases where heart failure is suspected. However, echocardiography has its limitations, including the need for a reliable ultrasound window and potential improvements in signal analysis for cardio-oncology diagnosis. The diagnosis of CTRCD is often based on a 2D LVEF decrease of more than 10% to below 53%, although absolute cut-off values remain controversial. The diagnostic accuracy of 2D LVEF is hindered by its test-retest variability of approximately 10%, which has been observed in both the general and oncological populations. The use of contrast agents can help mitigate this variability issue, but 2D LVEF still has limited sensitivity for detecting small changes in LV function due to visualization constraints, geometric assumptions, and its reliance on loading conditions. Guidelines have recommended 3D echocardiography to determine LVEF (3D LVEF) because it avoids geometric assumptions and offers better intra- and inter-observer reliability and test-retest variability. However, 3D LVEF may not always be feasible in cancer patients, especially those undergoing concurrent radiotherapy or surgical procedures affecting the chest. Additionally, changes in diastolic function and myocardial deformation (strain) measured by Doppler patterns and tissue Doppler imaging can precede systolic dysfunction and provide valuable insights into cardio-oncology patients' cardiac health.

Speckle-tracking echocardiography is gaining attention for its application in assessing other cardiac chambers beyond the left ventricle. Recent studies have demonstrated that anthracycline and trastuzumab therapy can lead to a reduction in right ventricular (RV) free-wall longitudinal strain in adult patients with breast cancer and lymphoma. This reduction in RV strain has also been observed in adult survivors of childhood lymphoma and acute lymphoblastic leukemia who were treated with anthracycline and radiation therapy. Another cardiac chamber of interest is the left atrium. Limited-scale studies have suggested that measuring left atrial strain may have the potential to identify patients at higher risk of developing chemotherapy-related cardiac dysfunction (CTRCD) after trastuzumab therapy. Additionally, left atrial strain has been explored in relation to atrial fibrillation in patients receiving the medication ibrutinib. These findings highlight the expanding role of speckle-tracking echocardiography in assessing various cardiac chambers for potential early detection and monitoring of cardiac issues in cancer patients undergoing specific treatments.

Stress echocardiography is another technique that plays a crucial role in the field of cardio-oncology. Much like its application in general cardiology, stress echocardiography is valuable for evaluating patients for coronary artery disease. However, in cardio-oncology, it takes on an additional role by assessing patients who are at an increased risk of cardiac ischemia due to specific anticancer therapies, including 5-fluorouracil, nilotinib, ponatinib, and sunitinib. Beyond evaluating coronary artery disease risk, stress echocardiography is also useful in assessing subclinical left ventricular (LV) dysfunction and contractile reserve in patients who have received cardiotoxic drugs. Additionally, it can be employed to evaluate valvular function in patients who have undergone radiation therapy. In this way, stress echocardiography contributes significantly to the comprehensive evaluation and management of cardiac health in cancer patients undergoing various treatments.

Recent advancements in cardiac MRI have introduced novel MRI sequences that offer multiparametric tissue characterization, addressing some limitations of traditional techniques. Traditional methods required additional acquisition time and the use of gadolinium-based contrast agents for each parameter. The introduction of native T1 and T2 mapping techniques has provided a significant advantage, allowing for the detection of tissue-specific changes while saving time and eliminating the need for gadolinium contrast. Another development is the establishment of fast-strain encoded cardiac MRI sequences, which have proven effective in detecting subclinical structural changes. These sequences are currently being tested for their potential in the early detection of cardiotoxicity. Additionally, high-quality cardiac real-time imaging is converging with strain detection, aiming for a "single-heartbeat" acquisition approach. This innovative approach not only has the potential to reduce costs but also promises broader application in cancer patients, making it a promising avenue for improving cardiac assessment in this population.

Cancer treatments, especially when chemotherapy is combined with radiation therapy in the mediastinal area, can increase the risk of developing coronary artery disease and valvular dysfunction later on. CT provides various assessment modalities for coronary, valvular, pericardial, and cardiac chamber structures. Nongated CT has been extensively studied for assessing coronary artery calcium (CAC), which serves as a predictor of future cardiovascular events. The amount of CAC is positively correlated with the likelihood of future cardiovascular events and allows for improved risk stratification, particularly in both low and high-risk patients. CT coronary angiography (CTA) goes further by evaluating obstructive coronary artery disease, including noncalcified plaque. It can be especially valuable in patients with hematological disorders, potentially eliminating the need for invasive procedures. In contrast to CTA, new techniques such as CT-derived fractional flow reserve (FFR) and CT perfusion imaging can identify hemodynamically significant coronary lesions. CT, either alone or in conjunction with echocardiography, has become a standard for assessing valvular heart disease. Current valvular guidelines establish specific calcium score thresholds for diagnosing severe aortic stenosis, particularly in cases of low-flow, low-gradient aortic stenosis. Multidetector CT (MDCT), which can rapidly capture images during precisely defined phases of the cardiac cycle, can be employed alongside echocardiography to assess mechanical heart valve structure and function, especially when valve thrombosis is suspected. CT is less affected by patient body habitus compared to echocardiography or fluoroscopy. However, it's important to note that while CT can be used to assess large vessels and cardiac structure, it provides less information about myocardial disease when compared to cardiac MRI. SPECT is a primary application is in detecting variations in myocardial perfusion. Besides its prognostic value in assessing cardiac ischemia, SPECT also plays a crucial role in guiding therapy. Recent advancements in SPECT technology, particularly the use of solid-state detectors based on cadmium−zinc−telluride (CZT), have significantly improved its sensitivity. CZT-based SPECT systems have shown an impressive sensitivity of 84% in detecting obstructive coronary artery disease. For SPECT imaging using CZT, the tracer of choice is often 201Tl because it has demonstrated superior physiological properties compared to tracers labeled with 99mTc. Recent studies have indicated that combining SPECT myocardial perfusion imaging (MPI) with coronary CT angiography can serve as a long-term predictor for major adverse cardiac events. However, the specific application of these modalities in cancer patients has not been thoroughly evaluated, despite many cardio-toxic events being associated with endothelial dysfunction. Therefore, further investigation and research are needed to assess the clinical utility of these imaging tools in evaluating vasculotoxic events in cancer patients.

^{18}F-FDG (Fluorodeoxyglucose) uptake by activated immune cells can be selectively visualized in the heart by suppressing cardiac glucose utilization through nutritional preparation. Consequently, ^{18}F-FDG uptake has become the primary

imaging technique for diagnosing active cardiac inflammation, particularly in conditions like sarcoidosis or device infection. When combined with cMRI, ^{18}F-FDG PET/MRI shows promise in improving the detection of cardiovascular inflammation beyond what either method can achieve alone. This approach merges structural and functional assessment of the heart with tracer-specific information about tissue-level changes, all within a single scan. MRI-driven correction for motion enhances the accuracy of PET images, making it a valuable tool in various scenarios. In the context of cardio-oncology, this approach holds potential for patients with myocarditis or vascular inflammation, such as those associated with immune checkpoint inhibition. Experimental models have also shown its effectiveness, with ^{18}F-FDG PET/MRI successfully detecting myocardial inflammatory infiltration in a canine model as early as 1 week after radiation exposure.

Continuous innovation in hardware and system design is expected to enhance the accuracy and reliability of cardiovascular imaging in the risk assessment of cardio-oncology patients. A significant limitation of nuclear medicine imaging is its limited spatial resolution, which has been partly addressed by combining SPECT and PET scanners with CT-derived data to correct for attenuation-related signal loss and artifacts. Reducing radiation exposure remains a critical goal, especially in cardio-oncology, where patients may undergo repetitive imaging during multiple cycles of potentially toxic therapies. The latest generation of systems includes hybrid PET/MRI scanners, which, as mentioned earlier, offer superior soft tissue contrast and the potential for decreased radiation exposure due to the inherent characteristics of MRI technology. However, these hybrid systems come with increased costs, longer scanning times, and technological challenges in combining the two modalities. Further research is needed to demonstrate their added value compared to standard workflows.

8.1.4.5 Molecular imaging

Pathological cardiac remodeling is closely linked to fundamental metabolic changes. Preclinical research suggests that these metabolic alterations precede adverse cardiac remodeling and could potentially serve as early or predictive markers for patients at risk [61]. In simplified terms, pathological cardiac remodeling involves a series of molecular events crucial for the development of left ventricular dysfunction [61–63]. Many of these underlying molecular mechanisms were initially identified in preclinical models of pathological cardiac hypertrophy. This hypertrophy is characterized by an imbalance between cardiomyocyte growth and angiogenesis, resulting in the loss of functional cells due to cell death and their replacement with fibrotic tissue [64–67]. This process is associated with a shift in energy generation from primarily using fatty acid oxidation to less efficient glucose metabolism. It also leads to various other pathological effects, including an increase in reactive oxygen species, unfavorable posttranslational modifications, and inflammation [66,68]. These effects are expected in cases of cardiotoxicity However, the exact timeline of these molecular events on the path to cardiac dysfunction is not yet clear. In the case of cardiotoxicity, the precise timing of the toxic event is known, and "rapid" molecular processes occur early on

[69–76]. Novel imaging modalities hold promise for identifying several of these early pathological events in the context of cardiotoxicity.

In terms of metabolic imaging, stable isotope spectroscopy with ^{31}P and [13] C labeled substrate were traditionally used for assessing metabolic processes [70–72]. With advancement in magnetic spectroscopy and spectroscopic imaging to assess metabolic processes in the myocardium, particularly in the context of cardio-oncology. Traditional methods for assessing metabolic processes using stable isotope spectroscopy have limitations due to low signal intensity and poor spatial and time resolution [77–87]. Hyperpolarized 13C spectroscopy enhances signal intensity significantly, allowing the detection of 13C signals despite their low abundance. This approach enables real-time, noninvasive monitoring of biochemical processes in the heart [88–91]. It has been applied in human studies to evaluate pyruvate dehydrogenase flux in healthy individuals and diabetes patients, providing insights into myocardial metabolic processes. In a rat model, the technique revealed a decrease in myocardial oxidative metabolism in cardiomyocytes after doxorubicin treatment, demonstrating a dose-dependent toxic effect [92–95]. Similar impairments in myocardial mitochondrial oxidative activity were observed in breast cancer patients treated with doxorubicin. This technology offers a valuable tool for understanding and visualizing myocardial metabolic changes in cardio-oncology [95].

Another use of molecular imaging is detecting inflammation. The use of ^{18}F-FDG PET or combined ^{18}F-FDG-PET MRI for detecting inflammation is nonspecific when it comes to identifying the type of inflammatory cells involved. However, in cases where inflammation involves specific subgroups of inflammatory cells, such as CD8-positive T-cells (seen in patients with immune checkpoint inhibitor-associated myocarditis), specific imaging methods can be valuable for diagnosis and monitoring. In animal studies, PET-CT tracers designed to target CD8$^+$ T-cells have been investigated for assessing inflammatory cells infiltrating tumors [95–99]. Among these tracers, 89Zr-labeled PEGylated single-domain antibody fragments (^{89}Zr-malDFO-169) hold promise as translational tools for diagnosing immune checkpoint inhibitor-associated myocarditis in patients.

Fibroblast-activated protein inhibitor (FAPI) imaging is another methods used to determine structural changes within the heart due to the activation of fibroblasts in the heart caused by elevated expressions of fibroblast activation protein (FAP). This activation of cardiac fibroblasts has been proposed as a common pathway for adverse cardiac remodeling in response to various stressors and is also a component of structural changes in the cancer microenvironment [88,89]. This remodeling is associated with subsequent cardiac dysfunction. A relatively new tracer, ^{68}Ga-FAPI, originally designed to image activated fibroblasts in oncological diseases, has shown promise in detecting pathological cardiac remodeling, cardiac inflammation, and potentially cardiotoxicity at an early stage [95–99]. Recent data suggest that ^{68}Ga-FAPI can identify these cardiac conditions, including cases like immune checkpoint inhibitor-associated myocarditis, where increased tracer uptake was observed in patients with clinical signs of myocarditis compared to those on immune checkpoint inhibitor therapy without such signs [80–89,100].

^{123}I-MIBG is another tracer that is capable of assessing sympathetic innervation and the reuptake of norepinephrine into presynaptic neurons. Myocardial sympathetic denervation, which occurs alongside systemic sympathetic hyperactivation, is a characteristic feature of heart failure. This is particularly significant in patients with heart failure and reduced left ventricular ejection fraction, as it allows for specific risk assessment. While I-MIBG has not yet been studied in cardio-oncology patients, it may be valuable because myocardial sympathetic denervation can occur before mechanical functional impairment [96,97]. This imaging technique has the potential to detect early signs of toxicity resulting from cancer therapies that are known to affect the peripheral nervous system and heart rate.

In the field of cardio-oncology, many imaging modalities provide abnormal findings, but the underlying molecular mechanisms leading to cardiovascular pathology often remain unclear [80−87]. To address this, there's a growing need for a "deep phenotyping" approach. This approach involves combining multiparametric tissue characterization with dynamic mechanical function data obtained from advanced cardiovascular imaging tools. This integration of data offers a more comprehensive understanding of the processes at play [95]. Furthermore, the translational application of innovative technologies capable of identifying early pathophysiological mechanisms that occur before structural cardiovascular changes become apparent could pave the way for new preventive strategies [89−98]. Shifting the clinical management focus toward visualizing the underlying root causes of diseases, rather than solely addressing downstream manifestations, in combination with high-throughput blood biomarkers for large-scale, cost-effective screening of early pathological stages, may offer the potential for novel early diagnostic strategies. The integration of machine learning into risk prediction models, data acquisition, and processing has the potential to enhance the definition of clinical tiers that necessitate testing. It can also improve the quality of data collection and reduce the variability in interpretation. These advantages can lead to several positive outcomes, including better test reproducibility, the need for fewer trial participants to reach conclusive results, and more precise and targeted application of imaging tools in clinical settings. Paradigm-shifting scientific discoveries have driven major transitions in therapeutic and diagnostic approaches in oncology, focusing on molecular and immunologic targets. This emphasis on understanding the intricate crosstalk between different aspects of cancer biology has revolutionized the field.

8.1.4.6 Artificial intelligence for optimizing translational imaging

The rapid advancement of AI in various industries, including healthcare and medical imaging, is driven by improved computing power, data availability, and machine learning techniques [101,102]. While initial expectations suggested that AI might replace some tasks performed by radiologists, experts generally believe that AI will complement radiologists and enhance patient care if used correctly [103−105]. However, there are concerns and challenges associated with AI in medical imaging [106]. The Department of Defense has highlighted the potential pitfalls of AI algorithms, emphasizing how easily they can be misled by introducing even minor noise, which could result in incorrect diagnoses or reduced confidence in results [107,108]. To ensure the successful integration of AI in healthcare, these challenges must be addressed, and AI algorithms must be reliable, safe, effective, and seamlessly integrated into physicians' workflows [95–99,101–108]. Additionally, issues related to interconnectivity, interoperability, and cybersecurity need resolution to maintain data integrity and implement AI in clinical practice. A workshop in 2018, involving stakeholders from academia, industry, and government, was convened to discuss AI in medical imaging and identify research priorities. The development of AI in healthcare involves data engineering, algorithm creation, and software integration, with foundational research driving progress in each step. The adoption of AI in healthcare is expected to be gradual, with machine intelligence complementing human intelligence in ways that improve patient outcomes. Similar to AI's progression in smartphones, its deployment in healthcare will become increasingly integrated into medical practice. Understanding the radiology information cycle is crucial in incorporating AI into medical imaging, as it encompasses clinical decisions, patient preparation, protocol determination, examination, interpretation, and care recommendations. While AI's interpretation phase receives significant attention, AI research and development are advancing in all areas, and subject matter experts are vital for converting ideas into AI use cases for various phases of the information cycle. Radiologists are encouraged to identify key areas for AI development. While the potential for AI to reach a level of general AI that mimics human capabilities exists in the distant future, current and foreseeable applications of AI in healthcare are more focused on solving specific challenges in medical imaging, such as detecting pneumothorax or classifying lung nodules. These narrow AI applications, even if not superhuman in performance, can still significantly benefit patient care as long as they outperform the lower end of radiologist performance standard.

The study conducted by Nekoui et al. utilized machine learning models to analyze raw cardiac MRI data from the UK Biobank cohort study [109,110]. They focused on defining different anatomical segments of the thoracic aorta and combining this information with genetic and health outcomes data for genome-wide association studies and clinical predictions. This approach aimed to provide insights into the biology of aortic segments and their relationship to clinical outcomes. The study found shared biological factors across the thoracic aorta and identified unique factors for specific segments [111]. Notably, the aortic root and proximal segments were associated with the risk of thoracic aneurysmal disease. This research offers new tools for predicting this condition, similar to screening for abdominal aortic aneurysms [112]. However, the authors emphasized the importance of approaching clinical applications with caution, especially regarding potential disparities in healthcare. They urged the need for inclusive data representation from diverse ancestral backgrounds to avoid creating new healthcare inequities. In summary, Nekoui and colleagues' study combined machine learning analysis of cardiac MRI data with genetics to uncover aortic biology, study epidemiological relationships, and develop clinical prediction tools for thoracic aneurysmal disease, emphasizing the importance of addressing healthcare disparities in the process [109–112].

8.1.5 Quality assurance management in translational imaging

Quality assurance management within the context of translational imaging is complex and agile due to the rapid adjustments quality control steps undergo as the intervention or imaging modality advances. For example, quality assurance in magnetic resonance imaging linear accelerator (MRL) systems used in radiation therapy could undergo several iterations of quality assurance procedures before and after implementation during the testing phase. These systems combine real-time MRI guidance with radiation therapy, allowing for precise tumor tracking during treatment. Two major vendors, Elekta Unity and ViewRay's MRIdian, offer such systems. Due to the presence of magnetic fields in MRL systems, QA is crucial for ensuring accurate treatment delivery. The American College of Radiology (ACR) and the AAPM have established guidelines for evaluating MRL system performance using dedicated phantoms. However, current QA processes are time-consuming and require manual analysis. A good quality control and assurance in this context is the potential use of the Magphan RT phantom, which comes with a web-based software called "Smári," as an alternative to the ACR phantom for periodic QA in low-field MRL systems. The goal is to develop a more efficient and automated QA process to save time while maintaining the precision required for radiation therapy. The Magphan RT 820 phantom consists of two modules: the top and bottom modules, allowing for the measurement of geometric distortion and uniformity over a specific volume. Over 100 spherical fiducials and other components filled with MRI-signal-generating liquid were used to evaluate the system's performance. Careful attention was paid to filling the phantom to avoid bubbles. The phantom includes various test objects and features, such as fiducial spheres for distortion measurements, slice thickness ramps, resolution apertures, noise rods, and uniform background fills. The study found that the phantom placement could disrupt the scanner's magnetic field as the gantry moves, leading to apparent shifts in the MR coordinate system. The T2-weighted images had artifacts that affected the distortion analysis, potentially causing measurement errors [113]. Quality Assurance plays a crucial role in identifying system issues proactively, reducing downtime. Existing monthly QA tests are typically conducted in MR-only mode, but it's essential to implement integrated testing for simultaneous MR scanner and linac use in clinical mode. This approach allows for the assessment of system reliability in online adaptive radiotherapy workflows. Using the Magphan phantom with its Smari software for analysis offers several advantages. It provides quick and fully automated results, standardizes the analysis process, and reduces the chances of manual errors compared to in-house or custom-tailored tools. However, there are limitations to consider, such as slice thickness requirements and signal-to-noise ratio (SNR) for T2-weighted images. The agreement between gantry angles may require further investigation into factors like shimming alignment and scanner mechanical alignment. Artifacts in the images can affect Magphan's ability to calculate certain parameters, particularly for T2-weighted images. The ACR phantom is sensitive to positioning and can impact results. Magphan provides efficient and reliable QA, reducing analysis time and improving workflow. It offers multiple parameters and 3D measurements with a single pulse sequence, eliminating subjectivity in the analysis. In conclusion, Magphan is a valuable alternative to the ACR phantom for evaluating low-field MRL performance. It offers speed and similar measurements, making it a practical choice for QA. However, keeping the ACR phantom as a backup for occasional analysis is advisable.

8.1.5.1 Clinical trials

Clinical trials play a crucial role in improving clinical care for oncology patients. However, the processes involved in data management and clinical trial investigation can be challenging, even for experienced investigators. These challenges include obtaining Internal Review Board (IRB) approvals, managing patient consent, handling data, and providing patient care throughout the study, from before its initiation to after its completion. These demands can sometimes be perceived as limiting clinical productivity when measured in relative value units (RVU). The complexity of data management and submission processes can also be seen as a barrier to protocol participation. This perception can impact how protocols are designed and how data is collected, managed, and archived by Quality Assurance (QA) centers. To encourage study accrual, compromises are often made by limiting the data acquisition process. This can result in reduced imaging submissions, elimination of real-time reviews, and a lack of oversight in trial management. While this approach has the immediate benefit of meeting study accrual goals, it comes with consequences. Limiting data acquisition may reduce confidence in the trial's outcomes. The experience at QARC (Quality Assurance Review Center) (now IROC RI) in managing Hodgkin lymphoma (HL) clinical trials illustrates how clinical trial processes have evolved to prioritize optimal trial management while addressing these challenges. Clinical trial 8725 in pediatric oncology, if conducted today, would be categorized as a study involving patients with intermediate and early high-risk Hodgkin lymphoma (HL). The trial's design involved a randomization process to determine whether radiation therapy (RT) after eight cycles of hybrid chemotherapy, including MOPP (mechlorethamine, vincristine, procarbazine, and prednisone) and ABVD (doxorubicin, bleomycin, vinblastine, and dacarbazine), would be beneficial for these patients. The RT treatment plan aimed to address all initial disease sites after the completion of chemotherapy. Response-adapted blocking techniques were employed, particularly for the mediastinum, to limit the radiation dose to the pulmonary parenchyma. CT images were used to confirm the volume of therapy that needed to be treated. Notably, the trial did not focus on the rapidity of response but rather on the response itself, and this aspect was not intentionally reviewed for protocol management. During this era, digital information was not readily available, and all RT-related information was collected by study investigators as a retrospective process after patients had completed their therapy. There was no real-time review of information by study investigators or Quality Assurance (QA) centers. In the original publication of the trial results, it was observed that there appeared to be no significant benefit to adding RT after chemotherapy for this specific patient population. A secondary analysis of the RT information from this study aimed to understand why the deviation rate from the trial protocol exceeded 30% and how the process could be improved for future Hodgkin studies. The analysis revealed the following key findings:

1. The deviation rate was primarily driven by radiation investigators who adjusted the volume of therapy and excluded segments of the original disease at the presentation from the RT fields. This was done based on the perception that limiting the treated volumes would reduce the risk of late side effects
2. Interestingly, the optimal outcomes were achieved when all sites of the original disease were included in the RT treatment field. The study showed that excluding segments of the original disease from the therapy field did not provide any statistically significant benefit

These findings held significant implications. It became evident to the leadership of the Pediatric Oncology Group (POG) that the application of RT in Hodgkin lymphoma (HL) by different investigators was inconsistent and had the potential to impact trial outcomes. Additionally, it was recognized that the retrospective review of RT plans was valuable, but the process needed adjustment if RT was to have a meaningful impact in clinical trials involving HL. As a result of these insights, the RT committee decided to implement a new approach for the next generation of studies. This approach involved obtaining pretreatment approval of RT treatment plans, aiming to standardize and improve the use of RT in clinical trials for HL patients. Children's Oncology Group (COG) Studies 9425 and 9426 were clinical trials focused on addressing intermediate and low-risk Hodgkin lymphoma (HL). Both studies incorporated RT as part of the consolidation management strategy, with the goal of including all soft tissue and bone sites of the disease at presentation. Response-adapted titration of mediastinal adenopathy, where disease extended into the pulmonary parenchyma, was also part of the treatment approach. In COG 9426, the low-risk study, response-adaptive titration of chemotherapy was included after a review of imaging following two cycles of chemotherapy. These trials were conducted before the digital era, but it was determined that reviewing RT treatment plans before therapy was feasible because RT would be administered after chemotherapy, allowing time for data submission and review. However, response imaging was conducted retrospectively. In COG 9426, the low-risk study, response-adaptive titration of chemotherapy was included after a review of imaging following two cycles of chemotherapy. These trials were conducted before the digital era, but it was determined that reviewing RT treatment plans before therapy was feasible because RT would be administered after chemotherapy, allowing time for data submission and review. However, response imaging was conducted retrospectively. Intermediate-risk COG AHOD0031 became the first study to integrate real-time review of imaging and RT objects into the protocol [116]. This study was designed to identify patients with rapid and slow early responses to chemotherapy, with separate treatment strata based on response. The study included anatomic and metabolic imaging for response assessment and digital RT objects for preplan review. A digital data transfer system was developed to facilitate data management and reminders to sites about due data. The study, involving nearly 1800 patients, was highly successful and resulted in important publications on the study process and outcomes. Real-time review of objects has since become a standard practice in the pediatric and adult clinical trials community. This approach has led to successful studies in limited-stage HL and investigations into volume titration with RT after comprehensive chemotherapy for advanced-stage patients. Reviewers have emphasized the importance of the QA process in providing confidence in the study outcomes [117].

8.1.6 Radiological technology advancement

Concurrently, advancements in computer hardware and software has continuously advanced the medical imaging interpretation providing practice enhancement to support Radiologists. Advancement in technology has enabled multiple software to process large quantities of image data that can be reconstructed and fused in different dimensions for the purpose of optimizing clinical and research practices. The picture archiving and communication systems (PACS) was developed to support some of this routine clinical and research imaging to store scans [118,119]. Multiple vendors have since developed similar systems with advanced image processing capabilities to ensure enable efficient and effective radiology reporting. The electronic health record (EHR) is a significant outcome of the digital revolution in healthcare. Radiologists now have the capability to access a patient's complete medical history, laboratory results, clinical notes, and comprehensive health information while they are reviewing or interpreting medical imaging studies. This integration has extended to include the radiology information system and hospital information system, which can now be connected with coding, billing, workflow dashboards, and computerized order entry, complete with decision support tools, in modern hospitals. This transformation has turned radiologists into knowledge integrators as they consider past medical history, previous medical studies, and lab results when offering a differential diagnosis during their readings. The digital revolution has significantly impacted medical imaging education. In the past, teaching materials were stored in analog film libraries, but now, digital technology has transformed this process. Today, educators can easily access and share case-based teaching materials through digital PACS systems and the internet. Additionally, the rise of social media and collaborative platforms has expanded the availability of a vast knowledge base for teaching and creating educational resources, offering unprecedented opportunities for medical imaging education.

8.1.7 Quality control challenges for the workforce

Financial concerns at the individual faculty level sometimes lead department chairpersons to hesitate in supporting junior researchers pursuing external funding opportunities like NIH career development grants (known as "K awards") or grants from professional organizations or companies. These grants typically require the recipient to allocate a significant portion of their time, often between 50% and 75%, toward research-related activities. Some objections to allocating academic time, despite being rooted in financial considerations, are often presented in clinical terms. There's concern that junior faculty members dedicating at least 50% or more of their time to research might become inadequate radiologists. However, this argument is countered by the success of colleagues in medical fields who excel clinically while conducting research. Furthermore, as imaging tools become more disease-specific and less hardware-dependent, radiology may need to embrace a similar approach to that of its clinical colleagues. This could involve promoting greater sub-specialization, especially within academic departments. By doing so, radiologist-scientists can maximize the value of their clinical work and deliver the highest possible level of patient care. Junior faculty members, despite their limited experience, face a pressing need for protected research time. They typically shoulder a heavy burden of clinical responsibilities and on-call schedules. Inefficient time management and the challenge of balancing clinical and scientific duties are common issues for these early-career researchers. Interestingly, these junior investigators, being freshly trained and up-to-date on clinical practices in radiology and related fields, are well-positioned to make significant breakthroughs, especially in areas that can benefit from advances in imaging-related techniques. Therefore, providing them with the necessary support and protected research time is crucial for fostering transformative discoveries. Moreover, the expensive nature of scanning time, coupled with the fact that clinical reimbursement is based on procedures rather than exam duration, leaves limited room in the clinical schedule for experimenting with new imaging sequences. This experimentation is a critical step in integrating new technology into routine clinical care and often occurs outside the standard hypothesis-driven scientific structure. Healthcare payors exhibit substantial resistance when it comes to reimbursing studies conducted using newer, more costly imaging techniques, even if these techniques have demonstrated their utility in research studies. An example is Brain MR spectroscopy, which offers valuable information for distinguishing recurrent tumors from radiation necrosis in brain tumor patients. Unfortunately, this technique currently lacks reimbursement from Medicare and Medicaid within the United States and is only sporadically covered by private insurance companies. This presents a significant obstacle to the widespread adoption of advanced tools that have the potential to greatly enhance patient care. Equally this procedure is available in limited hospitals across other parts of the world, especially in low-middle-income countries (LMICs). This also limits the use of this procedure or research projects that aim to include international to only a fraction, thereby introducing rate limiting issues to gather a statistically significant sample size.

Establishing the essential infrastructure for translational research within each department is a critical step toward building a translational research pipeline. Key elements include providing affordable or free scanning time for pilot projects, reducing scanning costs for researchers, offering professional support for lab management and grant writing, and developing effective mentorship programs. These measures are crucial for fostering a successful translational research environment. Radiologists should take a proactive role in establishing multidisciplinary research communities, acting as "centers of excellence" to drive advances in imaging for various diseases. This shift requires radiologists to lead research efforts rather than merely playing a technical support role in these groups. Institutional support can be fostered by creating additional platforms like retreats, speaker series, and journal clubs to facilitate meaningful collaboration between imaging scientists, disease biologists, and clinical radiologists. This collaborative approach can drive innovation in medical imaging. For example, translational research team in Multiple Sclerosis using MRI could benefit from Radiology expertise. This team comprises approximately 25 members with diverse backgrounds, including radiologists, neurologists, psychologists, physiologists, MR physicists, biomedical engineers, and molecular biologists. They collaborate regularly to develop innovative MR technology for diagnosing and monitoring patients with multiple sclerosis. This group demonstrated effective translation of knowledge from animal models regarding disease's pathogenesis to continue to a clinical phase. Additionally, they have optimized animal research studies to extract clinically relevant information. Close collaboration can be a quality control step that can the utility of skills and knowledge, producing value based research outcomes. Hence, multidisciplinary teams play a central role in advancing translational research in imaging [120].

8.2 Clinical radiology applications

The applications of radiology images can be categorized into diagnostic and functional systems and biomedical engineering. There are clear benefits to the patient when radiological investigations are used outweighing the low radiation risks. Even small radiation doses are not entirely risk-free. Although malignant diseases and genetic mutations can be attributed to background radiation, "*Diagnostic Medical Exposures*" use mainly man-made radiation. In the United Kingdom, the Ionizing Radiation (Medical Exposure) Regulations 2000 (IR(ME)R) and subsequent amendments (2006 and 2011) introduce a responsibility for organizations conducting imaging procedures to ensure that all exposures to ionizing radiation are justified, and that doses are optimized [11]. Thus, it is very important to know the role of Radiology and Nuclear Medicine investigations.

Imaging modality	Key features
Computed tomography	• CT images are generated by an X-ray tube rotating rapidly around the patient, producing a three-dimensional dataset that may be manipulated to examine different structures, in different planes with high resolution. • Oral and/or intravenous contrast medium can be administered to answer the clinical question(s). • Major indications are acute trauma and neurological syndromes, oncology, cardiothoracic, renal, and gastrointestinal disease.

Continued

Imaging modality	Key features
Magnetic resonance imaging	• MRI involves placing patients in a strong magnetic field and applying a series of radiofrequency pulses and time-varying gradients to generate images. • There is absence of any ionizing radiation (no radiation risk to the patient). • Major indications are evaluation of neurological syndromes and musculoskeletal disorders, together with oncological, hepatobiliary and gynecological disease. • contraindicated in patients with MRI noncompatible metallic foreign bodies
Interventional radiology	• There is use of image-guided therapies to treat nonvascular and vascular conditions. • Indications of nonvascular intervention are: drainage of urinary or biliary systems, drainage of abscess or fluid collections, biopsy of masses or lymph nodes and tumor ablation. • Indications of vascular interventions are: procedures for revascularization (angioplasty/stenting), treating aneurysms (stent grafting—abdomino-thoracic; coiling/flow diversion/portal vein occlusion [PVO]—cerebral), blocking blood vessels (embolization) to manage hemorrhage (e.g., GI bleeding/posttraumatic hemorrhage) and treating vascular tumors/malformations.
General nuclear medicine	• Functional approach to imaging of pathology by combining a physiological agent labeled with a radioisotope—commonly technetium-99m (Tc-99m). • Radiation dose is similar to, and often, less than for comparable anatomical studies. • Hybrid imaging: Includes SPECT-CT or SPECT-MR • Indications: bone scan for staging of cancer, renogram for assessment of renal function, and myocardial perfusion imaging for cardiac perfusion.
PET-CT	• (PET-CT) combines pathophysiological information, with anatomical localisation. • PET makes use of short half-life radioisotopes attached to pharmaceuticals • Indications are diagnosis, staging, follow-up and restaging of patients with cancer, pyrexia of unknown origin and paraneoplastic syndromes.

8.3 Clinical utility and quality standards of imaging

The RCR and College of Radiographers in the United Kingdom have worked collaboratively to provide guidance and roadmap for different Imaging departments to align their Quality Assurance matrices [8].

"The Patient" is the center of these quality assurance steps.

Imaging departments can also achieve accreditation by involvement in these Quality Standards Imaging (QSI) activities. These QSI then become an objective measure of patient experience and quality assurance [8].

The aim of these measures is to facilitate Clinical Radiology and Nuclear Medicine Departments support to clinicians and staff working in provision of care to improve the quality of care. Although, it is tempting to use these activities only for the purpose of accreditation, however Radiology and Nuclear Medicine Services should aim to work over these standards at all times and to reflect on feedback of peer review process as part of monthly Governance activities. The Royal College of Radiologists clearly state these as "minimum level of expectations rather than a ceiling of quality" [8].

8.3.1 Multifaceted nature of imaging and key steps for introduction of quality assurance model

Radiology and Nuclear Medicine modalities are capturing the disease processes at different stages. While guidance documents provided by Radiology and Nuclear Medicine scientific societies exist, the introduction of Quality Assurance model on top of stretched manpower becomes a problem. The basic key steps can be replicated in any department before structured documents are incorporated as part of Quality Assurance measure within local radiology quality management systems.

The Key Steps for the Introduction of the Quality Assurance Model (QAM) are as follow.

1. Setup Radiology and Nuclear Medicine Quality Assurance objectives
2. Clearly lay out Roles and Responsibilities in the Department
3. Plan the implementation without interruption of Clinical work
4. Clearly define the start date and end date at Clinical Governance Meeting
5. Review routine activities, unusual incidents and results of investigations
6. Disseminate findings at Clinical Governance Meetings.
7. Allow internal and external peer review
8. Discuss findings of peer review process with Clinical and Management Leadership

8.3.2 Defining the scope of quality assurance steps in radiology and nuclear medicine

Radiology and NM, being key support services, interact with almost all clinical specialities. Even within specialities there are special interests and subspecialities. The level of expectations to provide high quality diagnostic services is high. It is challenging to provide, incorporate as well as replicate Quality Assurance steps in Imaging Departments due to the way Radiology and Nuclear Medicine has evolved over the last few decades. Secondly, both modalities have (I am not sure this is the best verb to use) therapeutic aspects in addition to basic diagnostics. The multifaceted service faces the challenge of having unique nature of techniques, technology and professional practice. The scope of quality assurance steps thus should cover.

(A) Core spectrum of Quality assurance measures related to Radiology and Nuclear Medicine

(B) Specialized (unique) Quality assurance measures that require small individual quality statements

Term	Distinct role
Patient	An individual exposed to ionizing and nonionizing radiation as part of clinical investigation for diagnosis and treatment.
Carer	Person providing support to the patient while undergoing an imaging exposure.
Service user	Clearly defined in roles and responsibilities document, whether this term is for patient or clinician making referral. Avoid lack of clarity as the terms are interchangeable.

The RCR, UK provides structured and nomenclature approaches to deliver practices that are of quality standards. The "Quality Standard for Imaging" document have had several versions as it is updated part of quality improvement [121]. The salient points related to the structure are.

- **XR** is the prefix for generic quality standards.
- Specific additional quality standards are for five modalities
  - **(a)** Ultrasound
  - **(b)** Computed Tomography
  - **(c)** Magnetic Resonance Imaging
  - **(d)** Interventional Radiology
  - **(e)** Nuclear Medicine and Molecular Imaging

8.3.2.1 The reference number

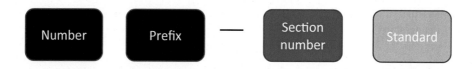

The standard name:
Three variables are defined as.

(a) Quality statement
(b) Outcome measure
(c) Indicative inputs

Modality Specific Quality Standards:
These include additional measures where the statement is related to a subdomain of imaging.

XR-1	Information and support for patients and carers
XR-2	Imaging workforce
XR-3	Scientific, technical and support for equipment
XR-4	Facilities and equipment
XR-5	Guidelines, protocols and clinical safety
XR-6	Service organisation and liaison with other services
XR-7	Governance
CT/IR/MR/NM/US-8	Modality specific standards

8.4 Clinical radiology for clinical research

The term clinical utility research relates to how the knowledge is developed and can improve clinical practice. There are many issues addressed by clinical utility research [9] such as.

- Access
- Sample specificity
- Uniqueness of each human condition
- Transferability

As Radiology and Nuclear Medicine modalities involve collaboration with different centers, clinical utility research bridges the gap between different geographical locations, cultures, settings of different imaging departments and problems unique to an individual setting. High impact factor journals with quality assurance standards promote controlled research with set standards in centers, which are devoted to the development of clinical service.

8.4.1 Efficacy research in radiology and nuclear medicine: basic concept

"Efficacy research" satisfies [9] the following.

(a) There is application of highly controlled
(b) Use of experimental designs
(c) Involves treatment of patients
(d) There is a narrow clinical problem for which an answer is sought.

These are generally guided by Randomized Clinical Trial (RCT) research designs that are considered high standard work. While Radiology and Nuclear Medicine journals have a major inclination toward dissemination of findings related to imaging manifestations of the disease process, the RCT research design is considered the best level of evidence.

8.4.1.1 Learning objective

The work by Hisham Mehanna related to PET-NECK [10] published in Health Technol. Assess. is a very good example of RCT involving PET-CT imaging which demonstrates the impact in clinical practice. The structured abstract of the work (PMID: 28409743) is as follows:

Background: Planned neck dissection (ND) after radical chemoradiotherapy (CRT) for locally advanced nodal metastases in patients with head and neck squamous cell carcinoma (HNSCC) remains controversial. Thirty percent of ND specimens show histological evidence of tumor. Consequently, a significant proportion of clinicians still practice planned ND. Fludeoxyglucose PET-CT scanning demonstrated high negative predictive values for persistent nodal disease, providing a possible alternative paradigm to ND. Evidence is sparse and drawn mainly from retrospective single-institution studies, illustrating the need for a prospective randomized controlled trial.

Objectives: To determine the efficacy and cost-effectiveness of PET-CT-guided surveillance, compared with planned ND, in a multicentre, prospective, randomized setting.

Design: A pragmatic randomized noninferiority trial comparing PET-CT-guided watch-and-wait policy with the current planned ND policy in HNSCC patients with locally advanced nodal metastases and treated with radical CRT. Patients were randomized in a 1:1 ratio. Primary outcomes were overall survival (OS) and cost-effectiveness [incremental cost per incremental quality-adjusted life-year (QALY)]. Cost-effectiveness was assessed over the trial period using individual patient data, and over a lifetime horizon using a decision-analytic model. Secondary outcomes were recurrence in the neck, complication rates and quality of life. The recruitment of 560 patients was planned to detect noninferior OS in the intervention arm with a 90% power and a type I error of 5%, with noninferiority defined as having a hazard ratio (HR) of no higher than 1.50. An intention-to-treat analysis was performed by Cox's proportional hazards model.

Settings: 37 head and neck cancer-treating centers (43 NHS hospitals) throughout the United Kingdom.

Participants: Patients with locally advanced nodal metastases of oropharynx, hypopharynx, larynx, oral or occult HNSCC receiving CRT and fit for ND were recruited.

Intervention: Patients randomized to planned ND before or after CRT (control), or CRT followed by Fluorodeoxyglucose PET-CT 10−12 weeks post CRT with ND only if PET-CT showed incomplete or equivocal response of nodal disease (intervention). Balanced by center, planned ND timing, CRT schedule, disease site and the tumor, node, metastasis stage.

Results: In total, 564 patients were recruited (ND arm, $n = 282$; and surveillance arm, $n = 282$; 17% N2a, 61% N2b, 18% N2c and 3% N3). Eighty-four percent had oropharyngeal cancer. Seventy-five percent of tested cases were p16 positive. The median time to follow-up was 36 months. The HR for OS was 0.92 [95% confidence interval (CI) 0.65 to 1.32], indicating noninferiority. The upper limit of the noninferiority HR margin of 1.50, which was informed by patient advisors to the project, lies at the 99.6 percentile of this estimate ($P = .004$). There were no differences in this result by p16 status. There were 54 NDs performed in the surveillance arm, with 22 surgical complications, and 221 NDs in the ND arm, with 85 complications. Quality-of-life scores were slightly better in the surveillance arm. Compared with planned ND, PET-CT surveillance produced an incremental net health benefit of 0.16 QALYs (95% CI 0.03 to 0.28 QALYs) over the trial period and 0.21 QALYs (95% CI -0.41 to 0.85 QALYs) over the modeled lifetime horizon.

Limitations: Pragmatic randomized controlled trial with a 36-month median follow-up.

Conclusions: PET-CT-guided active surveillance showed similar survival outcomes to ND but resulted in considerably fewer NDs, fewer complications and lower costs, supporting its use in routine practice.

8.5 **Quality assurance and organizational framework**

There are several internal and external stakeholders which directly or indirectly influence the process of QA in a Radiology or Nuclear Medicine facility. These may be local, regional, national or international. Due to multifaceted nature of Radiology and Nuclear Medicine, there is high likelihood of interactions between them with a common aim, that is, to streamline standards of local QA programs and provide road-map, which is reflective of ongoing processes rather than a single quality exercise.

It is of relevance to mention that in recent years, imaging accreditation programs, developed and managed by specialized scientific society, are part the overall local Quality Assurance programs in several countries in Europe and the United States. These imaging accreditation programs contribute significantly to raising the level of Quality Assurance programs, hence to the reputation of the services provided, especially in conducting high quality research imaging scans that are often required by large clinical trials sponsors. A famous example of this is the EARL/EANM accreditation of F-18 FDG PET/CT imaging services. More details of such an accreditation program can be accessed at: https://www.eanm.org/earl-research4life/

The flow chart captures some of the internal and external influencers.

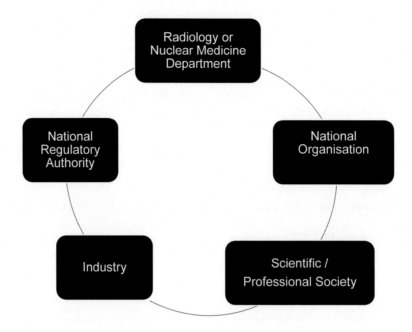

Key Stakeholders within the process are defined as below:

(a) Radiology or Nuclear Medicine Staff: Doctors, radiographers, technologists, medical physicists, nursing staff, allied health professionals (support staff), management and administration.
(b) Equipment manufacturer: Cameras, imaging and data storage management systems (Reporting workstation, PACS, RIS etc)
(c) National Organizations: National bodies, scientific societies and broadly including special interest user groups.

8.5.1 Health authority

These are national level bodies and work in association with government authorities at national and international levels along integrating the work of professional societies and organizations. In the United Kingdom, Health Research Authority oversees the research activities involving different bodies. Radiology and Nuclear Medicine modalities require special permissions, which are relevant to their respective regulatory bodies.

Health Research Authority, along with all other research activities also promotes Radiology and Nuclear Medicine research that improves people's health and wellbeing, and their main purpose is to protect and promote the interests of patients and the public in health and social care research.

To achieve this, the Health Research Authority ensures.

• Radiology and Nuclear Medicine research is ethically reviewed and approved
• Transparency in research involving Imaging Data sets

- Integrates different committees and services such as ARSAC
- Standardize research regulatory practice
- Facilitates independent recommendations on the processing of identifiable patient information where it is not always practical to obtain consent, for research and nonresearch projects.

Although Health Research Authority functions apply to research undertaken in England, they also work closely with the other countries in the United Kingdom to provide a UK-wide system. Health Research Authority is an arm's length body of the Department of Health and Social Care (DHSC), which means the Government has devolved some of its responsibilities to them.

The following table captures some essential elements.

Criteria	**(1)** Imaging requirements
	(2) Radiological equipment (image quality and exposure)
	(3) Acceptance requirements
	(4) Radiation protection
Testing	**(1)** Instruments
	(2) Staff
	(3) Standard operating procedures
Feedback mechanisms	**(1)** Continuous process
	(2) Mechanism for appropriate actions
	(3) Record keeping
Roles and responsibilities	**(1)** List of responsibilities
	(2) Quality assurance committee
	(3) Monitoring schedule
	(4) Maintenance of equipment
	(5) Budgetary provisions
	(6) Training of personnel
External bodies	**(1)** Equipment manufacturer
	(2) International bodies
	(3) National authorities
	(4) National organisations
	(5) Scientific/professional societies
Measurements	**(1)** Baseline quality assurance checks
	(2) Routine checks
	(3) Random inspections
QA involvement equipment	**1.** Latest guidelines at national and international levels compliance.
	2. Special recommendations between manufacturer and customer
	3. Acceptance testing
QA and national bodies	**1.** Setting of local QA programmes.
	2. Perform entire or part of QA program at local facility.
	3. Assess adequacy of local QA program.
	4. Provides code of practice.
	5. Provision of calibration facilities
	6. Facilitate (if required or requested) results of QA program
Scientific societies	**1.** Promote QA in meetings
	2. Collaborate with national organizations
	3. Training activities
	4. Provide guidelines

National authorities International bodies	Legislative measures General recommendations to different countries to adopt and coordinate QA activities.

In the UK Department for Business, Energy and Industrial Strategy regulates Radiological and Civil Nuclear Safety working as a government body. The UK Government has associated administration bodies with international bodies including International Atomic Energy Agency (IAEA), International Commission on Radiological Protection (ICRP), the Western European Nuclear Regulators Association (WENRA), the Heads of the European Radiological Protection Competent Authority (HERCA), and the United Nations Scientific Committee on the Effects of Atomic Radiation (UNSCEAR).

In the United Kingdom, both Radiology and Nuclear Medicine are heavily regulated so that ionizing radiation is used safely to protect patients from the harmful risks of ionizing radiation [12]. There are set out responsibilities for employers with regards to radiation protection and the basic safety standards that employers must meet. Protection of patients, individuals and carers and comforters for medical and nonmedical exposures are covered by the Ionizing Radiation (Medical Exposure) Regulations 2017 (IR(ME)R) in GB and the Ionising Radiation (Medical Exposure) Regulations (Northern Ireland) 2018 in NI.

For clinical as well as research involving ionizing and nonionizing radiation, the regulations provide legal means for.

- Minimizing unintended, excessive or wrong medical exposures
- Justifying each exposure to ensure the benefits outweigh the risks
- Optimizing radiation doses to keep them "as low as reasonably practicable" for their intended use.

Administration of Radioactive Substances Advisory Committee (ARSAC) advises the licensing authorities on applications from practitioners, employers and researchers who want to use radioactive substances on people [13].

For providing legislative support and compliance of Radiology and Nuclear Medicine procedures under IR(ME)R, employers who undertake medical and nonmedical exposures must appoint a Medical Physics Expert (MPE) for advice on complying with the regulations [14]. A comprehensive description of the updated regulations (since the United Kingdom left the European Union) can be found on www.gov.uk.

8.5.2 Clinical radiation expert, medical physics expert, and quality assurance

In the United Kingdom, the HRA provides a road map for standardization of research application approvals where radiation exposures are used by a clinical radiation expert (CRE) and medical physics expert (MPE). The MPE and CRE provides the appropriate scientific and clinical assessment of the radiological procedures and exposures included in a research study protocol. In addition, the CRE and MPE also provides a risk assessment to the participants and recommendations to the research ethics committees in regard to the use of radiology procedures. The overall CRE and MPE process serves several further steps such as below:

(a) Streamline the research approval process
(b) Minimize delays by identifying issues at an earlier stage
(c) Reduces duplication of work
(d) Provides a single point of contact for sponsors.

A research application submitted to HRA goes through a review process involving.

HRA Technical Assurances Manager

HRA Technical Assurances Officers

Clinical Radiation Expert Reviewers

Medical Physics Expert Reviewers

Four Nations Radiation Assurance Working Party

8.5.2.1 Medical physics expert

Within the United Kingdom, MPEs are Health and Care Professions Council (HCPC) registered Clinical Scientists. They are recognized by the RPA2000 (appointed by the DHSC to act as the authorized Assessing Body for MPE recognition) as meeting the criteria of competence specified by the DHSC. Their roles and responsibilities are described by IR(ME)R 14(2) and 14(3). MPEs deal with a wide range of medical exposures. They provide input to determine the level of hazard and risk from the procedure [15]. The scope of MPE is defined in their employer's procedures. Following implementation of IR(ME)R in 2018, the role of Medical Physics expert was considered an essential requirement to ensure protection of patients in all radiation-based diagnostic and therapeutic procedures. There is a legal requirement that a suitably qualified MPE must be appointment for all areas of Radiology and Nuclear Medicine exposures. The MPE should be involved in the whole chain of imaging of patients from discussing the suitable radiopharmaceuticals for specific scan, through developing and validating nonstandard scanning protocols to processing and assessing reconstructed image series.

In The Integrated Research Application System (IRAS) based research applications, MPEs perform radiation dose assessments on the basis of imaging examinations that are part of the research proposal. The assessment considers the type and number of standards of care (SoC) and nonstandard care (non-SoC) imaging scans. The assessment of radiation dose is an integral part of the scientific value and is essential to the ethical approval of clinical research proposals. It shall provide a clear indication of the level of exposure to ionizing radiation and associated risks to patients. The risks to patient shall also be explained in plain English in the patient information leaflet (PIL).

Full details and updates on submission and review process of research proposals via the IRAS could be found at: https://www.myresearchproject.org.uk/

The role of MP is illustrated in the two following examples.

1. Example of an MPE Radiation dose assessment carried-out for a clinical trial which included 5 F-18 FDG PET/CT scans (whole body scans), and five low-dose CT scans as part of the PET dynamic scan). This resulted in a total of 65 mSv effective dose. The estimated lifetime risk of inducing a fatal cancer in a healthy individual from the total research protocol dose was approximately one in 300.

   " ... ...

   The F-18 FDG-PET dynamic and whole-body scans with a low dose CT for attenuation correction is part of the total radiation dose due to participation in this study.

   The national (dose reference level) DRL for an F-18 FDG-PET scan for tumour imaging is 400 MBq, giving an effective dose of 8 mSv per scan (ARSAC, 2006). The participating patient will receive a total F-18 FDG PET radiation dose of 40 mSv (baseline, 12 weeks, 24 weeks and follow-up scans).

In a patient dose audit carried out locally, the low dose whole body CT protocol for PET attenuation correction at St Bartholomew's Hospital gave an effective dose of 4.5 mSv (ie approximately 0.5 mSv per PET bed position) for an average patient (using conversion factors in NRPB-W67, 2005).

The Total Research Protocol Dose in this study is therefore 65 mSv for average time spent in trial. The radiation dose from this study therefore falls into risk category III, as defined in ICRP 62 (effective dose > 10 mSv) and is considered a moderate level of risk.

The HPA have endorsed the ICRP recommendation that a nominal risk coefficient of 5×10^{-2} per Sievert is used as the approximate overall fatal risk coefficient (Documents of the HPA, RCE-12, 2009). From this it can be estimated that the lifetime risk of inducing a fatal cancer in a healthy individual from the total research protocol dose is approximately 1 in 300. The risk is age dependant and is increased for younger patients, decreasing with age. This should be compared with the natural incidence rate for cancer in the UK. These factors apply to healthy individuals and should be considered against alleviating the morbidity of the patient's long-term condition.

For comparison, the average annual natural background radiation dose in the UK is 2.2 mSv. The additional radiation dose incurred in this study can be compared to about 30 years annual background exposure.

… … … … … … … … … … …"

2. Example of PIL, which explain in plain English radiation risks to patient from being exposed to ionizing imaging scans (5 F-18 FDG scans, and five low-dose CT scans as part of the PET dynamic scan). The PIL section "***What are the possible disadvantages and risks of taking part?***" describing the procedures and risks to participating patients was written as follows

"… … … … … … … … … … ….

There are very few disadvantages of taking part in the study.

We will be obtaining imaging information about all parts of your body during the scan. You will already be having the whole body checked with standard imaging and, whilst this provides sufficient information to make choices on treatment the scans we are performing as part of the trial may highlight other areas not seen on the routine studies. Theoretically we may detect an incidental abnormality in a particular area of the body. The vast majority of such findings are of little importance but if we see something on the scan that is likely to affect your treatment, we will inform your doctor of the finding via a clinical report that is provided for all the scans we perform.

A PET/CT scan will be used to evaluate tissue abnormalities within the body organs performed to find out how well a treatment is working. A radioactive substance (radioactive chemical) is injected into a vein, and the image of its distribution in your body tissues is analysed to study disease characteristics, severity possible effects of therapy. There is no discomfort with the injection and there is no discomfort associated with the scan itself. This would be completed even if you were not taking part in this study. The PET/CT scan will include the area from your neck to your mid-thigh area. A low-dose CT scan uses X-rays and computer assistance to take detailed pictures of organs. You will be asked to lay on a special table that moves slowly into a large donut-shaped scanner for approximately 20 minutes immediately after injection and further 20 minutes.

The total radiation dose from PET/CT scans is approximately 30 times the natural yearly background radiation in the UK.

… … … … … … … …"

8.5.2.2 *Clinical radiation expert*

CRE's are registered clinical radiologists, clinical oncologists, dentists, or other medical practitioners who have clinical expertise in imaging or treatment method modalities, and provide clinical input related to justification of exposure. GMC registration is compulsory. They have expertise in the UK regulatory and clinical environment. They have experience of carrying out local IRMER Compliance review as CRE in the departments using Ionizing Radiation.

This study includes adult patients with resected (anonymised) carcinoma of the head and neck, who are at high risk for replapse and are ineligible for high dose Drug (Anonymised).

The participants in this study will receive additional radiation burden, which is above that anticipated in routine clinical care. These additional exposures are required to provide objective radiological disease assessmenet of treatment response in relation to specific time points.

However, participants in this study will also undergo radiotherapy treatment. The radiation dose incurred from the additional disease assessment exposures will be small compared with the dose incurred from radiotherapy. The highest radiation risk from inducing cancer will be incurred by the radiotherapy treatment (a known potential complication) and this risk will not be significantly altered by the inclusion of the additional exposures.

There is increasing emphasis on quality assurance in Radiology and Nuclear Medicine due to complexity of handling radioactive substances associated with performing Nuclear Medicine performing imaging scans and compliance with the relevant regulations. Royal College of Radiologists and Royal College of Physicians are actively involved in the process of revalidation and encourage members to follow the guidance provided by the General Medical Council for successful revalidation [16].

There are requirements for physicians to meet performance criteria [17] by following a range of evaluations. The overall feedback of quality assurance work is summed up in multisource feedbacks, which involve colleagues and patients. By default, and due to the nature of Radiology and Nuclear Medicine, the peer review process is an estimation of diagnostic accuracy. Moreover, punishing an individual's error is less important than optimizing group performance and it may be counterproductive to both error measurement and quality improvement.

There are several ways of classifying Radiology errors. Some examples are provided in table below.

Provenzal [19]	**(a)** Radiologist can fail to detect findings (miss) **(b)** Wrongly interpret a finding as abnormal (overcall) **(c)** Recognize an abnormality but dismiss it as normal or artifact (under-call) **(d)** Recognize an abnormality but assign an incorrect cause and fail to recognize technique limitations or fail to recommend another examination (next step).
Fitzgerald [20]	**(1)** Errors of technique **(2)** Perception **(3)** Knowledge **(4)** Judgment **(5)** Communication
Renfrew [21]	**(a)** Perceptual **(b)** Cognitive **(c)** Next step **(d)** Communication errors
Ramesh S. Iyer [17,22]	**1** concur **2** Discrepancy in interpretation not ordinarily expected to be made (understandable miss) 2a Unlikely to be clinically significant 2b Likely to be clinically significant **3** Discrepancy in interpretation should be made most of the time 3a Unlikely to be clinically significant 3b Likely to be clinically significant **4** Discrepancy in interpretation should be made almost every time; misinterpretation of the finding 4a Unlikely to be clinically significant 4b Likely to be clinically significant

The RCR has a very structured approach for Quality Assurance mechanism via Radiology Events and Learning Meetings (REALMs). The process involves review of anonymous studies which have been categorized as radiological discrepancy. As these errors can have a negative impact on reporters in busy resource stretched environment, it is also encouraged that excellent diagnoses are also discussed. RCR expects its members to follow a duty of candor process to be undertaken to improve trust of patients [23]. The RCR is currently working on guidance around the duty of candor and more advice on this topic will be published later this year. RCR has published a professional duty of candor guidance document, which sets standards for setting up and running REALM meetings [23]. A summary of set standards is as follows.

Clinical engagement	**(a)** Attendance at 50% of departmental radiology events and learning meetings.
	(b) Contribute at least one case a year to the REALM.
Organization of meeting	A minimum of six REALMs per year.
The chair	Recorded in the job plan as an 'additional NHS responsibility'.
The notifier	The radiologist who has detected a discrepancy or clinical incident (the notifier) has certain duties to record.
The cases	Anonymised and discussed for the purposes of education only.
The documentation	• Email sent to radiologists involved.
	• Learning points summarised and disseminated.
	• Attendance and contribution should be recorded.
Feedback and reflection	Encourage reflection.
	Identify patterns of errors.
The culture	Culture of respectful sharing of knowledge with no blame or shame.
Links with the RCR	Submit a case a year to REALM Newsletter

8.6 Artificial intelligence and quality assurance

AI in its most comprehensive definition is a subbranch of computer science that uses advanced algorithms to learn from experience and make decisions that normally require human intelligence. The term artificial intelligence was first coined by John McCarthy in 1956 and has not evolved much since due to lack of computing power and availability of big data [121,122].

Initially, AI methods, called expert systems or computer aided diagnosis software applications, were limited to the use of causal (cause-effect) relationships between different entities (e.g.,; patient symptoms, medical conditions, and patient history) to make human-like decisions [122–125]. With the availability and widespread use of electronic patient records through hospital information systems (HIS, radiology information systems (RIS) and PACS that incorporate manufacturer-independent data format (called DICOM image format), the nineties and 2000 decades noticed several developments of machine learning, natural language processing methods in different medical areas) [126,127]. Machine learning and natural language processing algorithms, in addition to the field of robotics are subbranches of AI that attempted to make the best use of large amount of data resulted from the widespread of hybrid imaging techniques and theragnostic treatment options [128–131]. This has led to an exponential increase of the number of AI-related scientific publications and help the education and training of junior scientists on the AI principles and algorithms that have been incorporated into the Radiomics pipeline since its inception in 2010 [127–133].

Radiomics is the science of extracting a large number of quantitative features from structured radiological and radionuclide images, unseen otherwise to the human eyes. Radiomics has proven to help tremendously in characterizing disease and identify disease patterns and hence offers sophisticated option to early diagnosis, effective follow-up and characterization of diseased tissues [134,135]. Unlike other "Omics" approaches such as, proteomics, genomics and transcriptomics that are of limited utility given their invasive nature, radiomics are fully noninvasive and are capable of extracting large amount of pertinent information to biopsies that are taken from a small fraction of tissue [136−141]. The use of AI techniques within the Radiomics pipeline has proven to ease the processes and extracting, selecting and identify disease-specific patterns [142−145].

AI has attracted most attention since 2016 with the significant increase in computing power and the introduction and better implementation of fully automated models, called Deep Learning models that have demonstrated unprecedented performance comparable to humans [144,145]. Recent advances in AI in the field of Radiology and Nuclear Medicine and their integration into modern software-based systems raise new challenges to the profession of radiologists and medical physics experts. The number of AI-based applications approved by the FDA are increasing exponentially. More than 70% of these AI imaging applications are in Radiology and Nuclear Medicine [145]. These AI applications cover a wide spectrum of activities: workflow, patient setup, data acquisition, image reconstruction, postprocessing and interpretation and perception of imaging scans. At present AI imaging applications/systems are outperforming radiologists in areas of Radiology and Nuclear Medicine, especially when speed and comparison to previous imaging scans are required.

Imaging AI applications are continuously evolving, which makes the assessment of their performance highly challenging. The deployment of AI in Radiology and Nuclear Medicine routine practice is a highly debatable due the current challenges such as generalizability, reproducibility, explainability of the AI models implemented AI applications. Data quality, large validation and ethical issues are yet to resolved.

Guidelines and best practices for developing, training, testing AI techniques are being developed and it will take a while to see AI applications fully adopted clinically and demonstrate its full potential in heath economics.

The use of AI in QA is an emerging area, which has not been well explored and requires a multi-disciplinary approach and close collaborations between medical doctors, radiologists, medical physics experts, and require close collaboration between healthcare professionals and research communities and the healthcare industry. Recently published papers stated that Quality in AI not a well-defined [130,131], while others focused on discussing the AI terminology and challenges in Quality Assurance with the AI applications to set a baseline for that purpose [138−145].

The authors believe that Quality Assurance of AI imaging applications and systems in Radiology and Nuclear Medicine will develop further in the coming years once regulatory bodies published clear and comprehensive regulations to make the use of AI safer, effective, and patient-centred for clinicians, radiologists and medical physics experts, and decision makers [135–140].

QA in Radiology and Nuclear Medicine is not just a stand-alone process but part of internal improvement assessment that make the best use of the latest technologies and effective use of relevant guidelines and best code of practices. It is expected to lead to service improvement and bring about an overall reduction in operating costs despite the time and money invested to fulfill the requirements of the QA program. Quality Assurance programs have stronger impact when used as part of a peer review exercise or in pursue of formal accreditation process. The regulatory bodies expect quality assurance standards to be maintained at all times to maintain patient safety and the quality standards of clinical care provided.

References

[1] Hussain S, Mubeen I, Ullah N, Shah SSUD, Khan BA, Zahoor M, et al. Modern diagnostic imaging technique applications and risk factors in the medical field: a review. BioMed Res Int June 6, 2022:5164970. https://doi.org/10.1155/2022/5164970. 2022.

[2] Berger D. A brief history of medical diagnosis and the birth of the clinical laboratory. Part 1—ancient times through the 19th century. Med Lab Obs 1999;31(7):28–30.

[3] Wilms G, Baert AL. The history of angiography. J Belge Radiol 1995;78:299–302.

[4] Wilk SP. Axial transverse tomography of the chest. Radiology 1959;72:42–50. https://doi.org/10.1148/72.1.42.

[5] All Nobel prizes in physics. Nobelprize.org. Nobel Media AB; 2014.

[6] Willemink MJ, Takx RAP, de Jong PA, et al. Computed tomography radiation dose reduction. J Comput Assist Tomogr 2014;38:815–23. https://doi.org/10.1097/RCT.0000000000000128.

[7] Kane D, Grassi W, Sturrock R, Balint PV. A brief history of musculoskeletal ultrasound: "from bats and ships to babies and hips". Rheumatology (Oxford) 2004;43:931–3.

[8] Kaproth-Joslin KA, Nicola R, Dogra VS. The history of US: from bats and boats to the bedside and beyond: RSNA centennial article. Radiographics 2015;35:960–70. https://doi.org/10.1148/rg.2015140300.

[9] Manbachi A, Cobbold RSC. Development and application of piezoelectric materials for ultrasound generation and detection. Ultrasound 2011;19:187–96. https://doi.org/10.1258/ult.2011.011027.

[10] Donald I, Macvicar J, Brown T. Investigation of abdominal masses by pulsed ultrasound. Lancet 1958;271:1188–95. https://doi.org/10.1016/S0140-6736(58)91905-6.

[11] Ligon BL. The mystery of angiography and the "unawarded" Nobel prize: Egas Moniz and Hans Christian Jacobaeus. Neurosurgery 1998;43:602–11.

[12] Hurst W, Heiss HW. Werner Forssmann: a German problem with the Nobel prize. Clin Cardiol 1992;15:547–9. https://doi.org/10.1002/clc.4960150715.

[13] Dababou S, Marrocchio C, Scipione R, et al. High-intensity focused ultrasound for pain management in patients with cancer. Radiographics 2018;38:603–23. https://doi.org/10.1148/rg.2018170129.

[14] Bergonie J, Tribondeau L. De quelques resultats de la radiotherapie et essai de fixation dune technique rationelle. C R Acad Sci 1906;143:983.

[15] Nias AHW. An introduction to radiobiology. 2nd ed. Chichester, England: Wiley; 1998. p. 4.

[16] Muller HJ. Artificial transmutation of the gene. Science 1927;66:84.

[17] Seeram E. Radiation protection. Philadelphia, PA: Lippincott; 1997. p. 74—92.

[18] Dowd SB, Tilson ER. Practical radiation protection and applied radiobiology. 2nd ed. Philadelphia, PA: Saunders; 1999. p. 118—20.

[19] Chapman JD, Stobbe CC, Gales T, et al. Condensed chromatin and cell inactivation by single hit kinetics. Radiat Res 1999;151:433—4.

[20] Raloff J. Panel ups RDAs for some antioxidants. Sci News 2000:244. April 15.

[21] Basic Review of Radiation Biology and Terminology Norman E. Bolus Journal of Nuclear Medicine Technology June 2001, 29 (2) 67-73;

[22] Ladou J. Occupational medicine. Norwalk, CT: Appleton and Lange; 1990. p. 197—8.

[23] Kasban H, El-Bendary MAM, Salama DH. A comparative study of medical imaging techniques. Int J Inf Sci Intell Syst 2015;4(2):37—58.

[24] radley WG. History of medical imaging. Proc Am Phil Soc 2008;152(3):349—61.

[25] P. Kazantsev, W. Lechner, E. Gershkevitsh, C.H. Clark, D. Venencia, J. Van Dyk, et al. IAEA methodology for on-site end-to-end IMRT/VMAT audits: an international pilot study.

[26] Abtahi SMM, Bahrami F, Sardari D. An investigation into the dose rate and photon energy dependence of the GENA gel dosimeter in the MeV range. Phys Med Eur J Med Phys 2023:106. https://doi.org/10.1016/j.ejmp.2022.102522.

[27] Schreiner LJ. Reviewing three dimensional dosimetry: basics and utilization as presented over 17 Years of DosGel and IC3Ddose. J Phys Conf Ser 2017;847. https://doi.org/10.1088/1742-6596/847/1/012001. Article 012001.

[28] Rousseau A, Stien C, Bordy J-M, Blideanu V. Fricke-Xylenol orange-Gelatin gel characterization with dual wavelength cone-beam optical CT scanner for applications in stereotactic and dynamic radiotherapy. Phys Med 2022;97:1—12. https://doi.org/10.1016/j.ejmp.2022.03.008.

[29] Babic S, Battista J, Jordan K. Three-dimensional dose verification for intensity-modulated radiation therapy in the Radiological Physics Centre head-and-neck phantom using optical computed tomography scans of ferrous xylenol—orange gel dosimeters. Int J Radiat Oncol Biol Phys 2008;70:1281—91.

[30] Rousseau A, Stien C, Gouriou J, Bordy JM, Boissonnat G, Chabert I, et al. End-to-end quality assurance for stereotactic radiotherapy with Fricke-Xylenol orange-gelatin gel dosimeter and dual-wavelength cone-beam optical CT readout. Phys Med September 2023;113:102656. https://doi.org/10.1016/j.ejmp.2023.102656. Epub 2023 Aug 23. PMID: 37625218.

[31] Matthews PM, Coatney R, Alsaid H, Jucker B, Ashworth S, Parker C, et al. Technologies Preclinical imaging for drug development. Drug Discov Today Technol 2013;10: e343—50.

[32] Cook D, Brown D, Alexander R, March R, Morgan P, Satterthwaite G, et al. Lessons learned from the fate of astrazeneca's drug pipeline: a five-dimensional framework. Nat Rev Drug Discov 2014;13:419—31.

[33] Leptak C, Menetski JP, Wagner JA, Aubrecht J, Brady L, Brumfield M, et al. What evidence do we need for biomarker qualification? Sci Transl Med 2017;9:417.

[34] Amuno S, Rudko DA, Gallino D, Tuznik M, Shekh K, Kodzhahinchev V, et al. Altered neurotransmission and neuroimaging biomarkers of chronic arsenic poisoning in wild muskrats (Ondatra zibethicus) and red squirrels (Tamiasciurus hudsonicus) breeding

near the city of yellow knife, northwest territories (Canada). Sci Total Environ 2019: 135556.

[35] Ferreira de Souza T, Quinaglia ACST, Osorio Costa F, Shah R, Neilan TG, Velloso L, Nadruz W, Brenelli F, Sposito AC, Matos-Souza JR, Cendes F, et al. Anthracycline therapy is associated with cardiomyocyte atrophy and preclinical manifestations of heart disease. JACC Cardiovasc Imaging 2018;11:1045–55.

[36] Willis MS, Parry TL, Brown DI, Mota RI, Huang W, Beak JY, et al. Doxorubicin exposure causes subacute cardiac atrophy dependent on the striated muscle-specific ubiquitin ligase murf1. Circ Heart Fail 2019;12. Article e005234.

[37] Zajac-Spychala O, Pawlak M, Karmelita-Katulska K, Pilarczyk J, Jonczyk-Potoczna K, Przepiora A, et al. Anti-leukemic treatment-induced neurotoxicity in long-term survivors of childhood acute lymphoblastic leukemia: impact of reduced central nervous system radiotherapy and intermediate- to high-dose methotrexate. Leuk Lymphoma 2018;59:2342–51.

[38] AlDhaleei W, AlMarzooqi A, Gaber N. Reversible metronidazole-induced neurotoxicity after 10 weeks of therapy. BMJ Case Rep 2018. https://doi.org/10.1136/bcr-2017-223463.

[39] Algahtani H, Shirah B, Ahmad R, Abobaker H, Hmoud M. Transverse myelitis-like presentation of methanol intoxication: a case report and review of the literature. J Spinal Cord Med 2018;41:72–6.

[40] Villamar MF. Acute methanol poisoning. Arq Neuropsiquiatr 2018;76:636–7.

[41] Grudzinski IP, Ruzycka M, Cieszanowski A, Szeszkowski W, Badurek I, Malkowska A, et al. Mri-based preclinical discovery of dili: a lesson from paracetamol-induced hepatotoxicity. Regul Toxicol Pharmacol 2019;108:104478.

[42] Bauckneht M, Ferrarazzo G, Fiz F, Morbelli S, Sarocchi M, Pastorino F, et al. Doxorubicin effect on myocardial metabolism as a prerequisite for subsequent development of cardiac toxicity: a translational (18)f-fdg pet/ct observation. J Nucl Med 2017;58:1638–45.

[43] Sarocchi M, Bauckneht M, Arboscello E, Capitanio S, Marini C, Morbelli S, et al. An increase in myocardial 18-fluorodeoxyglucose uptake is associated with left ventricular ejection fraction decline in Hodgkin lymphoma patients treated with anthracycline. J Transl Med 2018;16:295. https://doi.org/10.1186/s12967-018-1670-9.

[44] Ong G, Brezden-Masley C, Dhir V, Deva DP, Chan KKW, Chow CM, et al. Myocardial strain imaging by cardiac magnetic resonance for detection of subclinical myocardial dysfunction in breast cancer patients receiving trastuzumab and chemotherapy. Int J Cardiol 2018;261:228–33.

[45] Galan-Arriola C, Lobo M, Vilchez-Tschischke JP, Lopez GJ, de Molina-Iracheta A, Perez-Martinez C, et al. Serial magnetic resonance imaging to identify early stages of anthracycline-induced cardiotoxicity. J Am Coll Cardiol 2019;73:779–91.

[46] Ma RE, Ward EJ, Yeh CL, Snyder S, Long Z, Gokalp Yavuz F, et al. U. Dydak Thalamic gaba levels and occupational manganese neurotoxicity: association with exposure levels and brain MRI. Neurotoxicology 2018;64:30.

[47] Petroff R, Richards T, Crouthamel B, McKain N, Stanley C, Grant KS, et al. Chronic, low-level oral exposure to marine toxin, domoic acid, alters whole brain morphometry in nonhuman primates. Neurotoxicology 2019;72:114–24.

[48] Shimony JS, Rutlin J, Karimi M, Tian L, Snyder AZ, Loftin SK, et al. Validation of diffusion tensor imaging measures of nigrostriatal neurons in macaques. PLoS One 2018;13. Article e0202201.

[49] Criswell SR, Nielsen SS, Warden M, Perlmutter JS, Moerlein SM, Flores HP, et al. [(18)f]fdopa positron emission tomography in manganese-exposed workers. Neuro-toxicology 2018;64:43.

[50] Combalia M, Codella N, Rotemberg V, Carrera C, Dusza S, Gutman D, et al. Valida-tion of artificial intelligence prediction models for skin cancer diagnosis using dermo-scopy images: the 2019 International Skin Imaging Collaboration Grand Challenge. Lancet Digit Health 2022;4:e330e9.

[51] Daneshjou R, Barata C, Betz-Stablein B, Celebi ME, Codella N, Combalia M, et al. Checklist for evaluation of image-based artificial intelligence re- ports in dermatology: CLEAR derm consensus guidelines from the inter- national skin imaging collaboration artificial intelligence working group. JAMA Dermatol 2022;158:90e6.

[52] Daneshjou R, Smith MP, Sun MD, Rotemberg V, Zou J. Lack of transparency and po-tential bias in artificial intelligence data sets and algorithms: a scoping review. JAMA Dermatol 2021;157:1362e9.

[53] Elmore JG, Barnhill RL, Elder DE, Longton GM, Pepe MS, Reisch LM, et al. Pathol-ogists' diagnosis of invasive melanoma and melanocytic proliferations: observer accu-racy and reproducibility study. BMJ 2017;357:j2813.

[54] Esteva A, Kuprel B, Novoa RA, Ko J, Swetter SM, Blau HM, et al. Dermatologist-level classification of skin cancer with deep neural networks. Nature 2017;542:115e8.

[55] Guo LN, Lee MS, Kassamali B, Mita C, Nambudiri VE. Bias in, bias out: underreport-ing and underrepresentation of diverse skin types in machine learning research for skin cancer detection—a scoping review. J Am Acad Dermatol 2022;87:157e9.

[56] Han SS, Kim YJ, Moon IJ, Jung JM, Lee MY, Lee WJ, et al. Evaluation of arti- ficial intelligence-assisted diagnosis of skin neoplasms: a single-center, paralleled, unmasked, randomized controlled trial. J Invest Dermatol 2022;142. 2353e2362.e2.

[57] Harvey H, Glocker B. A standardised approach for preparing imaging data for machine learning tasks in radiology: opportunities, applications and risks. In: Ranschaert E, Morozov S, Algra P, editors. Artificial intelligence in medical imaging. Cham, Switzerland: Springer; 2019. 61e72.

[58] Hekler A, Kather JN, Krieghoff-Henning E, Utikal JS, Meier F, Gellrich FF, et al. Ef-fects of label noise on deep learning-based skin cancer classification. Front Med 2020; 7:177.

[59] Lester JC, Clark Jr L, Linos E, Daneshjou R. Clinical photography in skin of colour: tips and best practices. Br J Dermatol 2021;184:1177e9 [M Phung et al. Clinical Skin Image Acquisition in Translational Artificial Intelligence Research].

[60] Ly BCK, Dyer EB, Feig JL, Chien AL, Del Bino S. Research techniques made simple: cutaneous colorimetry: a reliable technique for objective skin color measurement. J Invest Dermatol 2020;140:3e12—e1.

[61] Moslehi J, Fujiwara K, Guzik T. Cardio-oncology:anovelplatformforbasicand transla-tional cardiovascular investigation driven by clinical need. Cardiovasc Res 2019; 115(5):819—23.

[62] Stoltzfus KC, Zhang Y, Sturgeon K, Sinoway LI, Trifiletti DM, Chinchilli VM, et al. Fatal heart disease among cancer patients. Nat Commun 2020;11(1). 2011.

[63] Cardinale D, Colombo A, Bacchiani G, Tedeschi I, Meroni CA, Veglia F, et al. Early detection of anthracycline cardiotoxicity and improvement with heart failure therapy. Circulation 2015;131(22):1981—8.

[64] Lipshultz SE, Colan SD, Gelber RD, Perez-Atayde AR, Sallan SE, Sanders SP. Late cardiac effects of doxorubicin therapy for acute lymphoblastic leukemia in childhood. N Engl J Med 1991;324(12):808−15.

[65] Cornell RF, Ky B, Weiss BM, Dahm CN, Gupta DK, Du L, et al. Prospective study of cardiac events during proteasome inhibitor therapy for relapsed multiple myeloma. J Clin Oncol 2019;37(22):1946−55.

[66] A.Y. Khakoo, C.M. Kassiotis, N. Tannir, J.C. Plana, M. Halushka, C. Bickford.

[67] Trent 2nd J, Champion JC, Durand JB, Lenihan DJ. Heart failure associated with sunitinib malate: a multitargeted receptor tyrosine kinase inhibitor. Cancer 2008;112(11): 2500−8.

[68] Ewer MS, Lenihan DJ, Khakoo AY. Sunitinib-related cardiotoxicity: an interdisciplinary issue. Nat Clin Pract Cardiovasc Med 2008;5(7):364−5.

[69] Hahn VS, Lenihan DJ, Ky B. Cancer therapy-induced cardiotoxicity: basic mechanisms and potential cardioprotective therapies. J Am Heart Assoc 2014;3(2):e000665.

[70] D.B.Johnson,J.M.Balko,M.L.Compton,S.Chalkias,J.Gorham,Y.Xu,M.Hicks, I. Puzanov, M.R. Alexander, T.L. Bloomer, J.R. Becker, D.A. Slosky, E.J. Phillips, M.A. Pilkinton, L. Craig-Owens, N. Kola, G. Plautz, D.S. Reshef, J.S. Deutsch, R. P. Deering, B.A. Olenchock, A.H. Lichtman, D.M. Roden, C.E. Seidman, I.

[71] Koralnik J, Seidman JG, Hoffman RD, Taube JM, Diaz Jr LA, Anders RA, et al. Fulminant myocarditis with combination immune checkpoint blockade. N Engl J Med 2016; 375(18):1749−55.

[72] Dorbala S, Cuddy S, Falk RH. How to image cardiac amyloidosis: a practical approach. JACC Cardiovasc Imag 2020;13(6):1368−83.

[73] Murphy KT. The pathogenesis and treatment of cardiac atrophy in cancer cachexia. Am J Physiol Heart Circ Physiol 2016;310(4):H466−77.

[74] Willis MS, Parry TL, Brown DI, Mota RI, Huang W, Beak JY, et al. Doxorubicin exposure causes subacute cardiac atrophy dependent on the striated muscle-specific ubiquitin ligase MuRF1. Circ Heart Fail 2019;12(3):e005234.

[75] J.C. Plana, M. Galderisi, A. Barac, M.S. Ewer, B. Ky, M. Scherrer-Crosbie J. Ganame, I.A. Sebag, D.A. Agler, L.P. Badano, J. Banchs, D. Cardinale, J. Carver, M. Cerqueira, J.M. DeCara, T. Edvardsen, S.D. Flamm, T. Force, B.P. Griffin,G. Jerusalem, J.E. Liu, A. Magalhaes, T. Marwick, L.Y. Sanchez, R. Sicari, H.

[76] Villarraga R, Lancellotti P. Expert consensus for multimodality imaging evaluation of adult patients during and after cancer therapy: a report from the American Society of Echocardiography and the European Association of Cardiovascular Imaging. Eur Heart J Cardiovasc Imag 2014;15(10):1063−93.

[77] Zamorano JL, Lancellotti P, Rodriguez Munoz D, Aboyans V, Asteggiano R, Galderisi M, et al. 2016 ESC position paper on cancer treatments and cardiovascular toxicity developed under the auspices of the ESC Committee for Practice Guidelines: the Task Force for cancer treatments and cardiovascular toxicity of the European Society of Cardiology (ESC). Eur Heart J 2016;37(36):2768−801.

[78] S.H. Armenian, C. Lacchetti, A. Barac, J. Carver, L.S. Constine, N. Denduluri, S. Dent, P.S. Douglas, J.B. Durand, M. Ewer, C. Fabian, M. Hudson, M. Jessup, L.

[79] Journal of Molecular and Cellular Cardiology 168 (2022) 24−32 Jones W, Ky B, Mayer EL, Moslehi J, Oeffinger K, Ray K, Ruddy K. ,D. Lenihan, prevention and monitoring of cardiac dysfunction in survivors of adult cancers: American society of clinical oncology clinical practice guideline. J Clin Oncol 2017;35(8):893−911.

[80] Thavendiranathan P, Grant AD, Negishi T, Plana JC, Popovic ZB, Marwick TH. Reproducibility of echocardiographic techniques for sequential assessment of left ventricular ejection fraction and volumes: application to patients undergoing cancer chemotherapy. J Am Coll Cardiol 2013;61(1):77—84.

[81] Jacobs LD, Salgo IS, Goonewardena S, Weinert L, Coon P, Bardo D, et al. Rapid online quantification of left ventricular volume from real-time three-dimensional echocardiographic data. Eur Heart J 2006;27(4):460—8.

[82] Santoro C, Arpino G, Esposito R, Lembo M, Paciolla I, Cardalesi C, et al. 2D and 3D strain for detection of subclinical anthracycline cardiotoxicity in breast cancer patients: a balance with feasibility. Eur Heart J Cardiovasc Imag 2017;18(8):930—6.

[83] Plana JC, Galderisi M, Barac A, Ewer MS, Ky B, Scherrer-Crosbie M, et al. Expert consensus for multimodality imaging evaluation of adult patients during and after cancer therapy: a report from the American Society of Echocardiography and the European Association of Cardiovascular Imaging. J Am Soc Echocardiogr 2014;27(9): 911—39.

[84] Thavendiranathan P, Negishi T, Somerset E, Negishi K, Penicka M, Lemieux J, et al. Strain-guided management of potentially cardiotoxic cancer therapy. J Am Coll Cardiol 2021;77(4):392—401.

[85] Farsalinos KE, Daraban AM, Unlu S, Thomas JD, Badano LP, Voigt JU. Head-to-head comparison of global longitudinal strain measurements among nine different vendors: the EACVI/ASE inter-vendor comparison study. J Am Soc Echocardiogr 2015;28(10): 1171—1181, e2.

[86] Ali MT, Yucel E, Bouras S, Wang L, Fei HW, Halpern EF, et al. Myocardial strain is associated with adverse clinical cardiac events in patients treated with anthracyclines. J Am Soc Echocardiogr 2016;29(6):522—527, e3.

[87] Negishi K, Negishi T, Hare JL, Haluska BA, Plana JC, Marwick TH. Independent and incremental value of deformation indices for prediction of trastuzumab-induced cardiotoxicity. J Am Soc Echocardiogr 2013;26(5):493—8.

[88] Zhao R, Shu F, Zhang C, Song F, Xu Y, Guo Y, et al. Early detection and prediction of anthracycline-induced right ventricular cardiotoxicity by 3-dimensional echocardiography. JACC CardioOncol 2020;2(1):13—22.

[89] Calleja A, Poulin F, Khorolsky C, Shariat M, Bedard PL, Amir E, et al. Right ventricular dysfunction in patients experiencing cardiotoxicity during breast cancer therapy. JAMA Oncol 2015;2015:609194.

[90] Bingcang A, Ramachandran K, Tzavara C, Charalampopoulos G, Filippiadis D, Kouris N, et al. Longitudinal changes of right ventricular deformation mechanics during trastuzumab therapy in breast cancer patients. Eur J Heart Fail 2019;21(4):529—35.

[91] Planek MIC, Manshad A, Hein K, Hemu M, Ballout F, Varandani R, et al. Prediction of doxorubicin cardiotoxicity by early detection of subclinical right ventricular dysfunction. Cardiooncology 2020;6:10.

[92] Christiansen JR, Massey R, Dalen H, Kanellopoulos A, Hamre H, Ruud E, et al. Right ventricular function in long-term adult survivors of childhood lymphoma and acute lymphoblastic leukaemia. Eur Heart J Cardiovasc Imag 2016;17(7):735—41.

[93] Park H, Kim KH, Kim HY, Cho JY, Yoon HJ, Hong YJ, et al. Left atrial longitudinal strain as a predictor of cancer therapeutics-related cardiac dysfunction in patients with breast cancer. Cardiovasc Ultrasound 2020;18(1):28.

[94] Singh A, ElHangouche N, McGee K, Gong FF, Lentz R, Feinglass J, et al. Utilizing left atrial strain to identify patients at risk for atrial fibrillation on ibrutinib. Echocardiography 2021;38(1):81—8.

[95] Yeh ET, Bickford CL. Cardiovascular complications of cancer therapy: incidence, pathogenesis, diagnosis, and management. J Am Coll Cardiol 2009;53(24):2231—47.

[96] Novo G, Santoro C, Manno G, DiLisi D, Esposito R, Mandoli GE, et al. Usefulness of stress echocardiography in the management of patients treated with anticancer drugs. J Am Soc Echocardiogr 2021;34(2):107—16.

[97] Ferreira VM, Piechnik SK, Robson MD, Neubauer S, Karamitsos TD. Myocardial tissue characterization by magnetic resonance imaging: novel applications of T1 and T2 mapping. J Thorac Imag 2014;29(3):147—54.

[98] S. Giusca, G. Korosoglou, M. Montenbruck, B. Gersak, A.K. Schwarz, S. Esch, S. Kelle, P. Wulfing, S. Dent, D. Lenihan, H. Steen, Multiparametric early detection and prediction of cardiotoxicity using myocardial strain, T1 and T2.

[99] Remnick D. Obama reckons with a Trump presidency. New Yorker 2016. Nov 28;28:3.

[100] Thavendiranathan P, Poulin F, Lim KD, Plana JC, Woo A, Marwick TH. Use of myocardial strain imaging by echocardiography for the early detection of cardiotoxicity in patients during and after cancer chemotherapy: a systematic review. J Am Coll Cardiol 2014;63(25 Pt A):2751—68.

[101] Hinton G. Geoff Hinton on radiology. Machine Learning and Market for Intelligence Conference, Creative Disruption Lab Toronto, Canada. Available at: https://www.youtube.com/watch?v1⁄42HMPRXstSvQ. Published November 24, 2016. Accessed May 1, 2019.

[102] Allen B, Dreyer K. The artificial intelligence ecosystem for the radiological sciences: ideas to clinical practice. J Am Coll Radiol 2018;15:1455—7.

[103] Thrall JH, Li X, Li Q, Cruz C, Do S, Dreyer K, et al. Artificial intelligence and machine learning in radiology: opportunities, challenges, pitfalls, and criteria for success. J Am Coll Radiol 2018;15:504—8.

[104] Perspectives on research in artificial intelligence and artificial general intelligence relevant to DoD (unclassified); JASON: JSR-16-Task- 003. January 2017 [Available at:].

[105] Herper M. MD Anderson benches IBM Watson in setback for artificial intelligence in medicine. Forbes. Zugriff im Juli; 2017. Feb.

[106] Langlotz CP, Allen B, Erickson BJ, Kalpathy-Cramer J, Bigelow K, Cook TS, et al. A roadmap for foundational research on artificial intelligence in medical imaging: from the 2018 NIH/RSNA/ACR/The Academy Workshop. Radiology April 16, 2019:190613.

[107] US Department of Health and Human Services. NIH videocasting and podcasting. Artificial intelligence in medical imaging (day 2). Available at: https://videocast.nih.gov/summary.asp?Live1⁄428180&bhcp1⁄41. Accessed April 14, 2019.

[108] Nekoui M, Pirruccello JP, di Achille P, et al. Spatially distinct genetic determinants of aortic dimensions influence risks of aneurysm and stenosis. J Am Coll Cardiol 2022; 80:486—97.

[109] Grafton F, Ho J, Ranjbarvaziri S, et al. Deep learning detects cardiotoxicity in a high-content screen with induced pluripotent stem cell- derived cardiomyocytes. Elife 2021; 10:e68714.

[110] Meyer HV, Dawes TJW, Serrani M, et al. Genetic and functional insights into the fractal structure of the heart. Nature 2020;584:589—94.

[111] Parlakgül G, Arruda AP, Pang S, et al. Regulation of liver subcellular architecture controls metabolic homeostasis. Nature 2022;603:736–42.

[112] Sohn JJ, Lim S, Das IJ, Yadav P. An integrated and fast imaging quality assurance phantom for a 0.35 T magnetic resonance imaging linear accelerator. Phys Imaging Radiat Oncol June 22, 2023;27:100462. https://doi.org/10.1016/j.phro.2023. 100462. PMID: 37449023; PMCID: PMC10338140.

[113] Dharmarajan KV, Friedman DL, FitzGerald TJ, et al. Radiotherapy quality assurance report from Children's Oncology Group AHOD0031. Int J Radiat Oncol Biol Phys 2015 25;91:1065–71.

[114] Weiner MA, Leventhal B, Brecher ML, et al. Randomized study of intensive MOPP-ABVD with or without low-dose total-nodal radiation therapy in the treatment of stages IIB, IIIA2, IIIB, and IV Hodgkin's disease in pediatric patients: a Pediatric Oncology Group study. J Clin Oncol 1997;15:2769–79.

[115] Friedman DL, Chin L, Wolden S, et al. Dose-intensive response-based chemotherapy and radiation therapy for children and adolescents with newly diagnosed intermediate-risk Hodgkin lymphoma: a report from the Children's Oncology Group Study AHOD0031. J Clin Oncol 2014;32:3651–8.

[116] FitzGerald TJ, Bishop-Jodoin M, Laurie F, Iandoli M, Smith K, Ulin K, et al. The importance of quality assurance in radiation oncology clinical trials. Semin Radiat Oncol October 2023;33(4):395–406. https://doi.org/10.1016/j.semradonc.2023. 06.005. PMID: 37684069.

[117] Huang HK. Medical imaging, PACS, and imaging informatics: retrospective. Radiol Phys Technol 2014;7:5–24. https://doi.org/10.1007/s12194-013-0245-y.

[118] Branstetter BF. Basics of imaging informatics: part 11. Radiology 2007;243:656–67. https://doi.org/10.1148/radiol.2433060243.

[119] Petrou M, Foerster BR, Reich DS. Translational research in radiology: challenges and role in a patient-based practice. Acad Radiol May 2009;16(5):593–6. https://doi.org/ 10.1016/j.acra.2009.01.017. PMID: 19345901.

[120] The Royal College of Radiologists. Guidelines for the management of the unscheduled interruption or prolongation of a radical course of radiotherapy. London: The Royal College of Radiologists; 2013.

[121] Henshaw ET. Quality assurance in diagnostic radiology—for its own sake or that of the patient. Qual Assur Health Care 1990;2(3–4):213–8.

[122] European Journal of Nuclear Medicine and Molecular Imaging [Internet]. Springer. [cited 2022 Dec 1]. Available from: https://www.springer.com/journal/259.

[123] Snapshot [Internet]. [cited 2022 Dec 1]. Available from: https://www.nema.org/about/.

[124] AAPM: The American Association of Physicists in Medicine [Internet]. [cited 2022 Dec 1]. Available from: https://www.aapm.org.

[125] Society of Nuclear Medicine and Molecular Imaging (SNMMI) [Internet]. [cited 2022 Dec 1]. Available from: https://www.snmmi.org/.

[126] General Information [Internet]. EANM. 2016 [cited 2022 Dec 1]. Available from: https://www.eanm.org/about/general-information-2/.

[127] The Quality Standard for Imaging (QSI) | The Royal College of Radiologists [Internet]. [cited 2022 Dec 1]. Available from: https://www.rcr.ac.uk/clinical-radiology/service-delivery/quality-standard-imaging-qsi.

[128] Beutler LE, Howard KI. Clinical utility research: an introduction. J Clin Psychol 1998; 54(3):297–301.

[129] Mehanna H, McConkey CC, Rahman JK, Wong WL, Smith AF, Nutting C, et al. PET-NECK: a multicentre randomised Phase III non-inferiority trial comparing a positron emission tomography-computerised tomography-guided watch-and-wait policy with planned neck dissection in the management of locally advanced (N2/N3) nodal metastases in patients with squamous cell head and neck cancer. Health Technol Assess April 2017;21(17):1−122.

[130] The Ionising Radiation (Medical Exposure) Regulations 2017 [Internet]. Queen's Printer of Acts of Parliament; [cited 2022 Dec 1]. Available from: https://www.legislation.gov.uk/uksi/2017/1322/introduction/made.

[131] How we regulate radiological and civil nuclear safety in the UK (webpage) [Internet]. GOV.UK. [cited 2022 Dec 2]. Available from: https://www.gov.uk/government/publications/how-we-regulate-radiological-and-civil-nuclear-safety-in-the-uk/how-we-regulate-radiological-and-civil-nuclear-safety-in-the-uk-webpage.

[132] Administration of Radioactive Substances Advisory Committee [Internet]. GOV.UK. [cited 2022 Dec 2]. Available from: https://www.gov.uk/government/organisations/administration-of-radioactive-substances-advisory-committe.

[133] Medical physics experts recognition scheme [Internet]. GOV.UK. [cited 2022 Dec 2]. Available from: https://www.gov.uk/government/publications/medical-physics-experts-recognition-scheme.

[134] Fraser L, Parkar N, Adamson K, Fletcher A, Julyan P, Kalirai C, et al. Guidance on medical physics expert support for nuclear medicine. BJR July 1, 2022;95(1135):20211393.

[135] Revalidation [Internet]. [cited 2022 Dec 2]. Available from: https://www.gmc-uk.org/registration-and-licensing/managing-your-registration/revalidation.

[136] Iyer RS, Swanson JO, Otto RK, Weinberger E. Peer review comments augment diagnostic error characterization and departmental quality assurance: 1-year experience from a children's hospital. Am J Roentgenol January 2013;200(1):132−7.

[137] Larson DB, Nance JJ. Rethinking peer review: what aviation can teach radiology about performance improvement. Radiology June 2011;259(3):626−32.

[138] Provenzale JM, Kranz PG. Understanding errors in diagnostic radiology: proposal of a classification scheme and application to emergency radiology. Emerg Radiol October 2011;18(5):403−8.

[139] Fitzgerald R. Error in radiology. Clin Radiol. December 2001;56(12):938−946. Renfrew DL, Franken EA, Berbaum KS, Weigelt FH, Abu-Yousef MM. Error in radiology: classification and lessons in 182 cases presented at a problem case conference. Radiology. 1992 Apr;183(1):145−946.

[140] RADPEER [Internet]. [cited 2022 Dec 2]. Available from: https://www.acr.org/Clinical-Resources/RADPEER.

[141] Standards for radiology events and learning meetings | The Royal College of Radiologists [Internet]. [cited 2022 Dec 2]. Available from: https://www.rcr.ac.uk/publication/standards-radiology-events-and-learning-meetings.

[142] Bouchareb Y, Moradi Khaniabadi P, Al Kindi F, Al Dhuhli H, Shiri I, Zaidi H, et al. Artificial intelligence-driven assessment of radiological images for COVID-19. Comput Biol Med September 2021;136:104665. https://doi.org/10.1016/j.compbiomed.2021.104665.

[143] Zhu S, et al. The 2021 landscape of FDA-approved artificial intelligence/machine learning-enabled medical devices: an analysis of the characteristics and intended

use. Int J Med Inf 2022;165:104828. https://doi.org/10.1016/j.ijmedinf.2022.104828.

[144] Borg M. The AIQ meta-testbed: pragmatically bridging academic AI testing and industrial Q needs. In: International conference on software quality. Process automation in software development; 2020.

[145] Felderer M, Ramler R. Quality assurance for AI-based systems: overview and challenges (introduction to interactive session). 2021. ArXiv, abs/2102.05351.

Further reading

[1] Selman J. Elements of radiobiology. Springfield, IL: Charles C. Thomas; 1983. p. 98.

[2] Academic radiology | The Royal College of Radiologists [Internet]. [cited 2022 Dec 1]. Available from: https://www.rcr.ac.uk/clinical-radiology/academic-radiology.

Case studies

9

Abstract

A maternity service was preparing for an announced mandatory inspection. This was one of many held in the past, some of which resulted in desirable outcomes.

Keywords: Inspection; Maternity services; Organization.

9.1 Resource influenced near misses-maternity

A maternity service was preparing for an announced mandatory inspection. This was one of many held in the past, some of which resulted in desirable outcomes.

9.1.1 Case presentation

This organization was registered under the national scheme, which required mandatory 2-year inspections. The organization had failed to adequately plan and prepare, by ignoring calls to engage more staff to assist with the actions, following completion of a gap analysis in relation to benchmarking against the set standards.

In the absence of a communications strategy to achieve buy-in from all key staff, the organization continued with limited human resources, which was not on par with the executive team's high expectations of the outcome. The postholder responsible for coordinating the process of accreditations continued to work according to their own plan with ad hoc support from a small team of clinicians.

Concerns were escalated following self-assessments against the expected standards, and this was escalated by the services accountable person in senior management. As the time approached, it became clearer that more staff members were required to assist with collating a particular type of evidence. This was envisaged to be extremely time-consuming, and while it required the deep involvement of midwives and doctors, there were significant parts of the process that fell neatly under the capabilities of administrative staff. This case was well thought out following an in-depth review by the coordinator leading the inspection. The coordinator continued with an extension of their working hours per day, with only two clinicians supporting by dedicating random 1 hour slots. Two days before the scheduled inspection, it had become clear that the organization would not be able to submit meaningful evidence to a major section of the standards. This would then invite a fail, as there was no allowance for flexibility.

9.1.2 **Learning objectives**

Managing a staffing issue is often perceived to be an operational issue. Resource-related issues go beyond the scope of operational responsibility, thus should be considered an operational and clinical issue. This case demonstrates a classical presentation of the disregard for the importance of a robust assessment of the appropriate resources when preparing for visits/inspections and that such a failure could leave the organization in a position where they would have to manage damage limitation.

Assessments of health services against national or local set standards are required to provide assurance of compliance, and all staff are actively working to achieve the common goal of patient safety at its highest level. While there are benefits to having a designated coordinator, leaders must give due regard to well-thought-out requests for appropriate resources.

Key learning objectives within this context include the following:

- One administrative staff member was employed to assist with the process a day before the inspection.
- Then the entire approach to the collation of evidence had to be amended to achieve maximum results.
- The 20 hours preceding the inspection were captivated by a shift pattern for volunteers to assist and complete various tasks.
- The maternity services believed there was nothing more that could be achieved and asserted that the unit was inspection-ready. The inspectors allowed for more time to gather further evidence during the inspection process.
- While there were minor gaps in the evidence, they had not crossed the threshold for a fail, and therefore, the unit celebrated a remarkable outcome.

9.2 **Inspection preparedness**

A maternity service was unprepared for an unannounced inspection visit of parts of services to women and their babies. This was following a recent successful routine inspection.

9.2.1 **Case presentation**

The role of compliance with policies and coordination of accreditations was devolved to managers and matrons following a recent restructuring of staff. During the consultation process, several suggestions were made to increase the governance team and give more support for demands relating to accreditations. The restructure culminated in the devolution of such responsibilities to managers and matrons, each assigned certain sections of a particular set of standards. Managers were given the autonomy to be creative in managing this responsibility, so far as to assign local champions and set up subcommittees. The channel for checking accountability was through an existing regular meeting, giving the managers and matrons the platform to update the team on progress with compliance, even in the absence of any known dates for formal inspections.

There was no requirement for managers to produce a written report, and the oral updates were included in a summary within the monthly meeting minutes. There was no checking-up process on the accuracy of the feedback, nor on any barriers to progress, further to the agreed actions at those meetings. The head of the department did not make the managers accountable, and the need to ensure compliance with set standards was not a priority. The unit's head did not make the focus on quality assurance a part of the governance framework within the unit, nor was there a demand by the executive team to ensure triangulation and confidence from the maternity services with the organizational-wide assurance framework.

After a period of time, it became obvious that the managers and matrons were no longer in touch with the last inspection report, in respect of lessons learned with actions, and that all became complacent, as they felt that the unit was in a safe place.

It was at one point during the monthly risk meetings that a report on complaints and incidents revealed that there were serious concerns that, if known to the inspecting body, may invite an unannounced visit.

9.2.2 **Learning outcomes**

A plan was immediately set out, which included forming a group with managers reporting to the unit's lead on a fortnightly basis on progress via action plans on compliance with standards and evidence of remedial actions taken to address themes in incidents and complaints. Concerns relating to medical staff were assigned to the Clinical Director, who was given the autonomy to adopt a suitable approach. Two weeks into the new plan, the maternity unit received an unannounced visit as they were notified of concerns regarding the number and gravity of incidents and complaints.

The manager advanced that there was regular discussion on compliance with the standards. When the managers and matrons fortnightly notes and the preexisting monthly meetings were submitted on the spot as evidence, they were deemed inadequate and unsatisfactory. The inspectors were of the impression that, at the management level, the safety of patients was not at the top of its agenda and that they had lost sight of the importance of delivering high-quality care and giving women and their families confidence in its services. The unit failed the inspection, its services were downgraded, and the report was made visible in the public domain.

This case demonstrates that leaders and senior and middle management must be convinced that quality of care is absolutely essential and that there must be checks and balances in place, all falling within the framework of quality assurance. A leader whose focus is the safety of patients must themselves be passionate, dedicated, a role model for staff to emulate, and take all measures to ensure public confidence.

9.3 **Risk mitigation**

The organization applied a flawed approach to registering risk on their corporate risk register.

9.3.1 **Presentation**

The organization highlighted that there were consistent reports of patient falls on a particular inpatient ward. These incidents were read out at the case/risk meetings on a weekly basis, with a brief discussion of the actions taken following the incidents. While these were largely different patients, there were particular themes and commonalities, especially around the patients diagnosis and staffing at night. Investigations into these incidents were usually brief, and on some occasions, when patients had sustained moderate to severe injuries, this did not necessarily trigger a detailed investigation. Upon a newly appointed governance team member joining the weekly meetings, they made an observation that the recurring theme in the incident reports at that meeting did not receive the appropriate response and attention.

There were a number of factors, including issues around the governance knowledge-base of some members who sat at the table on a fortnightly basis, as well as a denial and nonacceptance by key players of real risk and the need to undertake thematic reviews and formulate actions to mitigate and, where possible, control the risk. It was agreed by the majority that, owing to the fact that the incident reports were only focused on one clinical area, it would suffice for the ward manager to begin to review future incidents in more depth. Within a week of this decision, the clinical area reported a fatality following a patient fall. This was classified as a serious incident and reported to the Care Quality Commission.

9.3.2 **Learning outcomes**

The patient's death triggered a root-cause analysis and a detailed investigation by an independent qualified person. The investigation as dictated by the terms of reference also reviewed any possible themes in reported incidents of patient falls. It highlighted that over a 3-month period, there were in excess of 30 falls, mainly at night, of patients who were cared for by a number of agency staff, and most of these patients were receiving a particular sedative every night. It highlighted that there was a failure to undertake the appropriate risk assessments of patients and undertaking thematic investigations quite early on during the reporting process. This death was declared avoidable, as were a number of injuries sustained by some patients.

A decision was made to apologize to the families in adherence to the Duty of Candor policy. The organization, having given an undertaking to change the approach to reviewing incidents and having learned its lessons, implemented a robust process. The risk of falls for this vulnerable group of patients was accepted and placed on the departmental and corporate risk registers. Specific measures were put in place, including staff training and monitoring of rotas for an appropriate skill mix.

The process of incident reporting must not be viewed in isolation. It must be seen as an integral part of risk management, which assists organizations in gaining a better understanding of safety concerns. Further, while not all incidents will warrant an indepth patient safety incident investigation (previously root cause analysis), there must be clear guidelines as to which ones trigger a detailed investigation. Clusters of thematic incidents must be taken seriously, and careful approach and platform with the appropriate representation must be held to identify contributory factors to learn lessons towards meaningful improvements.

Further reading

[1] Johnston G, Crombie IK, Davies O, Alder EM, Millard A. Reviewing audit: barriers and facilitating factors for effective clinical audit. Quality in Health Care 2000;99:23—6 [Accessed 23 December 2019]. Available at: http://qualitysafety.bmj.com/.

[2] National Health Service Resolution (NHSR). National health service resolution overview. 2017 [Accessed on 11 June 2020]. Available at: https://www.nhs.uk/Services/Trusts/Overview/DefaultView.aspx?id=108356.

[3] Haslam D. What is the healthcare commission trying to achieve? J R Soc Med 2007; 100(1):15—8. [Accessed 11 June 2020].

[4] Health and social care act 2008 (regulated activities), as amended. 2014. Available at: cqc.org.uk. [Accessed 23 December 2019].

[5] The Kings Fund. The future of leadership and management in the NHS. Report from the King's fund commission on leadership and management in the NHS. London: The Kings Fund; 2011.

[6] Berwick D. Berwick review into patient safety. A promise to learn-a commitment to act. Improving the safety of patients in England. London: Department of Health and Social Care; 2013. Available at: https://assets.publishing.service.gov.uk/government/uploads/system/uploads/attachment_data/file/226703/Berwick_Report.pdf. [Accessed 5 December 2019].

[7] Kouzes J,M, Posner BM. The five practices of exemplary leadership. 2003 [pdf] Available at: http:www.pnbhs.school.nz/wp-content/uploads/2015/11/The-Five-Practices-of-Exemplary-Leadership.pdf. [Accessed 5 December 2018].

[8] National Health Service England (NHSE). Clinical audit. 2019. Available at: https://www.england.nhs.uk/clinaudit/. [Accessed 15 June 2020].

[9] Falup J, Ramsay A. How organisations contribute to improving the quality of healthcare. Br Med J 2019;(19):365.

[10] Gandhi TK, Kaplan GS, Leape L. Transforming concepts in patient safety: a progress report. Br Med J Qual Safe 2018;(27):1019—26.

[11] Jabbal J, Lewis M. Approaches to better value in the NHS: improving quality and cost. Kings Fund; 2018.

[12] Wedell-Wedellsborg M. The psychology behind unethical behaviour. Racial Equality Institute. Harvard Business Review; 2019. Available at: https://hhr.org/2019/the-psych. [Accessed 24 June 2020].

[13] NHS. NHS long term plan. 2019. Available at: https://www.longtermplan.nhs.uk/wp-content/uploads/2019/08/nhs-long-term-plan-version-1.2.pdf. [Accessed 24 June 2020]. www.longtermplan.nhs.uk.

[14] Scally G, Donaldson LJ. Clinical governance and the drive for quality improvement in the new NHS in England. Br Med J 1998;317(7150):61–5.

[15] De Jonge V, Sint Nicolas J, van Leerdam ME, Kuipers EJ. Overview of the quality assurance movement in health care. Best Pract Res Clin Gastroenterol 2011;(25): 337–47.

[16] NHS England (NHSE). Review of the friends and family test. 2014. Available at: https://www.england.nhs.uk/wp-content/uploads/2014/07/fft-rev1.pdf. [Accessed 1 July 2020].

[17] Kohn LT, Corrigan J, Donalson MS. To err is human: building a safer health system, xxi. Washington, D.C: National Academy Press; 2000.

Index

Note: 'Page numbers followed by *f* indicate figures and *t* indicate tables.'